T0261413

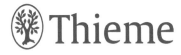

Pediatrics
A Case-Based Review

Michaela Kreckmann, MD

Private Practice
Saarbrücken, Germany

141 illustrations

Thieme
Stuttgart · New York ·
Delhi · Rio de Janeiro

Library of Congress Cataloging-in-Publication Data is available from the publisher.

This book is an authorized translation of the 2nd German edition published and copyrighted 2008 by Georg Thieme Verlag, Stuttgart. Title of the German edition: Fallbuch Paediatrie

Translator: Gertrude Champe, Surry, ME, USA

Names: Kreckmann, Michaela, author.
Title: Pediatrics : a case-based review / Michaela Kreckmann ; translator, Gertrude Champe.
Other titles: Fallbuch Phadiatrie. English
Description: Stuttgart ; New York : Thieme, [2019] | "This book is an authorized translation of the 2nd German edition published and copyrighted 2008 by Georg Thieme Verlag, Stuttgart. Title of the German edition: Fallbuch Paediatrie"-- Galley. | Includes index. |
Identifiers: LCCN 2019020002 (print) | LCCN 2019021658 (ebook) | ISBN 9783132053717 () | ISBN 9783132053618 (alk. paper) | ISBN 9783132053717 (e-ISBN)
Subjects: | MESH: Pediatrics | Diagnosis, Differential | Diagnostic Techniques and Procedures | Case Reports
Classification: LCC RJ50 (ebook) | LCC RJ50 (print) | NLM WS 100 | DDC 618.92/0075--dc23
LC record available at https://lccn.loc.gov/2019020002

© 2019 Georg Thieme Verlag KG

Thieme Publishers Stuttgart
Rüdigerstrasse 14, 70469 Stuttgart, Germany
+49 [0]711 8931 421, customerservice@thieme.de

Thieme Publishers New York
333 Seventh Avenue, New York, NY 10001, USA
+1-800-782-3488, customerservice@thieme.com

Thieme Publishers Delhi
A-12, Second Floor, Sector-2, Noida-201301
Uttar Pradesh, India
+91 120 45 566 00, customerservice@thieme.in

Thieme Publishers Rio, Thieme Publicações Ltda.
Edifício Rodolpho de Paoli, 25º andar
Av. Nilo Peçanha, 50 – Sala 2508
Rio de Janeiro 20020-906 Brasil
+55 21 3172 2297 / +55 21 3172 1896

Cover design: Thieme Publishing Group
Typesetting by Thomson Digital, India

Printed in Germany by CPI Books   5 4 3 2 1
ISBN 978-3-13-205361-8

Also available as an e-book:
eISBN 978-3-13-205371-7

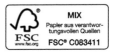

Preface

This casebook presents 85 disease patterns observed in daily pediatric practice. The intention is to make the preparation for examinations easier for the students. The descriptions of the medical histories and situations are as close as possible to clinical events as they have been encountered in the emergency department or reported by patients, parents, and nurses. Laboratory results, X-rays, and other diagnostic results are presented for analysis. This book explains the importance of why medical histories should be taken, diagnoses established, and treatment planned. In addition to everyday, easily diagnosed general pediatric and neonatal diseases, this book also presents misleading and easily misinterpreted symptoms that are intended to illustrate the special problems of pediatric diagnosis. Naturally, this book includes cases exemplifying classic emergency situations, which can be expected in everyday pediatric practice. Special problematic cases in social pediatrics and related fields are examined and discussed, such as pediatric surgery and child and adolescent psychiatry. The diagnosis and treatment described for such cases are based on the current guidelines of pediatrics associations and recommendations in the current specialized literature.

However, this book cannot and does not intend to replace a textbook. Rather, it is intended to encourage a critical approach to the, often dry, subject matter and to clarify and simplify problems by presenting them in a clinical context. It is also meant to help young colleagues in their first steps in clinical practice. For this purpose, it suggests simple and structured workflows for diagnosis and treatment and practical tips for interacting with little children, who are often frightened and uncooperative, and their parents. The student is trained to think and act like a doctor through case- and problem-oriented practice.

Last but not the least, this book would also like to show students the joy that work in pediatrics can bring, especially in light of the current public discussion of health policy. I myself have experienced most of these cases, or similar ones, as a resident in a hospital for children and adolescents in the Saarland, Germany. Every interested student and future colleague is warmly invited to take a look inside this book and enliven all the study of theory with a taste of clinical daily life.

This book would not have been possible without the help of many people. I owe a heartfelt thanks, first of all, to the children and parents who were willing to be photo models, and to Dr. Thomas Liebner, the head physician of the Clinic for Children and Adolescents in the Reinhard-Nieter Hospital, Wilhelmshaven, Germany, for his support and valuable advice. My thanks also to my colleagues for their encouragement and to the staff at Thieme Publishers, in particular Angelika-Marie Findgott, Joanne Stead, and Apoorva Gaurav Prabhuzantye, without whose active participation, constructive criticism, and persistent inquiries, this book would not have become what it is today. A lot of thanks to Gertrude Champe for her great translation. I also thank my family and all my friends for their patience, and especially my husband and children, who supported my work with thoughtful critiques and lovingly tolerated everything that they had to go through.

Michaela Kreckmann, MD

Table of Contents
By cases

Case	Page	Description
1	2	Six-year-old boy with high fever, vomiting, and headache
2	3	Child with barking cough and dyspnea
3	4	Child with high fever and seizure
4	5	Apathetic infant with persistent skin folds
5	6	Two-year-old girl with colic-like stomach pains and vomiting
6	7	Twelve-month-old boy comes for a health screening
7	8	Ten-year-old boy with painfully swollen knee
8	9	Girl with petechial dermatorrhagie
9	10	Infant with projectile vomiting
10	11	Young girl with recurrent shortness of breath
11	12	Fourteen-month-old toddler with "runny ear"
12	13	Three-year-old boy who has had contact with chicken pox
13	14	Five-year-old girl with a swollen jaw angle
14	15	Severely ill infant with cough and shortness of breath
15	16	Young girl with difficulty swallowing and fatigue

! = Difficult Case

16	17	Two-year-old boy with coughing fit and cyanosis
17	18	Twelve-month-old boy with screaming fit and swollen testicles
18	19	Eight-year-old boy with macrohematuria
19	20	Boy almost 1-year-old with failure to thrive
20	21	Macrosomal newborn after obstructed labor with shoulder dystocia
21	22	Ten-year-old girl with fever and headache
22	23	Eight-year-old boy with high fever and rash
23	24	Five-year-old girl after fall from jungle gym
24	25	Infant with high fever, sucking weakness, and vomiting
25	26	Toddler burned by boiling water
26	27	Five-year-old girl with abdominal pain and anal itching
27	28	Fourteen-year-old girl with weight loss and social withdrawal
28	29	Newborn whose mother has poorly controlled diabetes mellitus
29	30	Five-year-old girl with hematuria
30	31	Three-year-old boy with numerous pigment spots
31	32	Feverish 2-year-old girl with pustulent crusty rash
32	33	Hypotrophic newborn with abnormal phenotype
33	34	Five-year-old boy with knee pain and protective limping
34	35	Ten-year-old boy with scleral icterus
35	36	Fifteen-month-old child with an abrasion and no tetanus vaccination
36	37	Fifteen-year-old girl found unconscious with hypothermia
37	38	Two-year-old child who has ingested an unknown fluid
38	39	Five-day-old newborn with icterus and sucking weakness
39	40	Three-year-old girl refusing to eat
40	41	Newborn with morphological abnormalities
41	42	Two siblings with itching and eczematous changes on the skin of the neck and head
42	43	Consultation regarding "sudden infant death syndrome" (SIDS)

! = Difficult Case

43	44	Five-year-old boy with high fever and abdominal pain
44	45	Four-year-old boy with recurrent urinary tract infections
45	46	Seven-year-old boy with pneumonia and bone pain
46	47	Four-year-old boy with fever and exanthema
47	48	Four-year-old girl with facial swelling
48	49	Five-year-old girl with pale skin and splenomegaly
49	50	Seven-year-old girl with headaches and abnormal behavior
50	51	Four-year-old boy with pain in right lower abdomen
51	52	Three-year-old girl with protective posture of right arm
! 52	53	Ten-year-old boy with tingling paresthesia, speech disorder, and headache
53	54	Sixteen-month-old boy with undescended testis
54	55	Eight-year-old boy with abdominal pain and weight loss
55	56	Premature birth in the 28th week of pregnancy with shortness of breath and abdominal pain on pressure
56	57	Five-year-old boy with intense abdominal pain
57	58	Two-year-old boy with a high fever, rash, and swollen joints
58	59	Four-month-old screaming infant with inguinal swelling
59	60	Nineteen-month-old girl with bloody diarrhea, hematomas, and anuria
!! 60	61	Newborn with persistent cyanosis
61	62	Four-year-old boy with rattling breath and hypersalivation
62	63	Six-year-old boy with failure to thrive and recurrent pulmonary infections
63	64	Fourteen-year-old girl who collapsed on a school trip
64	65	Three-year-old boy with deteriorating general condition and gastroenteritis
65	66	Healthy newborn delivered by cesarean section
66	67	Eleven-year-old boy with high fever and joint pain
67	68	Newborn boy with conspicuous genitals
68	69	Six-year-old girl with abnormal appearance
69	70	Premature baby with acute deterioration of general condition

! = Difficult Case

70	71	Four-year-old girl with fatigue and difficulty concentrating
71	72	Exasperated parents with an 8-week-old screaming baby in the emergency department
72	73	Five-month-old infant with severe cough for the past few weeks
73	74	Fourteen-year-old girl with recurrent abdominal pain
74	75	Fifteen-year-old boy with no signs of progressing puberty
75	76	Two separate cases of infants following a fall from the changing table
76	77	Attention in the delivery room for newborns with congenital deformities
77	78	Newborn born in the 41st week of pregnancy after pathological CTG
78	79	Young boy with palpitations, reduced performance, and shortness of breath
79	80	Almost 2-year-old boy, with neurodermatitis
! 80	81	A young colleague during the pediatric admission examination
81	82	Five-month-old boy with therapy-resistant diarrhea
82	83	Thirteen-year-old school girl with petechiae in poor general condition
83	84	Fourteen-month-old boy with persistent nosebleed and hematomas
84	85	Uncontrollable 6-year-old boy with aggressive behavior
85	86	Twelve-year-old boy with painful swelling of the right foot

Appendix	273	
	274	Source of Images
	277	Forms of juvenile idiopathic arthritis (JIA)
	278	Childhood diseases
	280	Body mass index
	282	Important reference values
	291	Index

! = Difficult Case

Table of Contents
By topics

Development, Prevention, and Examination

Case 6 p.7   Case 42 p.43   Case 68 p.69   Case 80 p.81
Case 35 p.36

Nutrition and Eating Disorders

Case 71 p.72   Case 74 p. 75

Genetics

Case 32 p.33   Case 40 p.41

Neonatology

Case 20 p.21   Case 38 p.39   Case 65 p. 66   Case 77 p.78
Case 28 p.29   Case 55 p.56   Case 69 p.70

Metabolic Diseases and Water and Electrolyte Balance Disorders

Case 4 p.5   Case 54 p.55   Case 62 p. 63

Infectious Diseases

Case 7 p.8   Case 26 p.27   Case 39 p.40   Case 72 p.73
Case 12 p.13   Case 31 p.32   Case 64 p.65   Case 82 p.83
Case 15 p.16   Case 34 p.35   Case 66 p.67   Case 85 p.86
Case 22 p.23

ENT and Respiratory Organ Diseases

Case 2 p.3   Case 13 p.14   Case 21 p.22   Case 61 p.62
Case 10 p.11   Case 14 p.15   Case 43 p.44   Case 70 p.71
Case 11 p.12

Cardiac and Circulatory Diseases

Case 60 p. 61

Gastroenterology

Case 5 p. 6   Case 19 p. 20   Case 56 p.57   Case 73 p.74
Case 9 p.10   Case 50 p. 51   Case 58 p.59   Case 76 p.77

Urogenital Diseases

Case 17 p. 18   Case 24 p. 25   Case 47 p.48   Case 59 p.60
Case 18 p. 19   Case 44 p. 45   Case 53 p.54   Case 67 p.68

Hematological and Oncological Diseases

Case 8 p.9   Case 45 p.46   Case 49 p.50   Case 83 p.84
Case 29 p.30   Case 48 p.49   Case 81 p.82

Rheumatological and Immunological Diseases

Case 46 p.47   Case 57 p.58

Diseases and Injuries of the Postural and Motor Apparatus

Case 33 p.34   Case 51 p.52

Skin Diseases

Case 41 p.42   Case 79 p.80

Neuropediatrics

Case 1 p.2   Case 30 p.31   Case 52 p.53   Case 63 p.64
Case 3 p.4

Accidents and Poisoning in Childhood

Case 16 p.17   Case 25 p.26   Case 37 p.38   Case 75 p.76
Case 23 p.24

Psychiatry for Children and Youths

Case 27 p.28   Case 36 p.37   Case 78 p.79   Case 84 p.85

Table of Contents
Answers and Comments

1	88	Meningitis
2	91	Krupp syndrome
3	93	Febrile seizure
4	94	Severe exsiccosis/toxicosis in acute gastroenteritis
5	97	Invagination
6	98	Health screenings and the health log
7	103	Lyme borreliosis
8	105	Schoenlein–Henoch purpura
9	106	Hypertrophic pyloric stenosis
10	107	Bronchial asthma
11	111	Acute otitis media
12	112	Varicella (chicken pox)
13	114	Lymphadenitis colli
14	116	Bronchiolitis
15	117	Infectious mononucleosis
16	118	Foreign body aspiration

17	119	Testicular torsion
18	120	Post-streptococcal glomerulonephritis
19	122	Celiac disease
20	124	Injuries of birth trauma
21	126	Acute sinusitis
22	127	Childhood diseases: Scarlet fever, measles, mumps, pertussis
23	129	Cerebral concussion
24	129	Urosepsis/Urinary tract infection
25	131	Burns
26	133	Oxyuriasis
27	134	Anorexia nervosa
28	136	Diabetic (embryo-) fetopathy
29	138	Nephroblastoma (Wilms tumor)
30	139	Neurofibromatosis (von Recklinghausen disease)
31	141	Contagious impetigo in atopic dermatitis
32	142	Ullrich–Turner syndrome
33	143	Hip diseases in childhood
34	146	Hepatitis A
35	148	Immunizations
36	152	Alcohol intoxication and alcohol abuse
37	154	Intoxications
38	157	Neonatal icterus (Hyperbilirubinemia)
39	158	Gingivostomatitis herpetica (ulcerative)
40	160	Down syndrome (Trisomy 21)
41	161	Pediculosis capitis (Head lice)
42	163	Sudden infant death
43	165	Lobar pneumonia

44	167	Urinary tract infection and vesicoureterorenal reflux
45	169	Acute lymphatic leukemia
46	172	Kawasaki syndrome
47	174	Nephrotic syndrome
48	176	Spherocytosis (Hereditary spherical cell anemia)
49	177	Medulloblastoma
50	178	Acute appendicitis
!! 51	181	Chassaignac's paralysis
52	182	Migraine
53	184	Undescended testis
54	186	Diabetes mellitus Type I
55	189	Respiratory distress syndrome, retinopathy of prematurity, NEC
56	192	Constipation
57	194	Systemic juvenile chronic arthritis (Still syndrome)
58	196	Inguinal hernia
59	198	Hemolytic–uremic syndrome (HUS)
!! 60	199	Congenital heart defect
61	203	Tonsillitis, peritonsillar abscess, rheumatic fever
62	205	Cystic fibrosis
63	208	Epileptic seizure
64	210	Salmonella enteritis
65	212	First care and first examination of a neonate
66	217	Influenza (the flu)
67	219	Hypospadia
68	220	Normal and pathological development of puberty
69	223	Bacterial infections of the neonate
70	225	Adenoid hyperplasia

71	227	Counseling of parents of screaming child, breastfeeding, and nutrition
72	231	Tuberculosis
73	236	Cardinal symptom abdominal pain
74	240	Overweight and obesity
75	243	Falling from the changing table (craniocerebral trauma, child abuse)
76	247	Omphalocele and laparoschisis
77	249	Neonatal diseases caused by pre-birth injuries
78	252	Somatization syndrome
79	254	Neurodermitis
80	256	Anomalies in pediatric examination; neonatal reflexes
! 81	260	Neuroblastoma
82	262	Meningococcal sepsis/Waterhouse–Friderichsen syndrome
83	265	Idiopathic thrombocytopenic purpura (ITP)
84	267	Attention deficit hyperactivity disorder (ADHD)
85	269	Acute hematogenous osteomyelitis

Cases

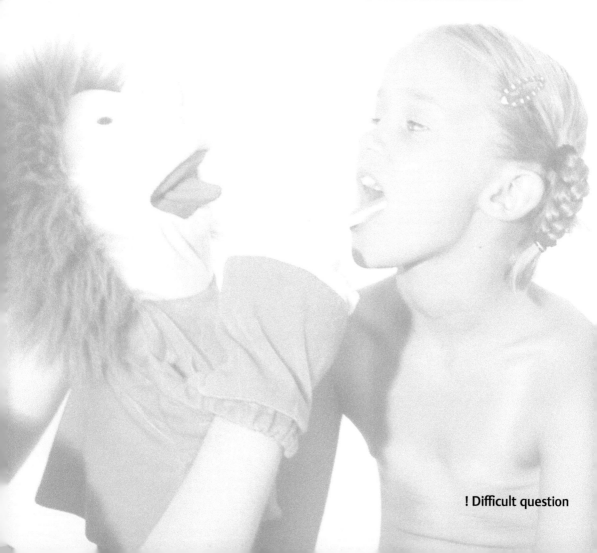

! Difficult question

| 1 | **Six-year-old boy with high fever, vomiting, and headache** |

A 6-year-old boy is presented to the emergency department as he has suddenly spiked a fever, between 39°C and 40°C since the day before, that could not be reduced with leg compresses and paracetamol. The boy is complaining of severe head and neck pain and has already vomited several times.

| 1.1 | What do you look for in the clinical examination to explain the high fever, the head and neck pain, and the vomiting in particular? |

Among other things, in the clinical examination you make the following observation (see Fig.).

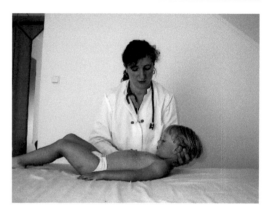

| 1.2 | Interpret the findings. What diagnosis do you suspect and what differential diagnoses can be considered? |

| 1.3 | What examinations do you perform to confirm the diagnosis? |

| 1.4 | Name the various forms of the disease and their causes. |

| 1.5 | Name typical cerebrospinal fluid findings by which the different forms can be distinguished. |

→ Answers and Comments Page 88

2 Child with barking cough and dyspnea

A 3-year-old girl awakes from sleep with a barking cough, inspiratory stridor, and dyspnea. The parents think that their child is suffocating and immediately bring the child to the emergency department. As you examine the pale and anxious girl. you notice a strong inspiratory (resting) stridor and marked inter- and subcostal retractions. The rectal temperature is 36.8°C.

2.1 What is your diagnosis? What important differential diagnosis are you considering?

2.2 Explain the etiology of the disease and define it for differential diagnosis.

2.3 Describe the different degrees of severity of the disease. What therapy is indicated for each?

Stage	Symptoms	Treatment
I		
II		
III		
IV		

→ Answers and Comments Page 91

3 Child with high fever and seizure

Late evening a 3-year-old girl is brought into the emergency department, who has just been brought in by ambulance. The child appears tired but otherwise has adequate reactions. The rectal temperature is 39.8°C. The parents are very upset. After you have reassured them, they tell you that the child has been fretful all evening. While they were telling her a bedtime story the child suddenly rolled her eyes and her arms and legs twitched for 3 minutes. She also turned blue. Thinking that the child was about to die, they immediately called the ambulance. By the time the EMTs arrived, it had all passed. They informed that no medical measures were required.

3.1   What is your suspected diagnosis? What do you explain to the parents in order to reassure them?

3.2   What immediate measures should you undertake?

3.3   What diagnostic measures should be initiated?

3.4   There are two forms of this clinical picture. Explain them.

→ Answers and Comments Page 93

Parents bring you their 6-month-old infant during the night shift. They report that since the day before, he has been suffering recurrent watery diarrhea and vomiting. In addition, he has a fever of up to 39°C. He is now apathetic, sleeps a lot, and neither eats nor drinks. The parents also noticed that since that night, his diaper has always been dry.

During the examination, you observe pale gray, mottled skin color and dry mucosa, dark circles under the eyes with infrequent blinking, and persistent skin folds (see Fig.). The fontanelle is depressed, pulse is 160 beats/ min, blood pressure 80/50 mmHg, and weight 7,200 g. The parents say that in the previous week, the boy still weighed 8,200 g.

In a blood study, among other things, you find the following values: sodium 158 mmol/L, potassium 5.2 mmol/L, and hematocrit 46%.

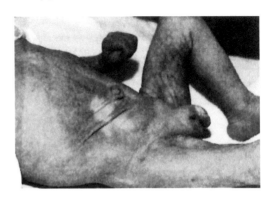

4.1   What is your diagnosis?

4.2   Explain the different forms and degrees of severity of this clinical picture. What form, with what degree of severity, does the infant have?

4.3   What treatment do you initiate?

4.4   What must you pay attention to during the treatment?

→ Answers and Comments **Page 94**

5 Two-year-old girl with colic-like stomach pains and vomiting

Three days ago, a 2-year-old girl became ill with symptoms of gastroenteritis, including diarrhea and vomiting. The symptoms improved on a low-fat diet. On the morning of admission, the girl again suffered an attack of vomiting. She screamed and hunched over with pain. Between the attacks, which were obviously painful, the child was rather quiet and seemed almost apathetic. In the admission examination, she appears pale. In the right, middle abdomen you palpate a cylindrical structure, painful on pressure. You then perform abdominal sonography and see the following findings in the right, middle abdomen (see Fig.).

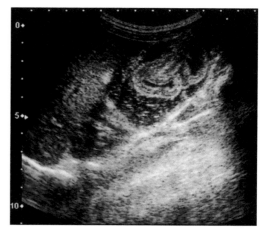

Abdominal sonography, right, middle abdomen

5.1 What is your suspected diagnosis?

5.2 What further measures will you undertake?

5.3 What complications must you watch for?

→ Answers and Comments Page 97

6   Twelve-month-old boy comes for a health screening

A 12-month-old boy born prematurely in the 29th week of pregnancy with a birth weight of 800 g, is brought for a health screening. It was determined in the previous screening that in spite of his premature birth, he developed quite well. However, there were a few deficits, especially in the motor area. For this reason, he was prescribed Vojta physiotherapy. The mother informed that she does not do the exercises at home because they make the boy cry, so, she agreed with the physiotherapist to continue the treatment by the Bobath method. During the conversation you notice that the boy is sitting on the floor and cheerfully playing with his older brother with the ball brought in from the waiting room.

6.1   What is the purpose of health screening? What is the health log?

6.2   Explain the usual course of a health screening.

The parents are principally interested to know whether the child has already made up for the delayed development caused by premature birth. When you ask, you are told that the boy has been able to sit for 4 weeks. His parents report that he can turn from his back to his stomach and vice versa and is making his first attempts at crawling. But when he does this he can only brace himself on his arms very briefly, as his arms are still quite weak. He forms chains of syllables like "wawawa" and understands speech well, i.e., he understands simple commands like "Give me the ball." He knows his family perfectly well and shows fondness for them where until 4 weeks ago he showed stranger anxiety. His parents say that he examines his toys intently with his fingers and his eyes, puts them in his mouth, shakes objects and uses them to pound with, and throws the ball when he plays with his older brother.

6.3   How would you assess the boy's developmental status?

6.4   What do you think about the fact that the mother does not perform the physiotherapeutic treatment as you prescribed?

→ Answers and Comments Page 98

7   Ten-year-old boy with painfully swollen knee

A 10-year-old boy is brought to the emergency department because of pain and swelling of the right knee.
There is no fever. The parents report that in preceding
weeks, the boy complained repeatedly of joint and
muscle pain in various locations; this was interpreted
as "growing pains." In addition, the mother describes
a skin rash that spread in rings but then disappeared
spontaneously. In the physical examination you also
observe a little redness and swelling on the right ear-
lobe (see Fig.).

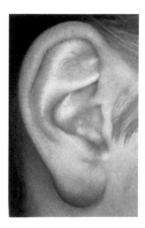

7.1   What is the most likely clinical picture here? What is the name of the skin finding shown in the
figure?

7.2   What further symptoms must be expected with this disease?

7.3   What treatment do you suggest for the patient?

→ Answers and Comments **Page 103**

A 4-year-old girl fell ill 2 weeks ago with a febrile respiratory infection. Now she has been brought to the emergency department because of a new maculopapular rash with individual petechial dermatorrhagie (see Fig.). The petechiae are located primarily on the extensor side of the lower leg and on the buttocks. The little girl also complains of abdominal pain.

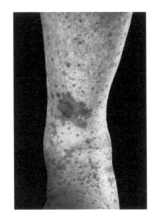

8.1 What is the most likely diagnosis?

8.2 Which differential diagnoses are you considering? Briefly characterize these diseases.

8.3 What treatment do you initiate?

→ Answers and Comments Page 105

9 Infant with projectile vomiting

A 5-week-old boy has been projectile vomiting after every meal for the past few days. He is increasingly restless and can barely be soothed. The parents bring him to the pediatrician who refers him to you for admission with suspected hypertrophic pyloric stenosis. An ultrasound image in confirmation of his suspicion is also sent along (see Fig.).

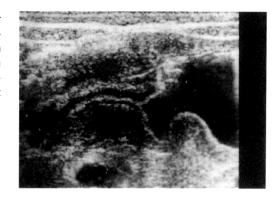

9.1 Describe what you see on the ultrasound image in the figure.

9.2 Explain the pathogenesis.

9.3 List the typical symptoms.

9.4 What treatment do you suggest?

→ Answers and Comments Page 106

A 14-year-old girl has been suffering for 2 years from shortness of breath in March and April. These symptoms occur primarily outdoors. Her primary physician has ordered an allergy test which showed significant reactions to the allergens of birches and hazel pollen as well as cat dander. Demand medication with a β2-sympathomimetic (metered dose aerosol) was initiated.

The girl's parents bring her to the emergency department of a hospital for children and adolescents because of shortness of breath and dry cough that has been increasing for the past 2 hours and is not improved by the medication. The admission examination reveals wheezing, from a distance, and on inspection massive thoracic retraction is found. Breath sounds are not audible over the lungs. The X-ray image shows the following finding (see Fig.).

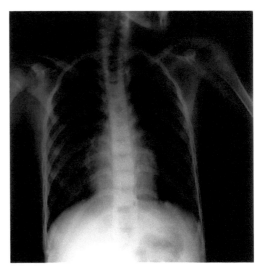

Thoracic X-ray

10.1 Describe the thoracic X-ray result. What do you notice? What is your diagnosis?

10.2 Explain the pathogenesis of this disease.

10.3 What acute treatment do you initiate?

10.4 What long-term treatment would you consider useful?

→ Answers and Comments **Page 107**

| 11 | Fourteen-month-old toddler with "runny ear" |

A 14-month-old boy, who has had a cold for a few days, is brought to the emergency department at night. The parents noticed a yellowish secretion running from the boy's right ear. During the day the child was very restless and repeatedly clutched his right ear. Physical examination yields the following pathological findings: serous rhinitis, tragus pain right, swollen lymph node in jaw angle right, reddened tonsillar ring, temperature 39.5°C. The following abnormalities are seen with the otoscope (see Fig.).

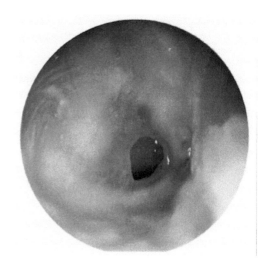

| 11.1 | Describe the otoscopic finding. What is your diagnosis?

| 11.2 | List the most frequent causes of this disease.

| 11.3 | What possible serious complications do you know of?

| 11.4 | What therapeutic procedure would you consider useful here?

→ Answers and Comments **Page 111**

12   Three-year-old boy who has had contact with chicken pox

A 3-year-old boy attends a kindergarten in which several cases of chicken pox have occurred in the past week. Fearing that their child could have become infected, the parents want to know what they should be looking out for.

12.1   Explain the typical symptoms of the disease to the parents.

12.2   In your opinion, how could the boy have become infected? When would you expect to see the first symptoms?

The parents are particularly concerned because the boy's mother is pregnant (32nd week of pregnancy).

12.3   Are there any dangers to mother and child at this stage of pregnancy? Would you have to expect complications if the mother were in another stage of pregnancy?

12.4   Is there any possibility of inoculation?

→ Answers and Comments Page 112

13 Five-year-old girl with a swollen jaw angle

A 5-year-old girl is brought to a pediatric hospital by her parents. She has severe swelling and redness in the right jaw angle that has increased massively since the day before (see Fig.). On examination, a unilateral lymphadenitis colli with incipient abscess and suppurative tonsillitis and a temperature of 38.9°C are diagnosed.

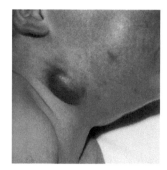

13.1 Name the possible causes of swollen neck lymph nodes.

13.2 What other studies do you order for this girl?

13.3 What treatment do you initiate?

In spite of 10 days of intravenous antibiosis, the local finding does not improve. On the contrary, the swelling has increased, and palpation reveals fluctuation.. The patient's general condition is not impaired. Repeated ultrasound examinations of the neck show an increasing number of necrotic foci. With the parents' agreement, the lymph node is excised in an ENT clinic. Microbiological examination of the abscess contents shows the following picture after staining (see Fig.).

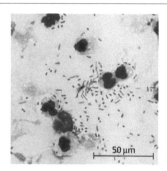

Ziehl–Neelsen stain

! 13.4 What pathological finding can you determine? What treatments does this require?

14   Severely ill infant with cough and shortness of breath

A 6-week-old infant has been suffering for 3 days from a cold, fever up to 38°C, and increasing dry cough. In the past few hours, the child became progressively worse. The child no longer drank, cried, clearly had severe shortness of breath, became increasingly pale, and seemed apathetic. At this point the parents called the emergency doctor. He immediately has the child transported to a pediatric clinic, with oxygen administration. The child is pale with nasal flaring, tachydyspnea, and massive thoracic retractions. On auscultation, bilaterally weakened breath sounds over the lungs and individual fine crackles and expiratory wheezing are heard.

14.1   What do you think causes these symptoms? What are your next steps?

You order a thoracic X-ray (see Fig.).

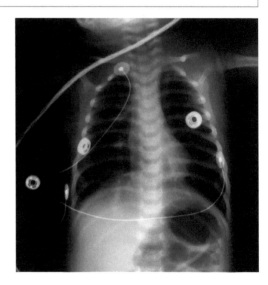

14.2   What is your diagnosis on the basis of the thoracic X-ray and the medical history? Describe the radiological changes typical for this clinical picture.

14.3   List the most frequent pathogens of this disease.

14.4   What therapeutic possibilities are available?

→ Answers and Comments Page 116

15 Young girl with difficulty swallowing and fatigue

A 15-year-old girl has had increasing throat pain for the past few days, difficulty swallowing, fatigue, exhaustion, and fever between 39°C and 40°C. She shows up with her mother during the day.

The girl reports a feeling of pressure, primarily in the right upper abdomen. The mother also reports a fine to moderately spotty skin rash on the day before that has now faded.

15.1 What is your suspected diagnosis?

15.2 With your suspected diagnosis, what examination findings do you expect?

15.3 List the most frequent causes of this disease.

15.4 What advice do you give the patient? When will the symptoms improve?

→ Answers and Comments **Page 117**

A 2-year-old boy playing alone in his playroom suddenly experiences a severe cough. When the mother comes in, the child is gasping for air and his face is reddish-blue. The mother suspects that the child has choked on something and tries to extract the foreign body by positioning the boy with his head down and pounding on his back. The cough improves but no foreign body appears.

The mother then takes the child to the emergency department of a nearby hospital.

16.1 What typical clinical symptoms and examination results do you expect if this is really a foreign body aspiration?

16.2 You order a thoracic X-ray (see Fig.). Describe the abnormalities.

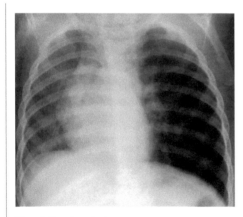

Thoracic X-ray in expiration

16.3 What treatment do you initiate if this is really an aspiration?

→ Answers and Comments Page 118

17   Twelve-month-old boy with screaming fit and swollen testicles

A 12-month-old boy is brought into the emergency department by his parents because for the past 2 hours, he has been crying without interruption and cannot be soothed. As he was changing the diaper, the father noticed redness and swelling of the scrotum. There is no fever. Examination reveals that the scrotum is reddish-livid in color. The right testicle is painful and coarsely swollen (see Fig.).

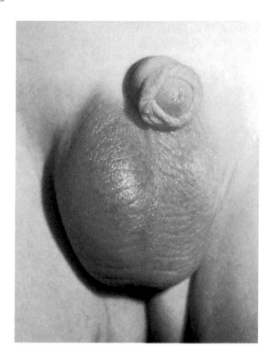

17.1   What is your suspected diagnosis? What differential diagnoses can be considered?

17.2   How do you confirm the diagnosis?

17.3   What are your next steps?

→ Answers and Comments Page 119

An 8-year-old boy's primary physician admits him to a pediatric hospital because of macrohematuria that has been present for 2 days. Physical examination reveals no abnormalities except a very high blood pressure (140/90 mmHg). The spontaneous urine is, in fact, stained red. The parents report a purulent tonsil infection 3 weeks ago which was treated for 10 days with penicillin.

18.1   What causes of macrohematuria do you know? What other causes are there for "red urine"?

18.2   What is your suspected diagnosis?

18.3   What is your diagnostic procedure?

18.4   How do you treat the boy?

→ Answers and Comments **Page 120**

An 11-month-old boy (see Fig.) is brought for health screening. The mother reports that the boy has been in an increasingly bad mood and cries a lot. She complains that there's not a thing she can do with him. Other mothers in the play group have noticed this.

What is more, he does not want to eat enough but nevertheless he produces voluminous, sour-smelling loose stools several times a day. Among other things, his body length and weight are measured, and the values are recorded in percentile curves (see Fig. percentile curves).

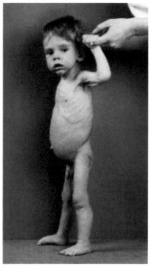

Eleven-month-old boy

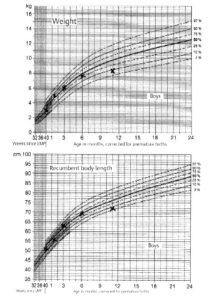

Percentile curves

| 19.1 | What is the purpose of percentile curves? What are somatograms? What important information do they provide? |

| 19.2 | What information do you derive from the percentile curves of the 11-month-old boy? |

| 19.3 | What is your suspected diagnosis on the basis of the medical history, the growth and weight development, and the external appearance of the boy? What differential diagnosis must you consider? |

| 19.4 | With your suspected diagnosis on physical examination, what further findings do you expect? |

| 19.5 | How do you confirm your suspected diagnosis? |

→ Answers and Comments Page 122

20   Macrosomal newborn after obstructed labor with shoulder dystocia

A few-minutes-old macrosomal newborn (birth weight 4,050 g) is presented for newborn examination. The child was delivered by vacuum extraction because of obstructed labor with shoulder dystocia. Physical examination reveals a soft high-parietal swelling on the right side of the head and a ring-shaped scrape on the skin of the head. The newborn does not move its right arm (see Fig.)

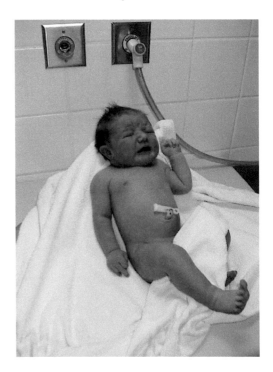

20.1   What could the soft swelling on the head be?
Name a typical differential diagnosis and distinguish the two clinical pictures from each other.

20.2   What is the most probable cause of the position of this newborn's arm?

20.3   List additional birth injuries.

→ Answers and Comments Page 124

21 Ten-year-old girl with fever and headache

A 10-year-old girl has had a cold and cough for a week. She was already recovering when she suddenly developed a high fever. Now she is also complaining of severe frontal headaches that are always particularly intense when she bends her head forward.

21.1 What is your suspected diagnosis?

21.2 What additional symptoms found on physical examination would confirm your suspected diagnosis?

21.3 List the most frequent causes of this disease.

21.4 What do you do next?

→ Answers and Comments **Page 126**

An 8-year-old boy visits his aunt on the weekend. After going on a bicycle ride with her, he suddenly no longer feels well and complains of a scratchy throat. Thereupon, the aunt takes his temperature. The boy's temperature is 39.8°C, so she treats her nephew's symptoms with paracetamol. The next day, the temperature is 38.9°C. The aunt now notices a skin rash all over the boy's body. She is concerned and immediately takes her nephew to the emergency department, suspecting that this is definitely "measles or mumps." Examination yields an exanthema with fine, slightly raised spots (see Fig.), red oral mucosa, and red tonsils.

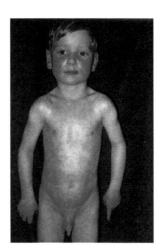

22.1 What is your suspected diagnosis? What are the grounds for this? Describe typical symptoms, incubation period, and treatment of the disease.

22.2 The aunt suspects "measles." What are the characteristic symptoms of measles?

22.3 Why can the disease not be mumps? Name the most important symptoms, incubation period, and treatment of mumps.

22.4 An additional children's disease is whooping cough. What are the clinical symptoms of whooping cough? How long is the incubation time? How would you proceed with treatment?

→ Answers and Comments Page 127

23 Five-year-old girl after fall from jungle gym

While playing at a playground, a 5-year-old girl fell on her back from a jungle gym, from a height of 1.80 m onto sandy ground. The mother found the child unconscious, lying on her back. A little laceration on the back of her head was bleeding. A short while later, the little girl regained consciousness but couldn't remember anything.

On the way to the hospital, she vomited several times. During her examination, the girl gives the impression of being tired but otherwise reacts appropriately. The retrograde amnesia persists. There are no abnormal findings except for the occipital laceration and a scrape on the left shoulder. There are also no abnormalities in the neurological examination.

23.1 What is your diagnosis? What are the grounds for your decision?

23.2 What further measures do you undertake?

23.3 List possible complications.

→ Answers and Comments **Page 129**

A 5-month-old male infant is brought to the hospital outpatient department. He is acutely ill with a high fever, vomits occasionally, and has increasing difficulty nursing. The parents also report that his diapers have been dry for the past 12 hours. He appears to be very sick.

The skin is pale and blotchy, the extremities are cold and the trunk is feverishly hot. The rectally measured body temperature is 39.6°C. When he is touched, he cries pitifully, but otherwise is limp and apathetic. On examination you cannot find a reason for the fever. You order blood and urine studies. The following patho-logical blood values are found: leukocytes 16,400/µL with marked left shift, CRP 95 mg/L, sed rate 90/145, creatinine 78 µmol/L, urea 8.6 mmol/L. Urinstix (bag urine) read: leukocytes +++, erythrocytes ++, nitrite +, protein +. Microscopic examination of the urine

sediment shows the following picture (see Fig.). You admit the child.

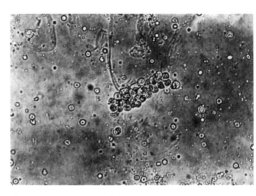

Microscopic examination of urine

24.1 Give the grounds for your decision to admit the child. What do you suspect?

24.2 How do you confirm the diagnosis?

24.3 List the most frequent causes of this disease.

24.4 What treatment do you initiate? Are any additional measures required?

→ Answers and Comments **Page 129**

25 | Toddler burned by boiling water

A 2-year-old girl has had a cold for a few days. The mother inhales with the child over a bowl of steaming water. In an unguarded moment, the girl pulls the bowl off the table and the hot water poured over the child's left arm, abdomen, and left thigh (see Fig.). The help-less mother immediately brings the loudly crying child to the clinic.

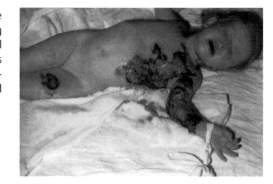

25.1 What should the mother have done immediately? What are the first-aid measures?

25.2 Determine the extent of the burns this child has suffered. Why is it important to determine the extent?

25.3 What do you do next?

25.4 What degrees of burn severity do you know?

→ Answers and Comments Page 131

26 Five-year-old girl with abdominal pain and anal itching

A 5-year-old girl is brought to you at night in the emergency department with abdominal pain. Palpation and auscultation of the abdomen reveal no abnormal findings. When the anal region is inspected, traces of scratches are found but there is no indication of eczema-like or inflammatory changes. The child tells that her "bottom itches so badly."

The status of other organs shows no other abnormalities.

26.1 What is your suspected diagnosis?

26.2 How do you confirm the diagnosis?

26.3 Explain the path of infection to the parents.

26.4 What treatment do you initiate?

→ Answers and Comments Page 133

27 Fourteen-year-old girl with weight loss and social withdrawal

A 14-year-old girl (see Fig.) has had an intended weight loss of 16 kg in the past year. Her body weight now is only 40 kg with a height of 160 cm. She says that she started her "diet" because at school they called her "fatty." All her girlfriends have "model figures." Even now, she feels too fat. Her parents observed increasing social withdrawal and the girl doesn't take part in family meals anymore. She would rather prepare "healthy" low-calorie food for herself (for instance, half apple or one carrot for breakfast, one low-fat yogurt for lunch, salad for supper).

The mother suspects that her daughter also secretly forces herself to vomit. Moreover, the girl works out several times a day on the family's home exercise machine. The rather hefty mother reports that she "simply can't get through to her daughter anymore." There is no conversation; the daughter thinks that everything is an attack on her "healthy" lifestyle.

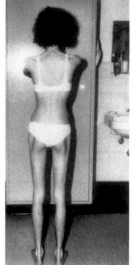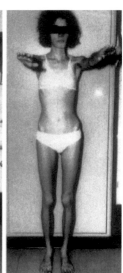

27.1 What is your suspected diagnosis?

27.2 List the most important diagnostic criteria.

27.3 List causes of this disease.

27.4 What do you do next?

→ Answers and Comments Page 134

A colleague in gynecology brings you a 3-hours-old newborn male, born by natural delivery, of a 32-year-old, poorly balanced Type 1 diabetic (HbA1$_c$ 7.5%) mother, for consultation.

The child's birth weight was 4,680 g, body length 58 cm, head circumference 38 cm, APGAR 8/9/9, navel artery pH 7.20. The postpartum blood sugar checks in the delivery room were 48 mg/dL (2.6 mmol/L) after 30 minutes and 45 mg/dL (2.5 mmol/L) after 1 hour.

In the nursery, the boy exhibited expiratory grunting, tachypnea, and acrocyanosis. The blood tests showed these values among others: blood sugar 32 mg/dL (1.8 mmol/L); serum calcium 1.7 mmol/L; capillary blood gas: pH 7.23, pCO$_2$ 58 mmHg, pO$_2$ 46 mmHg, HCO$_3^-$ 22 mmol/L; peripheral oxygen saturation 90%.

28.1 What clinical picture are you considering? Explain the pathogenesis of the child's clinical picture.

28.2 What symptoms can generally be expected in newborns with this clinical picture?

28.3 What measures do you undertake? As consultant, what do you recommend to your colleague in gynecology?

28.4 What prophylactic measures are recommended to women with Type 1 diabetes during pregnancy? What are the grounds for this?

→ Answers and Comments Page 136

29 Five-year-old girl with hematuria

A 5-year-old girl is brought to the emergency department by her parents because of intense abdominal pain, burning sensation during urination, and blood in the urine. The child was examined by a physician, who diagnosed urethritis and initiated symptomatic treatment as well as antibiosis with Cefaclor. The complaints disappeared with this treatment, but there is still blood in the urine.

The parents inform that the girl has often been tired and listless in recent days. In the physical examination, you observe that the girl's skin is pale. In palpating the abdomen, you feel a structure the size of a chicken egg in the right upper abdomen. Spleen and liver are not enlarged; the lymph nodes are not palpable. In the laboratory results, among other things, the following values are found: leukocytes 9,500/ μL, Hb 8.3 g/dL, hematocrit 25%, thrombocytes 320,000/ μL, CRP negative, sed rate 98/144; urine: leukocytes/erythrocytes/ protein positive, and nitrite negative.

Abdominal sonography shows the following findings in the right upper abdomen (see Fig.).

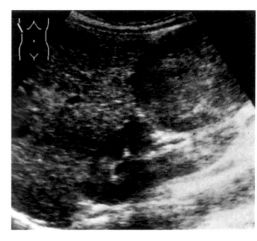

Longitudinal section in right flank

29.1 Describe the sonography result. What is your suspected diagnosis? What differential diagnosis must you consider?

29.2 How do you proceed?

29.3 What do you know about the prognosis for the disease you suspect?

→ Answers and Comments Page 138

A 3-year-old boy is brought to the clinic because while he was playing, a swing crashed into his head. The mother was concerned because of a large lump on the boy's forehead. The boy did not lose consciousness, did not vomit, or behave abnormally. The neurological examination is normal. Physical inspection showed about 12 large, brownish pigment spots of varying sizes (see Fig.) distributed over the whole body.

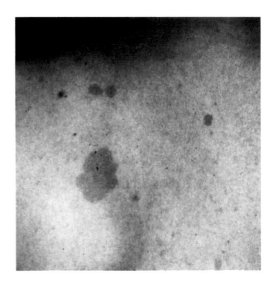

30.1   What is your suspected diagnosis regarding the skin changes?

30.2   What further clinical abnormalities/changes can be associated with this disease?

30.3   Which classification of this disease do you know of?

! 30.4   List other diseases in the same spectrum and give their characteristic symptoms.

30.5   The boy was brought in because of a blow to the head. What diagnostic and therapeutic procedures do you initiate?

→ Answers and Comments Page 139

| 31 | Feverish 2-year-old girl with pustulent crusty rash |

A 2-year-old girl has had atopic dermatitis since she was 6 months old. For the past few days, she has had pustulent, crusty, itching skin changes with a honey-colored crust, especially in her face (see Fig.) and the crooks of her arms. They now appear to be distributed over her whole body. Since the day before, the girl has had a fever up to 39°C. Her general condition is reduced.
Her brother, who is 2 years older, has similar perioral crusty skin changes.

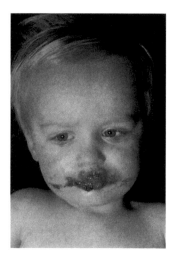

| 31.1 | **What is your suspected diagnosis?** |

| 31.2 | **What triggers the disease?** |

| 31.3 | **List one complication of the disease.** |

| 31.4 | **What treatment do you initiate?** |

→ Answers and Comments Page 141

32 Hypotrophic newborn with abnormal phenotype

A 3-day-old little girl is examined in the nursery. This is the first child of a 30-year-old woman, born at term. The child's birth weight was 2,550 g, body length 44 cm, head circumference 32 cm, APGAR 9/10/10, umbilical cord pH 7.28. The physical examination revealed the following anomalies: gothic palate, wide spacing between nipples, webbed neck, low hairline at the nape of the neck, and changes in the hands (see Fig.).

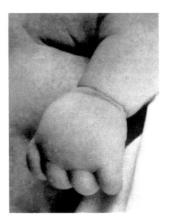

32.1 Which clinical picture do these symptoms suggest?

32.2 What other abnormalities do you expect?

32.3 How do you confirm the diagnosis?

32.4 What do you tell the parents about the course and prognosis of the disease? What therapy does the diagnosis call for?

→ Answers and Comments Page 142

33   Five-year-old boy with knee pain and protective limping

A 5-year-old boy has been complaining of pain in his right knee since the day before. The pain has gotten so intense that he can hardly walk. There is no fever. Anamnestically, he had a respiratory infection a week earlier and also has a distinct protective limping on the right side. Examination shows painful limitation of movement in the right hip joint. The joint is neither warm and swollen, nor red. All other joints, including the right knee joint, are freely movable. Ultrasound examination of the hip joint shows that compared to the other side, the intra-articular space is widened (see Fig.).

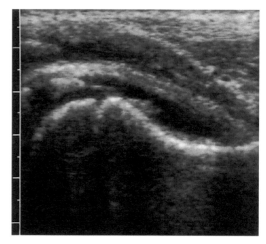

Sonographic longitudinal section of the proximal femur in the area of the femur neck

| 33.1 | What is your diagnosis? Justify your decision. |

| 33.2 | Explain the clinical picture of Perthes disease. |

| 33.3 | What do you know about slipped capital femoral epiphysis? |

→ Answers and Comments   Page 143

During vacation, a 10-year-old boy went camping with his family at a popular camp site that is no longer maintained daily by park rangers. The family has been home for 3 weeks. For the past few days, he has been complaining of upper abdominal pain, nausea, and lack of appetite. He feels listless and tired and has a slight fever (38.4°C). Since the day before, the mother has noticed yellowing of the sclera and so the boy is brought to the emergency department.

34.1 What diseases can be considered? What is the most likely diagnosis?

34.2 What diagnostic procedures do you order to confirm your suspected diagnosis? What findings would you expect?

34.3 Name additional clinical signs you would find if your suspected diagnosis is confirmed.

34.4 What do you know about the infectious pathway and incubation time of the disease? When may the boy return to school?

34.5 Do cases of this disease have to be reported?

→ Answers and Comments Page 146

| 35 | Fifteen-month-old child with an abrasion and no tetanus vaccination |

A 15-month-old child gets a scrape wound while playing on the playground. The wound is very soiled with earth. The child is brought to the emergency department. The parents, who up to now have refused all vaccinations for the child, are worried now and request an anti-tetanus vaccination.

| 35.1 | What are your first steps? |

The medical history reveals that the child has a cold at the moment. "... and actually, when someone has a cough and a cold, it's not right to give a vaccination," the parents inform.

| 35.2 | Are the parents right? Name the general contraindications for vaccination. |

The parents continue to be concerned that their child could suffer adverse effects from the vaccination. They have heard that there can be brain damage.

| 35.3 | What is meant by the adverse effects of vaccination? What is your reaction to the parents' assertion? What reactions to vaccination can the parents expect? |

You have answered the parents' questions and informed them. The parents give their permission.

| 35.4 | Must the parents' permission be recorded in writing? How do you proceed in vaccinating the child? |

| 35.5 | According to the recommendations of the United States Centers for Disease Control and Prevention (CDC), a 15-month-old child has normally already received various immunizations. What are they? List the ages at which these immunizations are normally given. |

→ Answers and Comments Page 148

EMTs bring in a 15-year-old girl in the early morning hours to the emergency department of a pediatric clinic. She was found unconscious in the city park by passers-by. She was lying in vomit and her clothes were completely wet. Using the personal data on a student ID that the girl was carrying, it was possible to inform the parents. The girl was invited on the evening before to a going away party for a classmate.

Examination reveals the following: unconscious patient, defense response to painful stimulus, no external signs of injury, distinct smell of alcohol, symmetrical proprioceptive reflexes, no pathological reflexes, pupils moderately large, prompt light reaction, auscultation of heart and lungs as well as abdominal palpation normal, blood pressure 100/70 mmHg, heart rate 60/min, body temperature (rectal) 35.1°C, and blood sugar 63 mg/dL (3.5 mmol/L).

| 36.1 | What is your suspected diagnosis?

| 36.2 | What acute measures do you initiate?

| 36.3 | What do you do next?

→ Answers and Comments Page 152

37   Two-year-old child who has ingested an unknown fluid

In your pediatric emergency department, you receive a phone call from an agitated father. His 2-year-old daughter was unattended for only a short time and during that time she swallowed almost all of a bottle of "some kind of medicine, he wasn't quite sure what it was."

37.1   The father asks you what he should do now. What additional information do you ask for on the telephone and what advice do you give the father?

About 45 minutes after the call, the father comes to the clinic's emergency department with his daughter. He has brought the almost-empty bottle along (see Fig.). The father informs that the bottle hadn't been quite full (5 mL syrup containing 200 mg paracetamol and 2.275 g sorbitol). The child weighs 11 kg. The little girl does not seem impaired; she is playing cheerfully with the teddy bear she brought along. The child's face and hands are still completely sticky with the syrup and there are also traces of the medicine on her T-shirt. Physical examination shows no abnormalities.

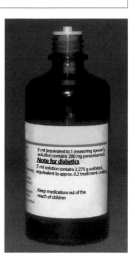

37.2   Approximately how much of the active agent has the little girl consumed? How do you estimate the toxicity of the active agent consumed?

37.3   What symptoms must you expect with paracetamol poisoning?

37.4   What measures do you initiate?

37.5   Give your reasons for the preferred use of activated charcoal for primary elimination of the poison. However, for what kinds of poisoning is activated charcoal without effect or contraindicated?

→ Answers and Comments **Page 154**

A 5-day-old newborn whose parents observed her yellow skin color and sucking weakness is brought to the pediatric clinic. The little girl is the second child of a healthy mother and is exclusively breastfed. The pregnancy was unremarkable and the outpatient birth was without complications. The birth weight was 2,980 g, body length 49 cm, head circumference 35 cm, APGAR 9/10/10, and navel artery pH 7.26. The mother's blood group is O Rh positive.

Examination shows the child's icteric skin color and scleral icterus. Moreover, the child appears listless and tired. The rest of the examination results are normal. In particular, you do not palpate hepatomegaly. Weight 2,780 g, temperature 36.8°C. The laboratory analysis of the child's blood shows the following values (see Fig.):

010403 Di 1:23 1882313	Analyte	Ref. / Therapeutic Range	Unit
	Complete blood count		
5.0	Leukocytes	5.0-20.0	/nl
5.61	Erythrocytes	4.0-6.0	/pl
21.2+	Hemoglobin	12.0-14.8	g/dl
59.0+	Hematocrit	28-42	%
37.8+	MCH	26-34	pg
35.9	MCHC	32-36	g/dl
105+	MCV	82-92	fl
143-	Thrombocytes	150-400	/nl
	Clinical chemistry		
144	Sodium	135-150	mmol/l
4.3	Potassium	3.8-5.0	mmol/l
3.8-	Calcium	4.0-5.3	mval/l
108	Chloride	95-108	mmol/l
41-	Glucose	70-125	mg/dl
33	Urea	to 44	mg/dl
0.6	Creatinine	to 1.3	mg/dl
20.7+	Bilirubin	to 1.3	mg/dl
0.5+	Direct bilirubin	to 0.2	mg/dl
<0.7	C-reactive protein	to 0.8	mg/dl
	GOT (AST)	to 17	U/l
	GPT (ALT)	to 23	U/l
	gamma-GT	to 37	U/l

Laboratory

38.1   What is your suspected diagnosis?

38.2   Explain the causes of the clinical picture to the worried parents.

38.3   What do you do next? What are the possible complications if the clinical course is unfavorable?

39   Three-year-old girl refusing to eat

A 3-year-old girl is brought to you because of a very high fever. Moreover, she has been refusing to eat for 2 days, hardly drinks anything, and salivates profusely. Examination shows that the child is in impaired general condition, with decreased skin turgor and rings around her eyes. She has foul breath. On the mucosa of mouth and tongue, there are multiple white-coated bubbles and ulcerations; the gums seem swollen and they are bleeding in spots (see Fig.). You palpate painfully swollen cervical lymph nodes.

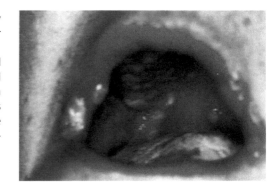

39.1   What is your suspected diagnosis?

39.2   Explain the etiology of the disease.

39.3   What further measures do you initiate?

39.4   The little girl's brother is 3 weeks old. The worried mother would like to know whether there is any danger for the little boy.

→ Answers and Comments   Page 158

While on night duty, you are called into the delivery room, where a little girl has just been born. The obstetrician has observed morphological abnormalities in the child.

On inspecting the newborn, you observe the following abnormalities: The eyelid axis slants upward toward the temple, there is a sickle-shaped skin fold at the inner, upper edge of the eyelid that extends to the lower lid and covers the nasal lid commissure. Excess skin at the nape, short, plump hands and feet, single transverse palmar crease on both sides, sandal gap (see Fig.).

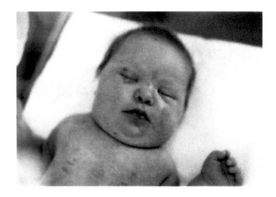

40.1 What is your suspected diagnosis? What other typical symptoms or findings do you look for?

40.2 What is at the basis of the clinical picture?

40.3 What do you know about the prognosis for this disease?

41 Two siblings with itching and eczematous changes on the skin of the neck and head

The mother of a 5-year-old boy notices that her son has been constantly scratching his neck and head for the past few days. She inspects the skin of his head and finds scratch marks and also eczematous skin changes, particularly behind the ears and on the neck. The mother also finds similar but milder changes in the skin of the older sister's head. The girl also complains of itching. The mother brings the children to the emergency department. Examination of the boy reveals the following changes on his head (see Fig.).

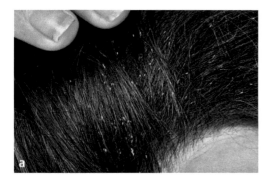

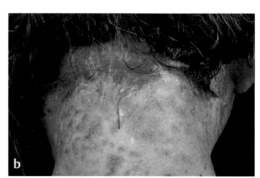

41.1 What is your suspected diagnosis?

41.2 How can you confirm the diagnosis?

41.3 What treatment do you initiate?

41.4 What additional recommendations do you give the family?

→ Answers and Comments Page 161

42 Consultation regarding "sudden infant death syndrome" (SIDS)

In the newborn nursery, you are caring for a little girl whose brother died because of sudden infant death syndrome at the age of 8 months. The parents of the newborn are very scared that they will suffer the same fate again.

42.1 What is meant by "sudden infant death?" What does the acronym "SIDS" stand for?

42.2 How is the risk for this newborn of sudden infant death assessed? What do you explain to the parents?

42.3 What diagnostic or treatment consequences result for the newborn?

42.4 What do you recommend to the parents in order to decrease the risk of sudden infant death?

→ Answers and Comments Page 163

43 Five-year-old boy with high fever and abdominal pain

A 5-year-old boy is presented to the emergency department with a high fever and intense stomach pain. The complaint began 2 days earlier and the boy got progressively worse. He coughed and vomited repeatedly and hardly ate or drank. Examination of the boy reveals the following findings (see Fig. for admission findings). The laboratory findings are as follows: leukocytes 27,800/ µL, Hb 10.6 g/dL, hematocrit 32%, thrombocytes 370,000/ µL, sodium 132 mmol/l, potassium 4.6 mmol/L, creatinine 1.0 mg/dL, GOT 12 U/L, GPT 8 U/L, γ-GT 20 U/L, CRP 38 mg/dL, and sed rate 180 mm in the first hour.

Condition on admission:	on: 12/18/03 at 18:30 age: 5y	Examining physician: Kreckmann Temp. 40.6° C	
Nursing status, general status, nutritional status	Very sick!		☐
State of consciousness			☒
Skin, hair, nails	Pale skin color, perspiring		☐
Skull, skeleton, Fontanelle			☒
Eyes, pupils			☒
Ears, eardrums	no inflammation		☐
Nose, mouth, throat	tonsillar ring and tonsils red no coating		☐
Neck, thyroid gland	no palpable lymph nodes		☐
Heart, pulse	clear and rhythmical heart rate 120/min		☐
Breathing, lungs dull sound on percussion	tachypnea, dyspnea, flaring nostrils, bronchial breathing right over upper and middle field, also moderate and fine crackles, vesicular breathing left		
Abdomen renal bed rectal examination	bloated, tense, diffuse pain on pressure paraumbilical p.m. lively peristalsis		☐
Genitals			☒
Neurology	no meningism reflexes symmetrical		☐

43.1 What possible diseases are you considering? What studies do you order to arrive at a diagnosis?

Among other things, you ordered a thoracic X-ray (see Fig.).

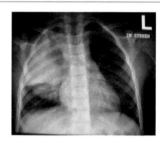

Thoracic X-ray

43.2 Describe what you see on the survey radiograph of the thorax. What is your diagnosis on the basis of the medical history, clinical picture, and diagnostic findings?

43.3 What pathogens do you suspect in the child? Which pathogens are quite commonly typical for the disease at this age? Which pathogens do you expect in newborns or school children?

43.4 Name additional forms of this disease. Which pathogens do you expect in these forms?

43.5 What treatment do you initiate?

→ Answers and Comments Page 165

A doctor in private practice refers a 4-year-old boy for admission because of an acute urinary tract infection. The boy has been sick with a high fever and abdominal pain since the day before. The examination in the doctor's office revealed leukocytes and erythrocytes in the urine. Nitrite was positive. In the past 2 years, the boy had been treated with antibiotics three times for urinary tract infections.

The child appears tired and sick. The rectal temperature is 39.8°C. Auscultation of the abdomen indicates normal peristalsis; on palpation the boy complains of diffused pain on pressure. Neither resistances, nor peritoneal inflammation of enlarged organs, can be palpated. Both renal beds are free. The remaining physical examination is normal.

44.1 What do you do next?

In further diagnostic workup, you order a micturating cystourethrography (MCU).

44.2 Explain the course of the examination.

44.3 Interpret the finding from the MCU (see Fig.). Explain the stage classification of the disease.

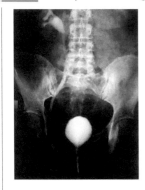

Micturating cystourethrography

44.4 What additional treatment do you recommend for this patient?

→ Answers and Comments Page 167

45 Seven-year-old boy with pneumonia and bone pain

A 7-year-old boy fell acutely ill 2 days earlier with cough, fever up to 40°C, and pain in the shoulder girdle. The pediatrician diagnosed bronchial pneumonia and tried to treat the patient with oral erythromycin. The child vomited the medication repeatedly so the pediatrician has now referred the boy for admission, for i.v. antibiotic treatment. The boy is in distinctly reduced general condition and can barely stand up. According to the mother, the boy hasn't been really "fit" for the past 2 weeks or so. He is constantly tired, noticeably pale, and has no appetite.

Examination reveals the following findings: reduced general condition, pale skin, tonsils somewhat enlarged without coating, tonsillar ring red, ear drums not inflamed, pronounced coarse cervical lymph node adhesions bilaterally; intensified breath sounds over the lungs bilaterally, individual moderately coarse crackles left more than right, and productive cough. The liver can be palpated 3 cm and the spleen 2 cm below the costal arch. No abdominal pain on pressure, abdominal peristalsis normal, neurological examination normal.

The laboratory tests include the following values: Hb 8.6 g/dL, MCV 82 fL, MCHC 30 pg, leukocytes 2LDH 27,000/µL (differential 60% lymphoblasts), thrombocytes 80,000/µL, LDH 720 U/L, uric acid 8 mg/dL, CRP 82 mg/L, sed rate 80/140 mm, normal value. A blood smear is ordered (see Fig.).

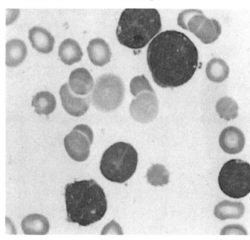

Blood smear

45.1 How do you interpret the findings?

45.2 What further diagnostic measures do you initiate?

45.3 How will this disease be treated if your diagnosis is confirmed?

45.4 Name additional risk factors that promote this disease.

→ Answers and Comments Page 169

A 4-year-old boy is brought in by his mother because for 3 days he has had fever, joint pain, and a rash with large, confluent spots. The clinical examination shows no pathological abnormalities other than swollen cervical lymph nodes and bilateral conjunctivitis.

46.1 What is your suspected diagnosis? What treatment do you initiate?

Four days later, the mother returns with the child. In the past 2 days, the fever had risen above 40°C and could only be reduced by about 1°C for a short time by administration of paracetamol. Examination of the boy yields the following findings: severely reduced general condition, morbiliform exanthema over the entire body, inner surface of hands and feet red and swollen, bilateral conjunctivitis, very red, slightly sensitive oral mucosa, ENT area otherwise normal, swollen lymph nodes in angle of jaw bilaterally, heart and lungs normal on auscultation, abdomen diffusely painful on pressure without protective tension, slight hepatosplenomegaly, normal peristalsis, neurological examination normal, in particular no meningism.

46.2 What diagnosis must now be considered?

46.3 What is the most likely diagnosis? What is the underlying cause? How do you confirm this diagnosis?

46.4 What complications should you expect if your suspected diagnosis is correct?

46.5 What treatment do you initiate if your suspected diagnosis is correct?

→ Answers and Comments Page 172

47 Four-year-old girl with facial swelling

A 4-year-old girl is brought to the pediatrician because in the past few days, her parents have observed increasing facial swelling (see Fig.). In particular, the eyelids are regularly "swollen shut" in the morning when she wakes up.

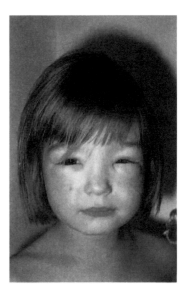

47.1 Make a suspected diagnosis. Name other findings and symptoms typical of your suspected diagnosis.

47.2 How do you confirm the diagnosis?

47.3 List the most frequent causes of this disease.

47.4 How do you treat the disease in this child?

→ Answers and Comments Page 174

A 5-year-old girl is brought to the pediatrician because of a 3-day-old febrile respiratory infection. During the physical examination, in addition to the pale skin and discrete scleral icterus, the pediatrician observed a markedly enlarged spleen. The blood tests run because of this showed these values among others: Hb 6.8 g/dL, MCV 65 fL, MCH 30 pg, MCHC 34 g/dL, reticulocytes 17‰, bilirubin 2.5 mg/dL. He refers the girl for admission to the children's hospital for a differential diagnosis. The child is admitted to the hospital and the medical history shows that as a child, the girl's father had "abdominal surgery for a blood disease."

48.1 Interpret the laboratory values. What causes associated with the medical history and clinical examination are you considering?

48.2 How do you confirm the diagnosis?

Subsequent diagnostic tests include the following result (see Fig.).

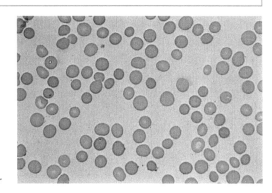

Blood smear

48.3 What is your diagnosis?

48.4 Explain the pathogenesis of the disease.

! **48.5** How can the disease be treated? What should be kept in mind here?

→ Answers and Comments **Page 176**

49   Seven-year-old girl with headaches and abnormal behavior

A mother brings her 7-year-old daughter to the emergency department of a children's hospital. The girl has been vomiting occasionally for a week, especially in the morning after she gets up. Since the day before, she has vomited five times and complains of headache. Her temperature is slightly elevated (38°C). The last stool, the day before, was of completely normal consistency. Examination reveals the following pathological findings: red tonsillar ring, intestinal peristalsis very active. An ordinary gastrointestinal infection is suspected. Suppositories for nausea, plentiful fluids, and a low fat diet are prescribed. The mother and child go back home for the time being.

During the night, the mother brings her daughter in again. In spite of Suppositories for nausea administration, the vomiting had become worse, and the girl vomited bile repeatedly. The child looks "miserable" and seems sicker than in the morning.

49.1   You examine the child once more in great detail. What do you look for in particular?

In discussion of the medical history, the mother now mentions, just in passing, that her daughter had recently been acting quite differently than usual. She had always been very nice and now she is often aggressive and impatient. Her performance in school had also deteriorated because she did not concentrate in class. In addition, the mother had observed a kind of clumsiness. She said that her daughter stumbled over her own feet, often dropped things, or knocked things over.

49.2   What differential diagnosis are you considering now that you have this new information? What diagnostic measures do you take to distinguish between the differential diagnoses?

49.3   An MRI of the skull with contrast medium is performed (see Fig.). Describe the result.

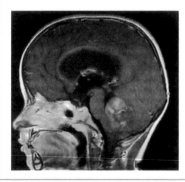

MRI

49.4   What will the further treatment be?

→ Answers and Comments Page 177

50   Four-year-old boy with pain in right lower abdomen

A 4-year-old boy is presented to the emergency department by his parents, in the early morning hours. Since the evening before, the boy has had acute abdominal pain with fever up to 39°C (rectal) and vomiting. In spite of symptomatic treatment (leg wraps, paracetamol), the fever could not be reduced, and in the course of the night, the abdominal pain kept increasing. The parents report that actually the boy "is otherwise not at all sensitive." He seldom complains of pain and up to now, he has never been really sick.

50.1   By questioning the parents and the child, try to narrow down the possible causes. What causes are you thinking of and what do you ask about?

In response to your questions, the boy reports pain all over his abdomen.

50.2   What diagnostic measures should you use next in order to establish a diagnosis?

You examine the little patient who is lying curled up on the examining table. The mother adds that the abdominal pain is particularly intense when her son urinates. You examine the abdomen very carefully while trying to distract the child, but the examination still seems to be painful. You palpate a distinct protective tension in the lower abdomen, right somewhat stronger than left. Lively peristalsis can be auscultated throughout the abdomen. In the rectal examination, the child resists vigorously but you cannot be sure this is caused by pain or the disagreeable examination.

50.3   What do you do next?

50.4   What complications should you expect if this is acute appendicitis?

50.5   What additional differential diagnoses would you have to consider if the patient were a 15-year-old girl?

→ Answers and Comments Page 178

51 Three-year-old girl with protective posture of right arm

Parents bring their 3-year-old daughter (see Fig. a) to the emergency department because for the past 2 hours she no longer wanted to move her right arm. On further investigation, you learn that earlier, while she was walking down the stairs holding her mother's hand, she slipped. The mother pulled her up by the hand, in order to prevent her from falling.

On examination, the arm seems to be painful and you cannot get her to raise the arm even with the incentive of a piece of candy (see Fig. b).

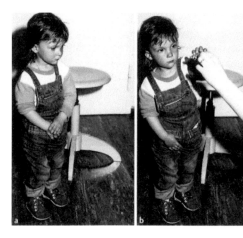

51.1 Justify your suspected diagnosis on the basis of the medical history and the clinical picture.

51.2 What other possible injuries should you be considering? How can you distinguish between these and your suspected diagnosis?

51.3 Explain the mechanism of injury for your suspected diagnosis.

51.4 What do you do next?

→ Answers and Comments Page 181

A 10-year-old boy is brought to the emergency department with the information that 1 hour ago he suddenly complained about flickering vision problems and a feeling of numbness first in the right arm and then in the right leg. The parents also observed blurred, "babbling" speech. After a few minutes, these symptoms disappeared, and instead, the boy was now complaining of strictly left-sided, intense headache and nausea. Bright light was unpleasant for him. This was the first occurrence of such an event. Anamnestically, the parents report that the little boy had febrile convulsions. His development has been normal.

You examine the boy, who is still complaining of left-sided headache and nausea. There are no other symptoms. The neurological examination and the remaining physical examination are normal.

52.1   Which differential diagnoses are you considering? What is the most likely diagnosis? What is your rationale?

52.2   What further tests would you consider useful?

52.3   What treatment do you initiate?

→ Answers and Comments Page 182

| **53** | Sixteen-month-old boy with undescended testis

During the night shift, a 16-month-old boy is brought in because of a febrile respiratory infection. In the physical examination, in addition to bronchitis, you make the secondary observation that only the left testicle has descended into the scrotum. Upon questioning, you learn that the right testicle has never been in the scrotum and that even while bathing it never migrates into the scrotum. Up to now, there has never been a diagnosis or a treatment.

| 53.1 | **What do you think about the fact that up to now there has never been a diagnosis or a treatment? What advice do you give the parents?**

| 53.2 | **What did you want to find out when you asked the parents whether the testicle is in the scrotum during bathing?**

| 53.3 | **Name and explain the different forms of undescended testis.**

| 53.4 | **What could cause undescended testis?**

| 53.5 | **What therapeutic possibilities are available for the treatment of undescended testis?**

→ Answers and Comments Page 184

54   Eight-year-old boy with abdominal pain and weight loss

An 8-year-old boy is brought to the emergency department because he has been complaining of abdominal pain and nausea for 2 days. On the previous night, though he vomited several times. diarrhea and fever were absent. Now he is increasingly sleepy. The parents informed that for the past 2 weeks the boy was tired, fatigued, and in a bad mood. In this time, he had lost a good 3 kg, although he was eating with good appetite and drinking a great deal. In addition, the parents observed that their son constantly needed the toilet. In fact, in the past week, the boy had even wet his bed on two nights.

54.1   **What is your suspected diagnosis on the basis of this medical history? What pathological findings might you gather in the clinical examination if your suspected diagnosis is correct?**

54.2   **What examinations do you perform to confirm the diagnosis?**

You examine the boy, who is sleepy but reacts when addressed. His breathing is markedly deep and his breath smells of acetone. Clear signs of dehydration are found: persistent skin folds, dry skin and mucosa, dry coated tongue, and sunken eyes. The abdomen is shrunken. It is soft on palpation and there is no defensive tension. You feel neither enlarged organs nor pathological resistances. Peristalsis sounds normal. Normal heart and lung sounds. In the neurological examination, reflexes are normal, and the pupillary light reflex is prompt. No signs of meningismus are found. The outpatient nurse measures pulse and blood pressure: Heart rate 110/min, blood pressure 90/50 mmHg.

54.3   **What acute treatment do you initiate? How do you proceed?**

54.4   **Explain the etiology of the disease.**

! 54.5   **What kind of diet should the child have with this disease? Explain and calculate the energy needs of the 8-year-old boy.**

→ Answers and Comments **Page 186**

55 Premature birth in the 28th week of pregnancy with shortness of breath and abdominal pain on pressure

In the premature ward, you are caring for an extremely small premature baby. The boy was born by cesarean section after 27 weeks and 5 days of pregnancy because of the mother's HELLP syndrome (special form of pre-eclampsia). The birth weight was 840 g, body length 30 cm, and head circumference 26 cm.
Postnatally, the boy adapted well at first, breathed spontaneously, and quickly became rosy with oxygen (2–4 L/min with mask). Six hours postpartum he showed symptoms of dyspnea, so much that he had to be intubated and ventilated (see Fig.).

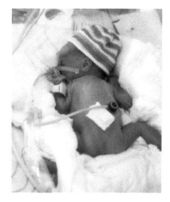

55.1 What are the symptoms of respiratory distress syndrome? Explain the etiopathogenesis of respiratory distress syndrome.

55.2 How is respiratory distress syndrome treated?

The parents have heard that ventilation can lead to "problems with the eyes."

55.3 What disease are the parents thinking of? Describe the clinical picture.

Two days later the child's general condition is dramatically worse. The child becomes septic: gray mottled skin, recapillarization time is extended to 5 seconds, the need for ventilation and oxygen has increased (FiO$_2$ = 0.7), the abdomen is swollen. The child vomits bile repeatedly and excretes bloody, mucous stools. Palpation of the abdomen clearly causes pain.

55.4 Which disease is it most likely? How can you confirm your suspected diagnosis?

→ Answers and Comments **Page 189**

A 5-year-old boy with intense abdominal and rectal pain is presented to the emergency department. The parents explain that the boy has not had a bowel movement for a week and can no longer go to the toilet because of the pain and hasn't vomitted. Occasionally, especially during the day, the boy would soil his pants; his underpants were often soiled. Often, the boy would have no bowel movement for days, but then have diarrhea. The mother already knows the symptoms; in the past 2 years, she has taken the child to the pediatrician more than once because of absence of bowel movements. It has not yet been possible to determine the cause of the complaints.

The boy, who is writhing with abdominal pain, is examined. The following clinical findings are observed: abdomen distended, diffuse pain on pressure, no defensive tension, resistances in lower abdomen bilaterally, active intestinal sounds, anus reddened perianally with traces of scratching. Rectal examination: painful, ampulla wide and filled with hardened stool, barely possible to insert finger, good sphincter tonus; remaining physical examination is normal.

57

56.1 How do you explain the alternation between stool retention and diarrhea? What is the cause of the boy's soiled underpants?

56.2 What is your suspected diagnosis? What are the general underlying causes of these symptoms?

56.3 What is your next diagnostic step?

The detailed diagnostic workup did not find a cause for the constipation.

56.4 What is your next treatment step?

→ Answers and Comments Page 192

A pediatrician refers a 2-year-old boy to the children's hospital. For 10 days he has had a high fever (about 39°C), lack of appetite, and a slightly transient skin rash with coarse spots (see Fig.). Since the day before, the little boy has not wanted to walk; the parents observed swelling in the left ankle. Similar symptoms, except for the joint swelling, occurred 3 months ago as well, which disappeared within a week on treatment with an anti-pyretic (ibuprofen). At that time, a suspected diagnosis of fifth disease was established.

The physical examination of the boy, who seemed to be very sick, reveals not only the maculopapulous rash already described and a hot, painful swelling in the left ankle, but also a generalized lymphadenop-athy and hepatomegaly. A blood study results in the following findings: Hb 9.6 g/dL, leukocytes 15,300/µL (differential: neutrophils 68%, banded neutrophils 11%, segmented neutrophils 13%, lymphocytes 8%), thrombocytes 635,000/µL, MCV 62 fL, MCH 20 pg,

CRP 27 mg/dL (270 mg/L), and sed rate 120 mm in the first hour.

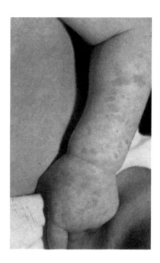

| 57.1   What is your diagnosis? What differential diagnoses are you considering?

| 57.2   What further tests would you consider useful?

| 57.3   How is the disease that you are suspecting generally treated?

→ Answers and Comments **Page 194**

A 4-month-old boy is brought into the emergency department by his parents at night because for the past 3 hours, he has been crying almost without interruption and cannot be soothed.

The screaming child has a right inguinal swelling and the rest of the physical examination reveals no pathological findings.

58.1 Name and justify your suspected diagnosis. What differential diagnoses must you take into account in case of an inguinal swelling?

58.2 There are two forms of this disease. List differences. What form is the infant most likely to have?

58.3 What do you do next?

58.4 List complications of this disease.

→ Answers and Comments Page 196

59   Nineteen-month-old girl with bloody diarrhea, hematomas, and anuria

An emergency doctor brings a severely ill, apathetic, 19-month-old little girl to the pediatric emergency department. The parents inform that the little girl has been suffering for 1 week from diarrhea and vomiting and has been passing bloody stools since the previous day. During the week that she has been ill, the girl increasingly refused all food and fluid and is no longer excreting urine. Examination reveals the following findings: apathetic

little girl with sallow, pale, icteric skin, individual hematomas and petechial skin bleeding on the trunk, persistent skin folds, circles around the eyes, protruding abdomen, lively peristalsis, liver and spleen not enlarged, no palpable resistances, heart 2/6 systolic murmur with maximum over Erb's point, lung sounds normal, no meningismus, temperature 36.5°C, blood pressure 90/50 mmHg, and pulse 120/min.

59.1   What diagnostic measures do you consider useful to initiate next? What are the grounds for·this?

The laboratory test had the following results, among others: leukocytes 12,300/μL, Hb 8.5 g/dL, MCV 86 fL, MCH 30 pg, thrombocytes 78,000/μL, reticulocytes 16‰, Quick 79%, PTT 20s, LDH 480 U/L, potassium 5.9 mmol/L, total bilirubin 5.3 mg/dL, creatinine 2.5 mg/dL, urea 22 mg/dL; blood smear (see Fig.).

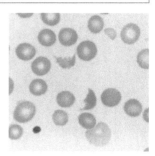

Blood smear

59.2   Interpret the laboratory values. What is your diagnosis?

59.3   Explain the pathogenesis of the disease.

59.4   How do you treat the girl?

→ Answers and Comments Page 198

A gynecologist calls a pediatrician, at night, to see a female newborn, born by spontaneous delivery a few minutes ago. With good spontaneous breathing and good tonus, the baby has persistent cyanosis that is not improved by administration of oxygen.

The pediatrician examines the child and confirms the cyanosis. No external deformity is found. The child's breathing is somewhat accelerated but there is no dyspnea. The physical examination is normal; in particular, auscultation of heart and lungs yields no pathological findings.

For better observation, the little girl is placed in an incubator and oxygen is introduced. But no matter how high the oxygen concentration, the oxygen saturation, measured with a pulseoxymeter, does not rise above 85% and the child remains cyanotic. Connatal pneumonia, which was considered as a differential diagnosis because of the tachypnea and the oxygen lack, was ruled out radiologically. Finally, a senior physician instructs to get an echocardiogram done.

60.1 What is your diagnosis on the basis of the clinical and echocardiographic findings? (see Fig.)

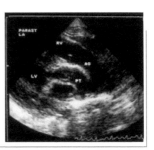

Echocardiogram

60.2 How is this deformity treated?

A few days later you do a newborn examination of a 5-day-old boy. According to the parents and the pediatric nurses, the postpartum course has been completely normal up to now. The child announces his hunger at volume and nurses well. On auscultation of the heart, a loud, hissing systolic heart sound is heard, with maximum point in the third and fourth intercostal space left parasternal.

60.3 What do you do next?

An echocardiography is performed (see Fig.).

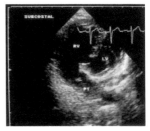

Echocardiogram

60.4 Diagnose the echocardiogram. What do you determine?

60.5 In many congenital heart defects, there is an elevated risk of endocarditis. In this connection, what is meant by endocarditis prophylaxis?

→ Answers and Comments Page 199

61 Four-year-old boy with rattling breath and hypersalivation

A 4-year-old boy was admitted 2 days earlier for febrile tonsillitis and complete refusal to eat. I.V. antibiotic therapy with amoxicillin was initiated.

At night, the boy has "rattling" breath and intense salivation. Moreover, he is complaining of earache in his left ear. When his throat is inspected, it is observed that the red and pus-coated left tonsil and the soft palate are arching forward into the throat and the uvula is displaced to the right. The lymph nodes of the left jaw angle are thickly swollen.

61.1 What is your diagnosis?

61.2 What do you do next?

61.3 Name and explain the complications of streptococcal angina.

61.4 What is meant by the Jones diagnosis criteria?

→ Answers and Comments Page 203

A 6-year-old boy has been suffering since birth from a failure to thrive. His body weight and length has always been below the third percentile. Currently, he weighs 17 kg and is 108 cm tall. In the process of diagnosing this failure to thrive, the private practice pediatrician performed an abdominal sonography and found the following abnormal sign in the liver (see Fig.). For further investigation, he admits the boy to the Hospital for Children and Adolescents.

During the detailed anamnestic conversation with parents and child, it was learnt that the boy always developed normally, except for his height. However, for 3 years, he has been suffering from bronchitis, and once, from pneumonia. In the previous year, it was determined that he has an allergy to house dust mites. Since then, the boy regularly inhales a combination preparation consisting of a glucocorticoid for inhalation and a long-acting β-sympathomimetic. In addition, the

parents report that the boy suffers from intense bloating and abdominal pain.

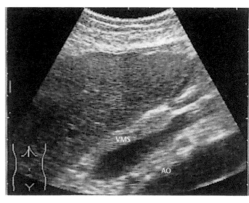

Liver sonography (SMV = superior mesenteric vein; AO = aorta)

! 62.1 Describe the abnormalities in the liver ultrasound findings. Which liver disease is probably present here?

62.2 In your opinion, what disease does the boy have? What is your rationale?

62.3 What pathophysiological changes underlie this clinical picture? Which organs are particularly affected by the changes?

62.4 What other studies do you order to confirm this diagnosis?

62.5 The boy's mother is expecting her second child. How great is the possibility that this child is also sick?

→ Answers and Comments Page 205

63   Fourteen-year-old girl who collapsed on a school trip

An emergency doctor was called to a fruit juice-pressing house where a 14-year-old schoolgirl had collapsed on a class trip. When he arrived, the girl was sleeping deeply and reacted inadequately when she was addressed or touched (pinching, cheek slap, tweaking). There was a great deal of excitement and no one could give any information as to what, precisely, had happened. The doctor started an infusion of Ringer solution and brought the patient by ambulance to the emergency department at a hospital for children and adolescents. During the transport, the girl woke up. Later on, she could not remember anything about this event. She reacts appropriately, and the vital signs, such as pulse, respiration, saturation, and blood pressure, are normal, and at 120 mg/dL, the blood sugar value is normal.

63.1   The emergency physician says: "That was certainly a seizure." What possible causes do you consider?

In the meantime, the classroom teacher and the patient's best friend arrive. The friend tells you that the girl cried out and then fell down. Then she got completely stiff and for a short time, twitched with her arms and legs. Her face was completely blue. Everything was terrible. She kept calling her friend by name and throwing cold water in her face, but the girl didn't wake up.

63.2   What is the most likely seizure type here? What do you look for in the physical examination?

63.3   What further measures do you suggest?

→ Answers and Comments **Page 208**

A 3-year-old boy was admitted 2 days ago with a sudden high fever (up to 40°C), colic-like abdominal pain, and bloody diarrhea. Up to now, he had been treated symptomatically, that is, the fever was lowered with paracetamol syrup; he was given a low fat diet and oral electrolyte solution as well as an accompanying infusion therapy, in order to compensate for the ongoing loss of fluid through diarrhea. His condition has become markedly worse than it was a few hours earlier. The boy is very restless. There is marked cyanosis of the lips, and the skin is blotchy over the whole body; the capillary filling time is extended (4 seconds). The breathing is rapid. A glance at the child's fever curve will give a better picture (see Fig.).

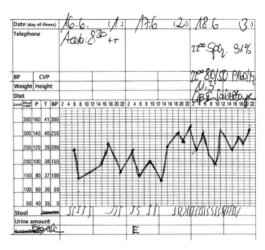

Fever curve

64.1   What information do you obtain from the fever curve? With what suspected diagnosis was the boy probably admitted?

Blood is drawn for analysis. In the meantime, the emergency laboratory provides the pathological findings (see Fig.).

160603 Mo	180603 We	Analyte	Ref./Therapeutic Range	Unit
		Hematology		
		Differential blood count		
66+	70+	Segmented cells	45-65	%
9+	7	Neutrophils	2-8	%
23	18	Lymphocytes	25-40	%
2	3	Monocytes	2-10	%
	2	Eosinophils	1-5	%
		Clinical chemistry		
136	129-	Sodium	135-150	mmol/l
3.6-	3.2-	Potassium	3.8-5.0	mmol/l
6.6+	47.3+	C-reactive protein	up to 0.8	mg/dl

Pathological laboratory results

64.2   Interpret the laboratory values. What do you do next?

One day later, the results of a stool culture are received. In addition, the microbiology lab informs that there were "rod-shaped bacteria" growing in the blood culture.

64.3   Explain the epidemiology of the clinical picture.

The boy's father has acute myeloid leukemia. Following a stem cell transplantation 2 years earlier, he has been in remission. But he continues to take immune-suppressive medications.

64.4   Is there a danger of contagion? What advice do you give the father?

→ Answers and Comments Page 210

65 **Healthy newborn delivered by cesarean section**

It is customary for obstetricians to ask the pediatrician to be present for first care of the newborn in cases of cesarean section and surgical delivery. The midwife calls the pediatrician for a cesarean section and provides the following information: "G2 P1, child at term, cesarean section when birth process was stalled, suspicion of malpositioning, CTG normal, section in 5 minutes."

65.1 **What is the meaning of the information the midwife gives you?**

In the OR, the mother has been given PDA (peridural anesthesia); she is awake and already positioned for the operation. The father is present for the cesarean section; he is already sitting at the head end, next to his wife. The resuscitation unit, suction equipment, and ventilation system function flawlessly; the Ambu bag is connected to the oxygen; and the radiant heater is turned on. Warmed blankets are fetched from the warming closet. In addition, the laryngoscope and tube of the right size are adjusted. The gynecologists operate and deliver a strong, rosy-looking boy.

65.2 **What do you do next?**

A few hours later, you are called to the delivery room for a birth. After the cord has been tied, the midwife brings you a boy who is not crying, but lying quite limp in her arms. The child's skin is cyanotic.

65.3 **What do you do next?**

The blood gas analysis on cord blood (umbilical artery) shows the following finding (see Fig.).

Date 23.10.	
pH	7.129
PCO2	56.9 mmHg
PO2	39.2 → 40 mmHg
HCO3	18.3 mmol/l
TCO2	20.0 mmol/l
BE	– 11.9 mmol/l
BEecf	– 9.7 mmol/l
O2sat	52.4 %

65.4 **What is the purpose of the blood gas analysis on umbilical artery blood? How do you interpret the values?**

→ Answers and Comments **Page 212**

It is the first holiday of Christmas and the emergency department is buzzing. Almost all the patients have the same symptoms as the 11-year-old boy who was just brought in by his father. He suddenly became ill the night before, with a high fever up to 40°C, joint pain, fatigue, and a feeling of being very ill. In addition, he complains of burning, painful eyes, head and throat pain, and a dry, irritating cough.

The boy appears to be very sick. He is pale, the conjunctivas are red, and the throat is very red. Auscultation of the lungs and the remaining physical examination reveal no pathological findings. The father reports that the boy's mother has been at home in bed with a high fever for the past 3 days.

66.1   What disease do you suspect as the source of the "epidemic"?

66.2   What do you know about the source of the clinical picture?

66.3   What complications of the disease are you familiar with?

66.4   What treatment seems useful to you?

→ Answers and Comments Page 217

| 67 | Newborn boy with conspicuous genitals

The genitals of a newborn boy, who was born by natural delivery a short time ago, has to be examined. Postnatal adaptation took place without a problem. At the first newborn examination, the examining gynecological colleague noticed a change in the external genitals of the little boy (see Fig.).

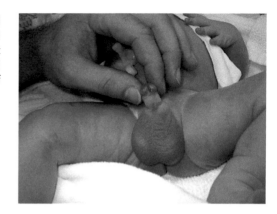

| 67.1 | Describe the finding. What is your diagnosis?

| 67.2 | What do you look for in particular in the clinical examination?

| 67.3 | What further diagnostic measures are necessary?

| 67.4 | What therapy do you recommend? When should the treatment take place?

→ Answers and Comments Page 219

68   Six-year-old girl with abnormal appearance

Parents bring in their 6-year-old daughter for admission. She was hospitalized by her ear, nose, and throat doctor for paracentesis and insertion of tympanostomy tubes to treat recurrent otitis. A pediatrician has to examine the child preoperatively and declare her fit for surgery (see Fig.).

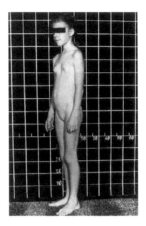

68.1   **What do you observe on examining the patient?**

A more detailed examination shows that in the pubic area there are already individual, long, darkly pigmented hairs growing.

68.2   **What is the stage of puberty, according to the Tanner classification?**

68.3   **What diseases should you consider for differential diagnosis?**

68.4   **What further diagnostic measures are necessary?**

68.5   **What therapy is indicated?**

→ Answers and Comments Page 220

69 Premature baby with acute deterioration of general condition

A boy, the second child of a 21-year-old woman in the 32nd week of pregnancy, was born by precipitate labor after a pregnancy that, until that time, had been normal. The following data were collected after the delivery: birth weight 1,880 g, body length 42 cm, head circumference 31 cm, APGAR 9/9/10, and umbilical artery pH 7.25.

In spite of the early birth, the child adjusted astonishingly well to postnatal conditions. An initial slight dyspnea syndrome (tachypnea, flared nostrils) was treated with oxygen in an incubator (max. 35% O_2 over a period of 3 days). Building up the nutrition with nutrients for premature babies proceeded without problems. The boy even drank large portions of his meals independently. The child was watched on a monitor. Breathing, heart rate, and blood pressure were always in the normal range.

Thirteen days after birth, an experienced pediatric nurse calls for a pediatrician as the child "really didn't look good to her." For the last little while, the monitor showed pauses in breathing and bradycardia and the skin was not as pink as usual. The boy also didn't want to drink anymore and vomited all of his last meal.

Examination shows that the child is pale gray, with blotchy skin, the recapillarization time is extended by more than 3 seconds, and the fontanelle is under tension. Moreover, expiratory grunting and tachycardia are also observed. Lungs and heart are normal on auscultation. The abdomen is distended and peristalsis is reduced. There are no signs of edema; skin turgor is not reduced. The body temperature is 37.2°C.

Then a series of breathing pauses is observed. The child has to be repeatedly stimulated and finally even briefly ventilated with the bag.

69.1 What do you do next?

For laboratory results, see Fig. The urine was normal, except for elevated urine osmolality (860 mosmol/L). Blood gas analysis: pH 7.23, pCO$_2$ 57 mmHg, BE −8 mmol/L.

Complete blood count

5.4	Leukocytes	6.0-17.5	/nl
4.03	Erythrocytes	3.0-5.4	/pl
15.0	Hemoglobin	13.3-16.5	g/dl
43.0+	Hematocrit	28-42	%
37.2+	MCN	26-34	pg
34.9	HCHC	32-36	g/dl
107+	MCV	82-92	fl
107-	Platelets	150-400	/nl

Clinical Chemistry

1217	Sodium	135-150	mmol/l
6.3+	Potassium	3.8-5.0	mmol/l
4.4	Calcium	4.0-5.3	mval/l
93-	Chloride	95-108	mmol/l
11.7+	C-reactive protein	to-0.8	mg/dl

Coagulation

57-	Quick	70-120	%
1.59	INR		
45+	PTT	up to 42	s
16	PTZ	17-24	s
636+	Fibringen	200-400	mg/dl
30-	Antithrombin III	80-120	%

Cerebrospinal fluid studies

Cerebrospinal fluid status

10400	Cell count in CSF		/3cells
<10	Glucose in CSF		mg/dl
461+	Protein in CSF	15-45	mg/dl
72+	Lactate in CSF	10-20	mg/dl

69.2 Interpret the laboratory values.

You receive the results of the blood culture—Group B β-hemolytic streptococci—3 days later.

69.3 Interpret the findings in the light of the clinical picture up to now. What do you know about this clinical picture?

! 69.4 In addition, the blood study shows hyponatremia. How do you interpret this electrolyte shift if you find out at the same time that the boy is gaining weight and excreting less?

→ Answers and Comments **Page 223**

Parents come to your pediatric practice with their 4-year-old daughter on the advice of a childcare worker who had noticed that the little girl was always tired in kindergarten and could barely concentrate on playing or doing crafts. The parents had also observed the marked tiredness and increased need for sleep; their daughter was hard to wake in the morning. They have no explanation for the little girl's tiredness since she goes to bed at 8:00 p.m. and falls asleep right away. They had only noticed that their daughter sometimes sweats a great deal at night. The parents are worried now and hope to have this cleared up.

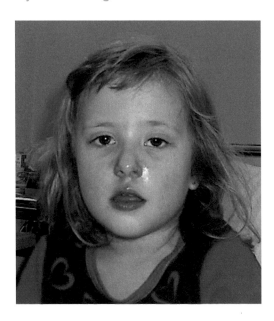

70.1   What do you observe on examining the patient (see Fig.)? What additional information from the medical history do you find interesting?

70.2   Make a suspected diagnosis. How do you confirm the diagnosis?

70.3   Explain the pathogenesis of the clinical picture.

70.4   What therapy is required?

→ Answers and Comments Page 225

71 Exasperated parents with an 8-week-old screaming baby in the emergency department

It is 3:00 a.m. Parents bring their sleeping, 8-week-old infant to the emergency department. They inform that the child was restless all day and that since early in the evening, he screamed almost without interruption, not allowing himself to be really calmed by anything. The parents have no idea of what else to do, and so they bring the child to the hospital. During the ride to the hospital, the child finally falls asleep. The mother informs that the infant has been restless since birth and has not found a rhythm either for sleep or for nursing. At night, he wakes up screaming, at the most after 2 to 3 hours, and only goes back to sleep after a lot of "back and forth." The baby cries a lot during the day and only sleeps occasionally "for a little hour," and then wakes up again, screaming. The neighbors are complaining already, especially because of the disturbance at night. The parents have already tried many things: tips from the grandparents, a friend, and the midwife, such as a warm sack of cherry stones on the stomach, stomach massage, wind oil (oil that is meant to help against flatulence), warm baths, carrying the baby around, pacifier, fennel tea, etc. These things have brought relief but no real solution to the problem.

71.1 How do you evaluate the parents' situation? What advice would you give the parents?

The mother wanted to breastfeed her child, but it seemed to her that she did not have enough milk, so after the child was 2 weeks old, on the midwife's advice, she added a complementary food.

71.2 What are the advantages of nursing? How long should the baby be exclusively breastfed? Are there situations in which the mother should be advised not to breastfeed?

After 4 weeks, the mother finally weaned the baby because of a "breast infection." The breast milk substitute did not seem to satisfy the child, so the mother switched to a "stage 1 baby food." From this time on, there were problems with the baby's stool. The child only had a bowel movement every 3 days. The pediatrician recommended adding lactose to the baby's food. This caused the stool to become softer and regular again. However, the child remained restless, and always pulled her legs to her stomach when she cried. A special food against flatulence was started. This did not improve the situation. At the moment, the parents are feeding a mixture of stage 1 and stage 2 formula with the addition of lactose.

71.3 What is meant by early stage, stage 1, and stage 2 food? How do these infant foods differ from each other? How do you evaluate the development of the child's diet up to now? What do you recommend to the family?

71.4 What should a nutrition plan for the first year of a child's life normally look like?

71.5 Do infants need nutritional supplements in addition to mother's milk or formula?

→ Answers and Comments **Page 227**

72 Five-month-old infant with severe cough for the past few weeks

A 5-month-old infant is presented to the emergency department. The boy has a cough that has been growing progressively worse over the past few weeks. He is almost always tired and listless, doesn't drink well, and vomits when he coughs. At night, the child is often wet with perspiration.

72.1 What are your next steps in establishing a diagnosis?

As part of the diagnostic workup, a thoracic X-ray is ordered (see Fig.).

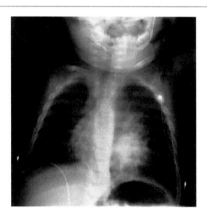

Thoracic X-ray

72.2 Describe what you notice on the thoracic X-ray. What is your suspected diagnosis, in light of the medical history, and how can you confirm it?

72.3 Give a brief picture of the course of this disease.

72.4 What do you know about the treatment of this disease?

A few days later a 5-year-old boy is presented to the emergency department. The mother is completely beside herself because a child in her son's kindergarten has tuberculosis. She demands that her son be given the inoculation that "everyone used to get."

72.5 What inoculation does the mother mean? Will you inoculate the child? What are the general recommendations for prophylaxis of this disease?

→ Answers and Comments Page 231

73 Fourteen-year-old girl with recurrent abdominal pain

A 14-year-old girl is brought to the emergency department. In the past 3 months, the patient was admitted twice to the Hospital for Children and Adolescents. As in the previous cases, the girl complains of severe epigastric and umbilical pain. The girl has repeatedly suffered from abdominal pain for the past half year, but no cause could be found. The girl's general condition is not significantly impaired and she has not lost weight. The girl is anxious.

73.1 What do you ask the patient?

73.2 What do you look for in the physical examination?

73.3 What are the possible causes of the patient's complaints?

73.4 What further tests do you consider necessary "basic tests" to differentiate between the causes of the complaints?

73.5 This time, you can again not find an organic cause for the complaints. What recommendations do you give the patient now?

→ Answers and Comments Page 236

A primary care doctor refers a 15-year-old boy for admission. The boy is in the ninth grade of high school. He was always among the tallest in his class (height 180 cm, weight 94 kg). Most of his classmates are already showing signs of progressing puberty, but in this 15-year-old, "nothing much is happening." The parents are concerned and the boy is suffering from his classmates' teasing. For this reason, his primary care doctor and his family would like to see this cleared up.

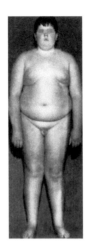

| 74.1 | Describe what you observe in the appearance of the 15-year-old boy (see Fig.).

| 74.2 | What do you find particularly interesting in the medical history?

| 74.3 | Calculate the BMI (Body Mass Index). How do you evaluate the result (see Appendix/BMI tables)?

| 74.4 | What do you particularly look for in the physical examination? What further tests would you consider useful?

| 74.5 | What is the most probable cause for the fact that puberty has not yet begun?

| 74.6 | What advice do you give the patient and his parents? What are the possibilities for planning therapy in the most efficacious way?

→ Answers and Comments Page 240

75 Two separate cases of infants following a fall from the changing table

In the middle of the night, parents bring their 5-month-old infant to you in the emergency department. He had fallen from the changing table a short while ago. "Florian has never turned over alone...!," the mother, in tears, gives an excuse for the accident. Fortunately, the child fell into the laundry basket standing on the floor next to the changing table. But the child hit his head on the edge of the laundry basket and cried terribly. Then the parents wrapped the boy in a blanket and set out immediately to the emergency department.

The infant is smiling in a friendly way and is busily trying to put his feet into his mouth.

75.1 What do you look out for during the examination?

75.2 Your examination does not uncover any abnormalities. What do you explain to the parents? What do you recommend? The child's mother is a nurse. She says she will monitor the child at home.

75.3 Is it possible to monitor the child at home? What are the grounds for your decision? What do you have to inform the parents about if they want to monitor the child at home?

A few hours later, a mother brings her 10-week-old infant. He had also fallen from the changing table. The mother describes how she only turned around for a moment and "then it happened." The child fell from the table to the shower mat, landing on his stomach. The infant did not lose consciousness, but right after that, he fell asleep. That didn't disturb the mother yet. But because 3 hours later, the infant vomited while he was asleep, the mother wanted someone to "take a look."

The infant is perfectly cheerful. Physical examination shows a sign of a contusion on the back of the head and, on his stomach, an extensive skin reddening measuring about 8 cm in diameter with five linear extensions that resemble a hand. On his buttocks, two smaller, obviously somewhat older hematomas are found. It seems something is not right.

75.4 What is disturbing about this case?

75.5 What do you do next?

→ Answers and Comments **Page 243**

You are called to a case in the delivery room. The little girl is already born and cries loudly as you enter the delivery room. "Thank God, the child is fine..." you think, yet you realize why you have been called (see Fig.).

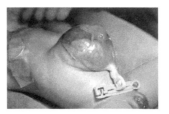

76.1   What is your diagnosis? What is involved in this deformity?

76.2   What steps do you take next? What does the postpartum care of the child require?

76.3   This deformity often occurs with a specific syndromal clinical picture. Name and explain this clinical picture.

76.4   List other deformities in the same spectrum.

→ Answers and Comments Page 247

A newborn is admitted to a newborn and premature ward at night. In the morning, the ward physician is informed that the boy was born by cesarean section after 40 weeks of pregnancy because of a pathological CTG. The child is doing well and his postpartum adjustment proceeded without problem (APGAR values 9/10/10). The birth weight was 1,830 g, body length 46 cm, and head circumference 33 cm.

| 77.1 | Enter the measured values in the percentile curve. Interpret the findings (see Fig.).

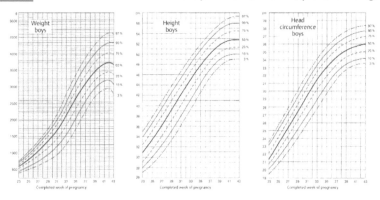

In the morning rounds the chief physician enquires about the reasons for the pathological findings, so the ward physician visited the child's mother to speak with her in detail once more and to see her pregnancy log.

| 77.2 | What do you ask the mother? What do you look for in the pregnancy log?

The mother reports that while she was pregnant, she smoked about 10 cigarettes a day. She reduced the number (earlier she used to smoke a pack of cigarettes a day), but didn't stop completely. She heard from acquaintances that it is bad for the child if smoking is stopped during pregnancy because the withdrawal could harm the child.

| 77.3 | What do you think of that?

| 77.4 | What problems related to nicotine abuse could arise in the child postpartum?

A particular obsession of the chief physician is connatal infections. Such infections can also be the cause of the pathological findings.

| 77.5 | Name the chief connatal infections, their pathogens, and the typical clinical symptoms in newborns.

→ Answers and Comments Page 249

A 15-year-old boy is presented to the emergency department at noon. He is accompanied by his mother. The boy paces nervously up and down as he reports the reason for coming in: For about the past 5 weeks he has been feeling less resilient than before. He repeatedly feels a sharp chest pain lasting a few seconds. Even with slight efforts, his heart beats so intensely that he can feel it in his throat. In those moments, his pulse, which he checks several times a day, is very fast. The values were seldom under 90 beats per minute. His primary care doctor, whom he has seen several times because of this complaint, has already done an ECG, a long-term ECG, and even an ultrasound examination of his heart. In addition, thyroid and blood studies have been done. But his doctor was not able to find a cause. That morning, in school, he had had one of those attacks again, and he could not get enough air either. He felt his hands tingling as a result. He felt really sick, and asked his classroom teacher to let his mother know.

78.1 Summarize the boy's complaints. What else interests you in the medical history?

78.2 What could be the organic causes of these complaints? What do you do next to rule out these organic causes?

78.3 How do you evaluate the boy's complaints?

78.4 Assuming that the examination results are all normal, how do you explain the boy's complaints to him?

→ Answers and Comments Page 252

79 Almost 2-year-old boy, with neurodermatitis

Among your acquaintances, there is a little boy who already had neurodermatitis when he was an infant. At the age of 4 months, cradle cap appeared for the first time. The eczema spread over his upper body. The child always seemed restless and cried a great deal. It was not rare to see bloody traces of scratches on his face. The parents consulted several doctors. They acquired numerous salves, creams, bath supplements, and diet plans, but nothing really helped. Cortisone had not been used yet. The parents are concerned about its side effects. Now the boy is almost 2 years old and the neurodermatitis persists, unchanged. The parents now come to you for help.

79.1 What do you do next to find out why, in spite of multiple attempts at therapy, there has been no improvement?

79.2 What therapy do you recommend to your acquaintances?

79.3 The parents are afraid of cortisone side effects. What is your opinion of using cortisone-containing medications?

→ Answers and Comments Page 254

At lunch, you meet a young colleague who has been working in the children's clinic with you. He seems quite exhausted and in a bad mood. You ask him cautiously why he looks so tired and disappointed. He replies that he has just gone through a difficult "initiation." A little infant, 11-month-old, "fought like a lion" and struggled against the examination. Neither auscultation nor abdominal palpation nor inspection of the ears was possible because "the boy screamed so hard that my ears were ringing."

And then it was time to draw blood. He had to intuit the veins on the back of the child's hands, rather than see them. But in spite of everything, he dared to try, but he failed. When he failed second attempt, the father lost it and the young colleague feared for his life.

At the next admission examination, you support the young colleague by accompanying him. You see a 2-year-old girl, with her doll in her arms, who absolutely doesn't want to be put down by her mother.

80.1 What do you do next?

Together you manage to get the little patient to cooperate in the examination.

80.2 Describe how you examine the child. What do you look for in particular?

At the end, it's time to draw blood. The little girl already suspects what lies ahead and clings frantically to her mother. She screams and kicks, and the mother has no idea what she should do.

80.3 What tips for taking blood can you give your colleague?

The pediatric examination mainly follows the same pattern for infants and toddlers. However, there are differences in the neurological examination. Newborns and infants have reflexes that cannot be demonstrated later on.

80.4 Describe the chief reflexes.

→ Answers and Comments Page 256

Five-month-old boy with therapy-resistant diarrhea

You are on admission duty in the emergency department. A colleague in private practice calls you to report about a 5-month-old boy he has seen during office hours. He was brought in because of recurrent diarrhea. At first he thought this was acute gastroenteritis and treated it accordingly. But there was no improvement, so he performed an abdominal sonography, during which he noticed the inhomogeneous echo structure of the liver. As a result, he immediately sent the child for admission.

A short time later, the parents arrive at the emergency department with the little boy.

During the physical examination you palpate the child's liver a good 2 cm under the costal arch. The spleen is not enlarged and no lymph nodes can be palpated. No further pathological findings can be determined.

Together with your senior physician you perform an abdominal sonography, first and the following observations are made in the right longitudinal flank section (see Fig.).

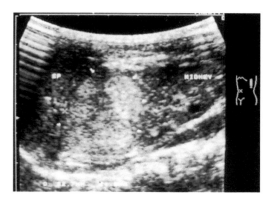

81.1 Your senior physician asks you which differential diagnoses you should consider with this finding.

The senior physician is of the opinion that with the abnormalities in the liver in association with the described clinical symptoms (therapy-resistant diarrhea), this is most likely to be metastases of a neuroblastoma.

81.2 What is meant by a neuroblastoma? What other examinations must you order to confirm your suspected diagnosis?

81.3 What clinical symptoms can a neuroblastoma cause? Can the persistent diarrhea also be ascribed to the neuroblastoma?

After all examination results have been completed, it is clear that the boy is suffering from a Stage 4S neuroblastoma.

81.4 What therapy does the tumor stage call for? What is the prognosis for the little patient? Are there factors that influence this prognosis?

→ Answers and Comments **Page 260**

A 13-year-old girl, who collapsed at a party, is presented to the emergency department. The patient comes in together with an emergency doctor and she is in a very bad general condition. The emergency physician reports that the girl suddenly felt ill during a party. She vomited and then collapsed. The hosts of the party immediately called the ambulance. When the EMTs came in, the girl was still unconscious. She was tachycardic at 120 beats/min, blood pressure stable at 110/80 mmHg, and temperature 40.1°C (measured in the ear). The emergency physician inserted a venous line on the spot. To stabilize the circulation the patient received an infusion of Ringer solution; to decrease the fever, paracetamol. The girl is examined. She is restless and reacts spontaneously but then fades away again. She is pale, tachycardic (110/min), and tachypneic (25/min). The rectal temperature is 39.1°C, and the percutaneous oxygen saturation is 97%. Petechiae are particularly distinct on arms and buttocks. Palpation of heart and lungs as well as abdomen reveals no pathological findings. No sign of meningismus. Inspection of the throat reveals a slightly reddened tonsillar ring and petechiae on the hard palate. Petechiae, rapid progression, bad general condition, and fever immediately call to mind a definitive, dreaded clinical picture.

82.1   What clinical picture is shown here? Please give a short definition and name the cause and prognosis of the clinical picture.

82.2   What differential diagnoses can be considered? What do you do next?

The emergency lab provides the following blood values: leukocytes 4,900/µL, CRP 50 mg/L, thrombocytes 132,000/µL, Quick 27%, PTT 135s, fibrinogen 129 mg/dL, and antithrombin III 72%.

82.3   How do you interpret the blood values? What supplementary studies must still be performed?

The news of the patient's severe disease quickly spreads. That same night you receive two calls from concerned parents whose children were at the same party. The parents want to know whether their children could have been infected.

82.4   Are there measures to prevent further spread of the disease?

→ Answers and Comments Page 262

83 Fourteen-month-old boy with persistent nosebleed and hematomas

On a weekend, a foster mother brings her 14-month-old foster child, who has been living in the foster family for the past 10 days, to the emergency department. The little boy has been suffering from nosebleed for almost 1 hour after falling down while trying to walk and bumping his nose on a chair. In spite of a cold washcloth on his neck, the nosebleed does not stop.

On admission, the boy is fine; he is rosy and in good spirits. The nose is bleeding from the left nostril. On his arms and legs, you observe numerous petechiae and hematomas of varying age. There are two small ones on his trunk and skull, right frontal. The tonsillar ring and the right eardrum are slightly red. On palpation, slightly enlarged lymph nodes are found in the angle of his jaw.

The remaining lymph nodes are normal, and spleen is not enlarged. Examination of the rest of the abdomen shows no abnormalities. When asked about the cause of the hematomas, the foster mother reports that she also had noticed the various "blue spots." At first, she attributed the hematomas to the abuse the child could have experienced. But later she observed that the little one also developed bruises after trivial traumas.

The bleeding nose is treated with a tamponade in the left nostril, using a swab dipped in xylomehazoline nose drops. The child only tolerates an ice bag on his neck for a short time. With this treatment, the nosebleed stops. But the boy's medical history and symptoms make you suspicious.

83.1 What important differential diagnoses should you consider in this case?

Blood is tested for a full blood count and to check coagulation. The blood picture shows an isolated thrombocytopenia of 30,000/µL. Leukocytes, hemoglobin, erythrocytes, and coagulation parameters (Quick, PTT) are within normal limits. The boy is admitted for further examination.

83.2 What causes of thrombocytopenia do you know? What further tests are necessary?

83.3 Can the symptoms—persistent nosebleed and hematomas—be attributed to the decreased thrombocyte count? Which symptoms can generally occur in thrombocytopenia?

83.4 Idiopathic thrombocytopenic purpura (ITP) is the most frequent cause of thrombocytopenia in children. Please speak briefly about the etiology, therapy, and prognosis of ITP.

→ Answers and Comments Page 265

The admissions nurse reports that a 6-year-old boy and his mother, who have been referred by a child psychiatrist, is brought to you in the outpatient department. "Please come right away, otherwise the child will take the place apart," she adds quickly. From far away you can already hear the loud dispute between the mother and son. The boy is berating his mother at the top of his voice, kicking and hitting against doors and the examining table. The outpatient nurse hands you the referral slip on which is only written "Request diagnosis before methylphenidate therapy." As you enter the examining room, the mother looks at you helplessly.

84.1   What can you do to quiet the situation down?

You have been able to calm down the boy to the point that he stops berating his mother and behaving aggressively, and you use the opportunity to talk to his mother. The little boy continues to be restless. He climbs upon the examining table, jumps back down, studies the desk, opens all the drawers, pushes the swivel chair around the room. The mother informs that her son has already been in trouble in pre-school because of constant activity, non-attentiveness, and fits of rage. Now the boy has been going to school for half a year and she and her husband have been asked several times to come to school for a discussion. They are told the boy is disturbing class, plays the clown, and displays aggressive behavior to his classmates. At home, life is getting more and more difficult: not a day goes by without quarrels and screaming, and homework is a daily battle.

84.2   What disorder seems to be present here? Please describe the clinical picture.

84.3   How is the diagnosis generally established?

84.4   What therapeutic possibilities are available?

84.5   The boy's grandmother considers hyperactivity "newfangled nonsense." "The boy's behavior is just a matter of bad upbringing," she says. What do you think of that statement?

→ Answers and Comments   Page 267

85 Twelve-year-old boy with painful swelling of the right foot

A 12-year-old boy, who is complaining about pain in his right foot, is presented for admission. While walking, the boy cannot put weight on his foot: he hops along on the healthy foot. He has been in pain since the day before and the pain is getting progressively worse. He has not hurt himself. In fact, in recent days he hasn't played any sports at all. On examining his right foot, it is found that the pain is located in the ankle and the heel. Even touching these spots causes the boy pain. The region seems slightly red and swollen. Passive movement of the joint is painful and only possible to a limited extent. No hematoma or skin wound is found. The remaining physical examination shows no abnormality. However, at 38.3°C, the body temperature is high.

| 85.1 | The boy says there was no trauma. What else could be the cause of the complaint? What do you do next? |

His mother, who accompanied the boy, asks to speak to you alone. She tells you that a few weeks ago, one of the boy's classmates was diagnosed with bone cancer. Now there is great fear that her son's complaints could also be due to bone cancer.

| 85.2 | Is the mother's fear justified? Please give a brief overview of the two most frequent malignant bone tumors. |

In the meantime, the laboratory results have become available. The leukocyte count is elevated to 17,600/μL and the remaining blood picture is normal. The CRP value is 7 mg/dL, the sed rate in the first hour is 70 mm, liver and kidney values are in the normal range. The X-ray you ordered shows no abnormalities.

You discuss the case with your senior physician. He advises you to order an MRI of the right foot.

| 85.3 | Please describe and interpret the abnormalities in the findings (see Fig.). What is your diagnosis now? Are any further studies necessary? |

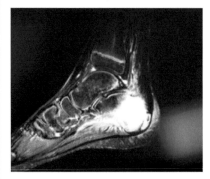

MRI right foot

| 85.4 | How is the disease treated? |

→ Answers and Comments Page 269

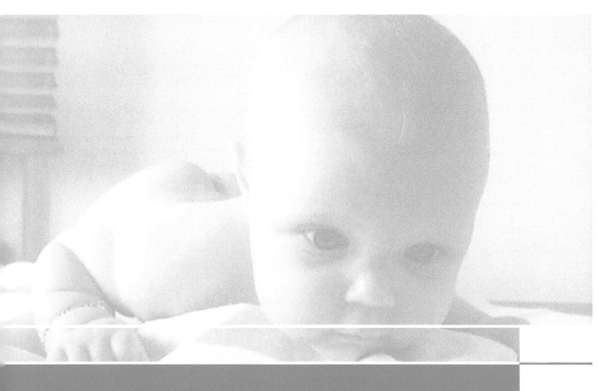

Answers and Comments

1.1   What do you look for in the clinical examination to explain the high fever, the head and neck pain, and the vomiting?
- **Fever:** Determine general condition (signs of severe acute infection, sepsis, dyspnea), pulse and blood pressure (shock), skin (turgor, color, temperature, recapillarization time, mottling, efflorescences, petechiae), lymph nodes (enlarged, pressure causes pain), examination of throat (redness, enanthem, coating, tonsillar swelling, postnasal drip), examination of auditory canals and eardrums (redness, injected blood vessels, bulging, retraction, tragus pain, secretion), thorax (evidence of bronchial pneumonia, e.g., dyspnea, tachypnea, cough, moist rattling sounds), heart (evidence of endocarditis, heart murmurs), abdomen (pressure causes pain, [painful] resistances, pain on percussion of renal beds, peritonism, organ enlargement, intestinal sounds), joints (limited range of motion, swelling, redness)
- **Head and neck pain:** Examination (position of head, mobility, swollen lymph nodes, signs of contusion, pupils), pressure causes pain (mastoid in suspicion of mastoiditis, exit points of the trigeminal nerve in suspicion of sinusitis, muscle tension), pain on percussion, bulging, stepping or depression of the skullcap (hematoma, trauma), test for meningism (Brudinski sign, Kernig sign, Lasègue sign, stiff neck)
- **Vomiting:** Quality of the vomitus (presence of blood, mucus, or bile), abdomen (pressure causes pain, resistances, intestinal peristalsis), signs of cerebral pressure (meningism, vigilance, difference of pupils, pupillary reaction to light), signs of dehydration (skin turgor, moist mucosa, rings around the eyes, frequency of blinking), smell of acetone in expired breath (indication of acetonemic vomiting as differential diagnosis of the vomiting: slender children with infections [among other things due to poor eating and drinking behavior] tend to form ketone bodies [hunger metabolism]. Acetonemia triggers vomiting [acetonemic vomiting]. Acetone can be smelled in the expired air.)

1.2   Interpret the findings. What diagnoses do you suspect and what differential diagnoses can be considered?
The figure illustrates a test for meningism (**Brudzinski sign**). The head is passively tipped forward, which elicits the pain reflex (meninges have sensory innervation) in meningeal inflammation: flexion of the hips and knees (positive Brudzinski sign, see Fig. for Case 1). High fever, vomiting, head and neck pain, and a positive Brudzinski sign suggest the suspected diagnosis of **meningitis**.
Differential diagnoses: Encephalitis, meningeal irritation, e.g., in other, similar infections (otitis media, sinusitis, mastoiditis) or sun stroke; intracranial bleeding, intracerebral space-occupying lesion.

1.3   What examinations do you perform to confirm the diagnosis?
- **Possibly examination of the ocular fundus (if it can be performed immediately without the significant delay of lumbar puncture):** Papilledema (indication of elevated cerebral pressure)
- **Lumbar puncture:** Most important diagnostic measure; **not** performed in case of elevated cerebral pressure (dilated, fixed pupils, paralysis of cerebral nerves III/IV, hemiparesis, pathological respiration such as phases of apnea or Cheyne–Stokes breathing), blood clotting disorder (thrombopenia < 40,000/μL), cardiovascular instability. For puncture technique, see Comments. For typical findings, see answer to question 1.5.
- **Diagnosis of cerebrospinal fluid:**
  - Evaluation of appearance: Color (purulent in bacterial infection, presence of blood [artificial, status post cerebral bleeding]), cloudiness (bacterial infection, elevated protein), clots (status post cerebral bleeding), coloration (for instance, xanthochrome in status post cerebral bleeding)
  - Determination of cell count
  - CSF cytology: microscopic examination of the CSF, in suspicion of bacterial meningitis, Gram staining for differentiation of the pathogen
  - Pandy test: qualitative confirmation of protein in the CSF
  - Determination of sugar in the CSF (CSF glucose/blood glucose ratio), electrolytes, lactate (normal values up to 1.9 mmol/L)
  - Preparation of a CSF culture: diagnosis of pathogen, antibiogram
- **Laboratory:** Blood panel (leukocytosis with left shift with bacterial infection; leukocytopenia with lymphocytosis with viral infection), inflammatory parameters (CRP, sedimentation rate elevated in bacterial infection), blood sugar, electrolytes, coagulation, blood culture (confirmation of bacterial pathogens), viral serology

1.4   Name the various forms of the disease and their causes.
- **Purulent (bacterial) meningitis:**
  - Newborns: *E. coli, B. streptococci*, rarely *Listeria*
  - Infants and toddlers *Meningococci, Pneumococci, Hemophilus influenzae*
  - School children, adolescents: *Meningococci, Pneumococci*
- **Serous (aseptic) meningitis (meningitis serosa):**
  - Viruses: Frequently echo and coxsackie viruses (enteroviruses); rarely mumps, tick-borne encephalitis, adeno, polio viruses among others
  - Bacteria: *Borrelia burgdorferi, Mycobacterium tuberculosis*
  - Fungi, protozoa

88

Case
1

- Drug side effects such as non-steroidal antiphlogistics, contrast medium, various antibiotics
- **Secondary meningitis:** In spreading purulent sinusitis, otitis, mastoiditis, CSF fistulas after traumatic brain injury, brain abscess; various triggers

1.5 **Name typical cerebrospinal fluid findings by which the different forms can be distinguished.** See Table.

	Bacterial meningitis	Serous meningitis
Appearance	Pus cells: turbid	Clear
Cell count	Usually > 1,000/μL, esp. neutrophil granulocytes	Usually < 1,000/μL, chiefly mononuclear cells (lymphocytes)
Protein	↑ > 1 g/L (positive Pandy test)	(usually) ↓ (Pandy test negative)
CSF/ blood glucose ratio	< 0.6	Usually ≥ 0.6; in tuberculosis, borreliosis, listeriosis ↓
Lactate	↑	Normal

Comments

Definition and forms: Meningitis is an acute inflammation of the meninges on the surface of the brain, triggered by a bacterial, viral, fungal, or other pathogen. A distinction is made between purulent meningitis, serous meningitis, and secondary forms of meningitis (see answer to question 1.4).

Etiopathogenesis: Depending on the age of the child, the frequency of certain pathogens varies (see answer to question 1.4). The spectrum of pathogens can vary in patients with certain predisposing factors (for instance, immune suppression, asplenia). In patients with asplenia, *Pneumococci, Meningococci,* and *Haemophilus influenzae* type B are the predominant pathogens while in patients with ventriculoperitoneal shunts, *Staphylococcus aureus* and *epidermidis* predominate. Most cases of bacterial meningitis are primary (hematogenous) meningitides. Bacterial meningitis is often preceded by a respiratory infection. After colonization of the nasopharynx, the pathogen invades the blood and enters the CNS. But hematogenous dispersion can also result from other infectious foci (for instance, osteomyelitis, endocarditis). Secondary bacterial meningitides occur post-traumatically (traumatic brain injury), postoperatively (after neurosurgical interventions), or as transmitted meningitides (in mastoiditis or sinusitis).

Clinical aspects: The typical clinical symptoms are **fever, reduced general condition, headache, vomiting,** and **stiff neck**. Possible additional symptoms are: general sensitivity to touch, photophobia, altered mental state, seizures, paralysis of cerebral nerves, possibly also skin bleeding, in infants a bulging fontanelle, symptoms of sepsis.

The onset of symptoms can be insidious, peracute, or acute. Newborns and patients with lowered resistance or after neurosurgery often exhibit slight or atypical symptoms.

Diagnosis: In addition to the general clinical examination, the patient is screened for signs of meningism. In addition to the **Brudzinski sign** (see answer to question 1.2), the **Kernig sign** (bending the extended legs at the hip leads to reflex bending of the knees) can be positive. The **Lasègue sign** is positive if bending the extended leg at the hip up to 90° is impossible because of pain.

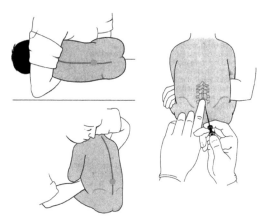

Holding a toddler or school-age child in recumbent or sitting position for lumbar puncture

To confirm the diagnosis, a **lumbar puncture** must be performed as soon as there is a suspicion of meningitis (see answer to question 1.3, Fig.).

The puncture is performed on the recumbent or seated patient after the puncture point (between L4 and L5) is numbed, for instance, with a dressing covered with anesthetic cream. The most disagreeable

89

Case

1

aspect of lumber puncture is not necessarily the puncture but can be the position in which the child's body is held. Depending on the child's age (it is easier to explain the procedure to older children and adolescents) or in case the patient is very frightened, sedation shortly before the puncture (for instance, chloral hydrate 20–50 mg/kg body weight, rectally) can make the procedure more bearable for the child and the examiner. An experienced person should hold the child. It is important to hold the spine such that it does not bend to the side. Palpation to find the puncture site is repeated (an imaginary line between the two iliac crests intersects with the spine at the level of L3/L4 and the optimal puncture point is one interspinal space below that) and marked, for instance, with the fingernail. Then, using aseptic technique (sterile gloves, mouth covering, puncture point ideally disinfected three times with a dyed disinfectant and sterile pads, working outward from the center) the puncture is performed, that is, the puncture needle is pushed forward toward the navel. When the ligamentum flavum is pierced, the "give" may be felt. After this the stylet is withdrawn, and usually, the CSF is allowed to flow into three sterile tubes (one tube for CSF culture and Gram staining, one tube for clinical-chemical analysis and microscopy, and one tube for possible further examinations, such as serology, PCR, etc.). Important information is already obtained during the puncture process: Color, possible turbidity of the CSF. This information, together with the microscopic examination (cell count, differentiation of the cells, detection of bacteria), the determination of CSF sugar to blood sugar ratio, and the Pandy test (evidence of albumen), help decide whether the illness is a bacterial or serous meningitis (see answer to question 1.5). There are also bacterial meningitides with only slight pleocytosis. In such a case, the pathogens are usually *Borrelia* or *Mycobacteria* among others. In such cases (especially in mycobacterial infections) there is often a severely lowered CSF sugar.

Since the Pandy reagent is highly poisonous, an albumen test strip can also be used to detect the protein.

Treatment: In **purulent meningitis**, in addition to stabilization of vital functions, **immediate antibiotic treatment** with a broad spectrum antibiotic such as ceftriaxone or cefotaxime must be instituted, over a period of at least 7 days. For newborns, the antibiotic treatment must also be effective not only against B-streptococci but also Listeria and Gram-negative pathogens. For this reason, the combination of a third-generation cephalosporins with ampicillin or piperacillin and an aminoglycoside must be considered. Possible modification of therapy depending on the results of the antibiogram.

Dexamethasone should be administered 10–15 minutes before the start of antibiotic therapy to prevent a possible Jarisch–Herxheimer reaction. It also acts as prophylaxis against brain edema. Recommendations about this point are not all in agreement. Clinical and animal model studies have shown that administration of cortisone has a positive effect on cerebral circulation, thus decreasing the occurrence of neurological deficits, especially hearing loss. This is particularly true of meningitis triggered by *Haemophilus influenzae* type B.

Symptomatic and supportive therapy consists of intensive monitoring and administration of antipyretics such as paracetamol, infusion therapy, and, if necessary, anticonvulsive agents. **Aseptic** or **serous meningitis** is treated **symptomatically** with bed rest, antipyretics if necessary, and analgesics. If herpes viruses are detected, acyclovir is added.

Mandatory reporting: Reporting meningococcal meningitis to the appropriate local health authority or health agency is mandatory.

Prognosis: The lethality of purulent meningitis in newborns is 15%; in older children, 5%. In 30% of newborns and 15% of older children, recovery is only partial, with secondary pathologies such as seizures, hearing loss, hydrocephalus, and impaired intelligence.

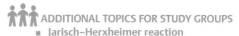 ADDITIONAL TOPICS FOR STUDY GROUPS
- Jarisch–Herxheimer reaction
- Complications of meningitis
- Prophylaxis (immunization, infection prophylaxis for contact persons)
- Encephalitis

2.1   What is your diagnosis? What important differential diagnosis are you considering?
- **Diagnosis: Krupp syndrome** (formerly: Pseudokrupp); rationale: clinical characteristics (barking cough on awaking, inspiratory wheezing, inter-/subcostal retractions)
- **Differential diagnosis:** acute epiglottitis (Syn.: epiglottitis)

2.2   Explain the etiology of the disease and define it for differential diagnosis.
- **Krupp syndrome:** Usually a viral infection (parainfluenza, influenza, RS-, rhino-, or adenovirus) with inflammatory, stenosing swelling of the respiratory mucosa of the vocal cords and to caudal
- **Acute epiglottitis:** Acute infection of the epiglottis (see Comments), usually triggered by *Haemophilus influenzae* type B

2.3   Describe the different degrees of severity of the disease. What therapy is indicated for each?
See Tab.

Stage	Symptoms	Treatment
I	Barking cough, occasionally hoarseness, soft inspiratory stridor increasing with agitation	Calming cold fresh air, fetch ice from the refrigerator and have the patient lick it.
II	Stridor at rest, incipient dyspnea, jugular retractions, anxious facial expression, perioral paleness	Calming, administration of prednisolone (100 mg rectally), if there is no improvement, inhalation of adrenaline (1: 1,000; 0.5 mL/kg body weight [max. 5 mL] diluted with 0.9% NaCl) or micronefrin (epinephrine racemate, 0.5 mL to 5 mL 0.9% NaCl)
III	Resting dyspnea, marked inter- and subcostal retractions, tachycardia	From stage III, admission to hospital, otherwise treatment as in stage II, possibly administration of oxygen
IV	Intense dyspnea with cyanosis and incipient respiratory failure ranging to bradycardia and somnolence, danger of suffocation	Additional sedation (*caution*: respiratory depression), intubation

Comments

Definition and etiopathogenesis: Formerly, the so-called "croup" indicated membranous laryngotracheitis in diphtheria. All other forms of croup, such as subglottic laryngitis, were grouped under the term "pseudo-croup." Since diphtheria has practically disappeared in the Western developed countries, thanks to introduction of immunization, the croup syndrome subsumes three acute diseases:
- Viral croup
- Spasmodic or relapsing croup
- Malignant laryngotracheobronchitis (bacterial tracheitis, pseudomembranous laryngotracheobronchitis)

Barking cough, **hoarseness**, and **inspiratory stridor** are symptoms that these have in common. The cause is inflammatory swelling of the respiratory mucosa extending primarily subglottally from the vocal cords to the trachea. For pathogens, see answer to question 2.2. The swelling is most intense in the region of the cricoid cartilage, the narrowest portion of the child's upper respiratory tract. Severe air pollution, weather conditions, and passive smoking can promote (but not trigger) this condition. A secondary bacterial superinfection is possible. Children are most frequently affected at preschool age; children younger than 6 months or older than 6 years of age are seldom affected. A seasonal increase of cases is observed in the months from October to March.

Clinical aspects: **Viral croup** usually begins with the general symptoms of a respiratory infection such as fever, sore throat, runny nose, and fatigue, but these symptoms can also be absent. The inflammatory mucosal swelling usually leads acutely to the typical symptoms of barking cough, hoarseness, and inspiratory stridor. This occurs chiefly in the early morning hours because of the falling cortisol level during the night. Depending on the severity of the respiratory pathway obstruction (classified into degrees I to IV, see answer to question 2.3) there is also dyspnea with jugular, sub- and intercostal retraction. The transition to a life-threatening clinical picture with danger of suffocation is rare, but possible at any time. During the day, the symptoms improve or even disappear completely, but sometimes return the following night. The illness lasts between 3 and 7 days.

The rarer **spasmodic or recurrent croup** is characterized by recurrent appearance (3–50 episodes) of the symptoms without signs of a virus infection. Here too, the attacks occur principally at night and last between 1 and 6 hours. Affected children exhibit above-average occurrence of a hyperreactive respiratory system, atopia, and transition to bronchial asthma.

The rarely **malignant laryngotracheobronchitis** is caused by bacterial pathogens (*Staphylococcus aureus, Haemophilus influenzae*, Pneumococci, Streptococci) and is characterized by massive mucosal swelling with mucopurulent exudate and occasional pseudomembranous coating of the tracheal mucosa. In 5% to 10% of cases, this disease can have a fatal outcome.

Diagnosis: Usually the diagnosis is easily established on the basis of clinical signs.

Differential diagnoses: The most important differential diagnosis is **acute epiglottitis**, usually triggered by *Haemophilus influenzae* **type B**. Since introduction of the Hib immunization, it has become very rare. But acute epiglottitis can occur even in immunized children, since this clinical picture can also be caused by other pathogens, such as *Staphylococcus aureus*, pneumococcus, and hemolytic streptococcus. A seriously ill child, usually with a **high fever**, exhibits inspiratory stridor, **difficulty swallowing** with flowing saliva, thick speech, and increasing dyspnea. The child is conspicuously quiet and pale; the **barking cough is usually absent**. The child must be immediately brought to the nearest pediatric clinic, in seated position with oxygen insufflation. The throat should only be inspected in preparation for resuscitation and intubation, since there is a high risk of reflex cardiac arrest or asphyxiation. If the diagnosis is confirmed, the patient is intubated or a tracheotomy may even be necessary, and antibiotic treatment, for instance, with cefotaxime, is instituted.

Laryngeal diphtheria ("real croup"), caused by *Corynebacterium diphtheriae,* is another differential diagnosis. Since introduction of immunization, the number of cases occurring in the United States has decreased from nearly 100,000 in 1980 to 4,700 cases in 2013. Increasing hoarseness, barking cough, dyspnea with inspiratory stridor, attacks of cyanosis, and marked restlessness are characteristics. Loosened pseudomembranes (= confluent, difficult to loosen, gray-white coating on the tonsils) can cover

the entry to the larynx and thus lead to life-threatening attacks of asphyxiation. In addition to treatment with penicillin for 14 days, treatment with **diphtheria antitoxin** must be started **immediately** in order to prevent life-threatening organ complications such as myocarditis, polyneuritis, nephritis, vascular damage with tendency to diffuse bleeding.

Treatment: Treatment depends on the degree of severity of the disease (see answer to question 2.3). It is of great importance to remain **calm** and to calm the child and the parents. A very anxious child may have to be sedated (for instance, with chloral hydrate).

Even before the physician comes to the child, home care by having the child inhale cool, moist air can be suggested to the parents. One can ask the child to get ice out of the freezer chest. This has a calming effect on the child and the parents, and **inhaling cold air brings relief** to the child.

Invasive measures (inspecting the throat, taking blood, etc.) should be avoided because any excitement (almost every child cries and pulls back from throat inspection and blood drawing) increases the child's shortness of breath. **Glucocorticoids and inhaled adrenaline** to reduce swelling of the mucosa are the **treatment of choice**. The effect of nebulized adrenaline or epinephrine sets in after about 10 minutes but declines again after approximately 30 minutes. Thus after the first hours of the croup attack, symptoms can reappear. Therefore the indication for hospital admission should be rather freely made.

If there is accompanying rhinitis, decongestant nose drops can be helpful. The increased effort of breathing with a stuffy nose reinforces the croup symptoms by collapsing the upper respiratory tract, which is already narrowed by inflammation. This pathological mechanism can be avoided with the use of decongestant nose drops.

If there is indication of a bacterial superinfection, antibiotic treatment, for instance, with cephalosporins, should be instituted.

Prognosis: The prognosis is good if adequate treatment is begun on time and maintained. Intubation and ventilation are very rare since treatment with glucocorticoids and adrenaline inhalation has become routine.

ADDITIONAL TOPICS FOR STUDY GROUPS
- Diphtheria

3.1   What is your suspected diagnosis? What do you explain to the parents in order to reassure them?

- **Febrile seizure**, basis patient's age, infection with high fever, tonic–clonic seizure
- **Informing and counseling the parents:** First explain to the parents that this is a febrile seizure. It is always important to name and explain the diagnosis. Since "seizure" sounds terrible to the parents and immediately makes them think of severely handicapped children, reassurance is very important: Febrile seizures are usually harmless. With a high fever, the threshold for seizures declines. Children who have a predisposition can have a seizure. A seizure almost always occurs with a rapid rise in fever. In fact, it is often the first symptom. Parents often do not notice in advance that their child has a fever. It is only very rarely that febrile seizures have a severe or complicated outcome. They almost always stop spontaneously after a few minutes and usually remain without consequences!

3.2   What immediate measures should you undertake?

- **If the seizure episodes or the susceptibility to seizures persists** (= a restless child is one who does not react appropriately when addressed, has a fixed, distant stare, fiddles around, makes smacking sounds; the symptoms can vary—take particular notice if parents say they "don't recognize their child"): Administration of antipyretics such as paracetamol supp. 10–20 mg/kg body weight, anticonvulsive agents, for instance, diazepam rectal (5 mg for children < 15 kg body weight, otherwise 10 mg). If attack does not end after 10 minutes, clonazepam i.v. (0.05–0.1 mg/kg body weight). If treatment continues to be unsuccessful, phenobarbital i.v. (10–20 mg/kg body weight)
- **When attack has already stopped:** Take temperature, always rectally. If temperature > 38.5°C, **reduce fever**:
  - **Paracetamol:** 10–20 mg/kg body weight, rectally or as syrup; at most every 6 hours. Administered more frequently, there is a danger of paracetamol poisoning. If in addition the child has gastroenteritis, the syrup is preferable. If the last dose of paracetamol was administered more recently than

6 hours, the alternative is **ibuprofen** (10–20 mg/kg body weight, as syrup)
  - Loose clothing, light blanket, room temperature at 20°C

3.3   What diagnostic measures should be initiated?

- **Hospital admission** since the risk of recurrence within the first 48 hours is at its highest (especially if the fever is rising, which parents recognize too late, since they are still in shock) and appropriate diagnosis is only possible in this way
- **Look for cause of fever:** Physical examination (among other things, screen for meningism) and medical history (third party medical history: similar events)
- **Laboratory:** Inflammation parameters (CRP, sed rate), complete blood count, blood sugar, electrolytes, blood gas analysis, possibly blood culture, urine (test strips, infection)
- **Lumbar puncture:** In infants, complicated febrile seizure (see question 3.4), meningism to rule out an inflammatory disease of the CNS
- **EEG:** Not until 24 hour temperature < 37.5°C, since otherwise there will always be EEG variations, ideally 7 to 10 days postictal to rule out underlying epilepsy; *Exception:* complicated febrile seizures (to rule out a febrile focus), in this case, an immediate EEG

3.4   There are two forms of this clinical picture. Explain them.

- **Simple febrile seizure:**
  - Generalized, tonic–atonic or tonic–clonic febrile seizure
  - Duration ≤ 15 minutes
  - Peak frequency between the ages of 14 and 18 months
- **Febrile seizure with complications** (at least one criterion must be met):
  - Focal seizure or focal onset of seizure
- Previous cerebral damage
- Duration > 15 minutes
- Postictal paresis
- > One attack within 24 hours
- > Four recurrent attacks
- Persistent changes in EEG
- Age < 6 months or > 6 years

Comments

Definition and forms: Febrile seizures are among the occasional epileptic seizures that occur in infants and toddlers in association with fever. For forms, see answer to question 3.4.

Etiopathogenesis: The pathogenesis has not yet been elucidated. Fever lowers the individual seizure threshold. This seizure threshold is age-dependent and

presumably genetically determined, since familial clustering has been observed. In approximately 3% of cases, epilepsy develops in the further course.

Clinical aspects: See answer to question 3.4.

Diagnosis: See answer to question 3.3. Not all cerebral seizures associated with fever are febrile seizures. In particular, symptomatic seizures in inflammatory diseases of the CNS (meningitis, encephalitis) must be ruled out. For this reason, in a presumptive diagnosis, a lumbar puncture must be performed. In case of a febrile seizure in the first year of a child's life, a lumbar puncture must always be performed to rule out meningitis, since infants do not always exhibit specific symptoms of meningism.

Treatment and prophylaxis: Febrile seizures usually stop spontaneously after a few minutes. No causal treatment is known. Fever and the cause of the fever are treated symptomatically. The attack is interrupted by rectal administration of diazepam, if necessary in combination with clonazepam and phenobarbital i.v. (see answer to question 3.2). Subsequent febrile seizures are prevented by early lowering of the fever (for instance, with paracetamol or ibuprofen) if it is higher than 38.5°C. Intermittent diazepam prophylaxis over a period of 72 hours should be added (0.3–0.5 mg/kg body weight every 8 hours) if there is an increased risk of recurrence (febrile seizures in the medical history).

For home care, the parents are advised to take early antifebrile measures (with drugs, see answer to question 3.2). However, this is often impossible, since seizures can be the first symptom of a rapid rise in temperature. The pediatrician prescribes diazepam suppositories for emergencies. In case of recurrent or complicated febrile seizures and corresponding pathological signs in the EEG, anticonvulsive prophylaxis should be considered.

Prognosis: The prognosis is usually good. After the age of 6 years, febrile seizures become very rare. The risk of a recurrent febrile seizure is about 30% and is elevated in association with a positive family history, attacks in the first year of a child's life, and changes in the EEG. Epilepsy develops in 3–4% of cases. With a positive family history, previous brain damage, complicated and repeated febrile seizures, as well as constant pathological changes in the EEG, there is an elevated risk.

 ADDITIONAL TOPICS FOR STUDY GROUPS
- Epilepsy (focal, generalized attacks; treatment)
- EEG
- Meningitis, Encephalitis
- Lumbar puncture (technique; diagnosis of the cerebrospinal fluid)

4　Severe exsiccosis/toxicosis in acute gastroenteritis

4.1　What is your diagnosis?

Severe dehydration in acute gastroenteritis = toxicosis (infant enteritis with toxic symptoms); rationale: massive fluid loss due to recurrent vomiting, watery diarrhea, and fever resulting in dry skin/mucosa, pale gray, blotchy skin color, sunken eyes, weight loss, apathy, rare blinking, skin tenting, tachycardia, lowered blood pressure, hypernatremia, elevated hematocrit, oliguria

4.2　Explain the different forms and degrees of severity of this clinical picture. What form, with what degree of severity, does the infant have?
- Forms of dehydration:
  - *Isotonic dehydration:* Loss of water and electrolytes in the same ratio as in serum, for instance, in gastroenteritis, blood loss, → sodium values normal
  - *Hypotonic dehydration:* Electrolyte loss greater than fluid loss, for instance, in cystic fibrosis, preterminal kidney failure, adrenogenital syndrome, acute gastroenteritis, inadequate infusion therapy → hyponatremia (Na < 132 mmol/L)
  - *Hypertonic dehydration:* Water loss greater than electrolyte loss, for instance, in refusal to eat, hyperpyrexia, diabetes mellitus, diabetes insipidus, lack of food/fluids → hypernatremia (Na > 145 mmol/L)
- Degrees of severity of dehydration:
  - *Mild dehydration:* Weight loss < 5% of body weight; clinical: Thirst, skin turgor normal to ↓, mucosa still moist
  - *Moderate dehydration:* Weight loss 5–10% of body weight; clinical: reduced general condition, skin turgor markedly reduced, mucosa dry, sunken eyes, oliguria
  - *Severe dehydration:* Weight loss > 10% of body weight; clinical: Shock (blood pressure ↓, tachycardia), somnolence to loss of consciousness, skin tenting, mucosa very dry, oliguria to anuria.
- The infant has severe hypertonic dehydration, since the sodium concentration > 145 mmol/L and the weight loss is more than 10%.

4.3　What treatment do you initiate?
- Infusion therapy: Basic need + deficit + continuing losses:
  - *Basic need:* Depends on the child's weight; consists of a total of the individual recommendations
    - for the first 10 kg: 100 mL/kg body weight/d

- for the next 10 kg: an additional 50 mL/kg body weight/d
- from the 21st kg: an additional 25 mL/kg body weight/d
- for instance, 25 kg body weight: 1,000 mL + 500 mL + 125 mL = 1,625 mL
- *Deficit:* Weight loss in per cent
- *Continuing losses:*
  - Fever: for every 1°C (> 37°C) an additional 10% of the basic need
  - Diarrhea/vomiting: Estimate, for instance, by weighing the diapers
- **This gives the following calculation for the patient in the present case:**
  - Basic need: 8.2 kg × 100 mL/kg body weight/d = **820 mL/d**
  - Deficit: 12% of the original body weight, i.e., 12% × 8.2 kg = 984 g or mL; *caution:* Compensate for the water loss slowly (see answer to question 4.4), distribute this amount over 48 hours, that is 984 mL: 2 = **492 mL/d**
  - Continuing losses: 10% of the basic need/1°C temperature elevation = 82 mL × 2 = 164 mL; in case of continuing vomiting/diarrhea: Estimate losses and add
  - A total of 1,476 mL/d; rounded up, the replacement will be 1,500 mL/d.
- **Treatment of gastroenteritis in infants:** Breastfed infants should continue to be breastfed, more often and for shorter periods of time; breast milk is well tolerated even with gastroenteritis. Formula-fed infants should be given their usual infant formula, in small amounts and often; formula should *not* be diluted. Immediate increase in nourishment is important because a prolonged diet causes further damage to the intestinal mucosa, and there is a risk of postenteritis syndrome with chronic diarrhea and failure to flourish. Rehydration is oral but in

moderate and severe dehydration, additional i.v. fluid is added (electrolyte-glucose solutions)
- **Pathogen identification (= controversial from one hospital to another):** However
  - this is always done when the infant cannot be kept isolated in the hospital
  - always if there is blood in the stool
  - always when the infant develops the enteritis while in intensive care and was previously in a room with other children.
- **Antibiotic therapy:** Only indicated in exceptional circumstances, for instance, a serious septic course in salmonella infection, confirmation of *Campylobacter, Shigella,* amoebas, and *Giardia lamblia* in the stool in children with compromised immunity. Selection of the antibiotic is determined by the antibiogram. Treatment is intravenous. In salmonella and shigella, ampicillin (50–100 mg/kg body weight/d), in campylobacter, erythromycin (30–50 mg/ kg body weight/d), and in confirmation of *Giardia lamblia,* metronidazole (30 mg/kg body weight/d) are administered.

4.4 What must you pay attention to during the treatment?

- Try to compensate for water and electrolyte loss within 48 hours, not sooner. *Caution:* to prevent cerebral edema in hypernatremic dehydration, compensate for water loss relatively slowly. The serum sodium concentration may only fall at a maximum of 1 mmol/L/h. Therefore, initially infuse isotonic saline solution (NaCl 0.9%) and in the course of treatment, half-normal saline (NaCl 0.9%: glucose 5% = 1:1) until the sodium value is normalized
- Laboratory tests (electrolytes, BGA) every 4 to 8 hours in severe dehydration/acidosis
- Potassium replacement (if needed) not until urine excretion begins.

Comments

Definition and classification: **Dehydration** is the loss of body water through increased renal, gastrointestinal, pulmonary, or percutaneous excretion without equivalent ingestion. Toxicosis is the most severe form of infantile diarrhea with dehydration, acidosis, and symptoms of disorientation or confusion. Forms of dehydration are assessed according to the form and degree of severity (see answer to question 4.2).

Etiology: See answer/examples for question 4.2. The causes of acute diarrhea in children are viral gastrointestinal infections (for instance, rotavirus, enteral adenovirus, norovirus), bacterial infections (for instance, intestinal pathogens *E. coli, Salmonella, Shigella),* or parasites (for instance, *Cryptosporidium*). In addition, they can occur in food poisoning (for instance, toxins of *Staphylococcus aureus, Clostridium perfringens*), disturbed intestinal flora after antibiotic

therapy, eosinophilic gastroenteritis from alimentary causes (for instance, hyperosmolar beverages, fruit juices) as well as associated with focal (for instance, osteomyelitis, mastoiditis) or general infections (for instance, of the respiratory or urogenital tract).

Pathogenesis: Newborns, infants, and toddlers are at particular risk of acute dehydration because they have a relatively large daily water turnover. For this reason, they react very quickly to fluid loss (for instance, diarrhea, vomiting, polyuria, fever) or reduced intake (for instance, refusal to drink) with clinical symptoms.

Hypovolemia can lead to **shock.** In this situation, the reduced volume, with reduction of heart minute volume, leads to increased secretion of catecholamine, resulting in compensatory peripheral vasoconstriction, tachycardia, tachypnea, and redistribution of the remaining blood volume from muscles, the viscera, skin, and kidneys to the heart and brain (macrocirculation disorder, centralization stage). The result is peripheral tissue hypoxia and acidosis. Without adequate treatment, this first shock phase moves into the second shock phase of microcirculation disorder. Tissue acidosis causes precapillary vasodilation and elevated vascular permeability with resulting fluid, protein, and electrolyte loss into the interstitium (tissue edema). This reinforces the cell hypoxia and hypovolemia (vicious circle) with falling blood pressure, heart failure, unconsciousness, and disturbed renal function. Shock lung develops (ARDS) with pulmonary edema and respiratory failure. Without treatment, this stage moves into the third, irreversible phase of shock with multiorgan failure.

Clinical aspects: Typical symptoms of toxicosis are rapid **weight loss, sunken eyes, dry skin and mucosa**, slowly fading or persisting skin tenting, pale skin color, oliguria to anuria, possibly tachycardia with falling blood pressure as far as shock. In addition, in infants a depressed fontanelle. In long-term disease, acidosis develops, with deep thoracic breathing (so-called Kussmaul breathing). The clouded consciousness is characterized by a fixed, empty stare with infrequent blinking, decreased reaction to external stimuli, but also shrill crying, hypo- or hyperreflexia and susceptibility to seizures.

Diagnosis: In addition to the medical history and the clinical examination, in which skin (turgor and color), mucosa, circulatory parameters (pulse, blood pressure), and state of consciousness are assessed, determine the severity of dehydration, ideally through determination of weight loss, and the form of dehydration through determination of the **serum sodium concentration.**

Laboratory tests should include determination of electrolytes (Na, K, Cl), hematocrit, creatinine, blood gases, and blood sugar, and in gastroenteritis, identification of the microbiological pathogens.

Treatment: For formula-fed infants, see answer to question 4.3. In **mild dehydration** (weight loss < 5%), **oral rehydration** with electrolyte solutions (ORS) is preferable. In refusal to drink, rehydration can be achieved with a feeding tube. Especially for infants, conducting the rehydration requires care and patience. The oral rehydration solution (for instance, pedialyte, G2) should ideally be chilled and administered with a spoon or a syringe every few minutes. Even if the child has to vomit during rehydration, it is important to continue, since fluids are absorbed in the stomach in spite of vomiting. Home remedies such as cola drinks are not recommended since colas are hyperosmolar and draw additional water from the body. The same applies to other homemade

remedies intended to promote rehydration since mistakes in mixture ratios are common. In addition, **moderate and severe dehydration require infusion therapy** under hospital conditions. During this treatment, care must be taken to compensate for the fluid loss slowly (see answer to question 4.4). The rapid inflow of water associated with excessively rapid rehydration can lead to swelling of the brain cells with formation of cerebral edema (clinically: loss of consciousness, cerebral seizures). **After successful rehydration** (recognizable through normal skin turgor, normal laboratory values, and clinically improved child), prompt buildup of oral nutrition (to avoid damage to the mucosa with postenteritis syndrome) and simultaneous reduction and termination of infusion therapy. Realimentation already begins on the first day with grated apple and banana (constipating action) as well as zwieback and pretzel sticks. On the second day, a low fat bland diet such as soup, noodles, or rice with small amounts of sauce, boiled potatoes, and on the third day a largely normal but fairly lean diet can be given.

In support of this regimen, probiotics to prevent diarrhea can be helpful: *Saccharomyces boulardii* (a strain of baker's yeast) has proven effective in clinical studies, among other things in prevention of antibiotic-associated diarrhea. The lactic acid bacterium *Lactobacillus GG* shortens the duration of diarrhea (in studies on children with rotavirus gastroenteritis) by 1 day, reduces the stool frequency, and shortens the excretion of the rotavirus with the stool.

Shock therapy, in addition to treating the cause of the shock, is based on volume replacement in order to maintain the heart's pumping function, thus ensuring sufficient circulation and oxygen supply to the tissues. This requires the largest venous access possible. Placement of a venous access device is difficult even with a healthy child, but the vasoconstriction caused by shock can make it impossible. Placement of a central venous access device in the subclavian and jugular veins of a child, particularly in an emergency situation, has the potential for complications (pneumothorax), and it is time-consuming. If a peripheral venous access cannot be achieved in a maximum of 5 minutes, intraosseous infusion therapy is recommended. The bone marrow has a rich circulation, making rapid rehydration and administration of medications possible. The optimal puncture site is at the proximal tibia, medial, approximately 2 cm below the tibial tuberosity, and alternatively on the medial malleolus of the tibia. Entry into the cortical bone is obtained by boring with turning motions and increasing pressure, at a 45° angle, with an intraosseous needle or a bone marrow puncture needle. If the puncture is successful, dark red bone marrow can be aspirated. The needle is firmly seated and it can now be used to inject medications and replace fluids or electrolytes. Volume replacement and stabilization of the circulation can then be done by administration of crystalline solutions (for instance, isotonic saline or Ringer lactate, 10–20 mL/kg body weight over a period of 10–20 minutes, repeated if necessary), alternatively, or if unsuccessful with colloidal solutions (for instance, 5% human albumin, dextran; for severe volume deficiency 10 mL/kg body weight as a bolus, otherwise 5 mL/kg body weight over a period of 10–20 minutes). *Note:* Resuscitation without fluid replacement is completely useless. In addition, take supportive measures such as shock position (head down, legs up). It may become necessary to intubate and ventilate. If volume replacement alone does not stabilize the circulation, medicamentous therapy with catecholamines such as dopamine (2–5 µg/kg body weight/min), dobutamine (5–10 µg/kg body weight/min), (Nor-) adrenaline

(0.01–5 µg/kg body weight/min) becomes necessary Catecholamines may only be administered over a central or intraosseous port.

Prognosis: The prognosis is good. Most children admitted with this clinical picture can be discharged from the hospital after 2–3 days. For patients in shock, the prognosis depends on complications such as cerebral edema or seizures.

ADDITIONAL TOPICS FOR STUDY GROUPS
- Hyperhydration conditions
- Acidosis, alkalosis
- Disturbance of electrolyte balance (for instance, of potassium metabolism)
- Shock
- Acute hyperpyretic toxicosis

5   Invagination

5.1   What is your suspected diagnosis?

Invagination; rationale: suddenly occurring attacks of pain/vomiting; in pain-free intervals, child is apathetic; palpable, mid-abdominal cylindrical tumor; prior gastroenteritis, sonography (**pathological target sign** in cross section where the different structures surround each other like rings on a target; centrally invaginated intestinal loop, externally enveloping intestinal loop [see Fig.])

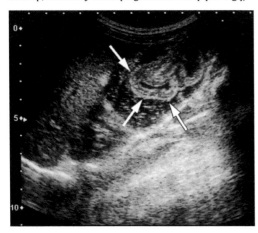

5.2   What further measures will you undertake?

- Hospital admission and infusion therapy (electrolyte-glucose- or Ringer solution) to compensate for fluid loss (for calculation of infusion amount, see case 4)
- For attempt at hydrostatic repositioning under sonographic or radiological monitoring (sedation!), see Comments
- Surgical intervention: if conservative treatment fails, laparoscopic and manual repositioning. In case of infarction, partial intestinal resection

5.3   What complications must you watch for?

- Shock
- Intestinal infarction with subsequent intestinal gangrene
- Perforation and peritonitis after late diagnosis
- Risk of perforation during hydrostatic repositioning

Comments

Epidemiology: In children, the incidence of invagination is relatively high at 3 out of 1,000. Ninety percent of cases occur up to the end of the third year of a child's life.

Etiopathogenesis: In 80 to 90% of cases, the cause of the invagination remains unclear. However, there is frequently a history of (usually viral) gastroenteritis (see case) or a respiratory infection, but mechanical impediments (for instance, lymphomas, Meckel diverticulum, polyps, fecal stones) as well as Schoenlein–Henoch purpura can be triggers.

In an invagination, a proximal section of the intestine folds into a distal section. Intestinal peristalsis pulls the invaginated section further toward the anus; ileus results. The most frequent location of the invagination is the ileocecal junction, where the ileum folds into the cecum. Often the mesentery is also pulled in, so that the mesenteric vessels are compressed. This venous blockage leads to mucosal edema and bleeding; the arterial blockage leads to ischemia with necrosis of the intestinal wall and possibly perforation and peritonitis.

Clinical aspects: The clinical symptoms in the current case were described very classically. But children can behave completely normally between attacks, playing and even laughing. Rectal excretion of bloody mucus is a late symptom.

Diagnosis and Treatment: The next step toward establishing a diagnosis, after taking a comprehensive medical history and performing a clinical examination (always digital examination of the rectum; if invagination has been present for some time, traces of blood on the finger cot), is **abdominal sonography**. Here, at first, many fluid-filled intestinal loops with little intrinsic peristalsis are noted (because of inflammatory participation of the intestine and possible ileus). The invaginated portion appears as a target-like double structure ("pseudo-kidney"), usually in the right middle or lower abdomen (see Fig.). *Note:* if sonography shows a great deal (and not only air), then one should look for an invagination.

Even during sonography, it is already possible to try hydrostatic devagination by instillation, for instance, of Ringer-lactate solution (2–3 L, warmed)

through a bladder catheter, placed into the rectum and blocked. The child must be sedated for this procedure (for instance, with midazolam) or even anesthetized. Usually the outcome of the treatment can be clearly monitored sonographically. Sonographic devagination should always be tried first. It if does not succeed, the invaginated portion can be seen as a conical interruption of the contrast medium column by visualizing the colon with water-soluble contrast medium, and the contrast enema can be used therapeutically in order to reposition the invaginated section. *Caution:* In attempting to devaginate hydrostatically, there is a risk of perforation. It is essential to inform the Surgery Department in advance.

If repositioning is unsuccessful or if the attempt to reposition ends in perforation, the only remaining possibility is laparotomy with manual repositioning. A partial intestinal resection cannot always be avoided in this procedure.

Sometimes the invagination resolves spontaneously. In that case, in spite of the classical medical history, the invagination can no longer be seen sonographically. Because there is a danger of recurrence, meticulous in-patient observation for 2 to 3 days is urgently recommended.

Prognosis: The prognosis is good but there is a high risk of recurrence (10% in the first 48 hours). In that case, a laparotomy is usually necessary.

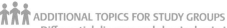 ADDITIONAL TOPICS FOR STUDY GROUPS
- Differential diagnoses abdominal pain in children
- Ileus in childhood
- Volvulus
- Schoenlein–Henoch purpura
- Meckel diverticulum

6 Health screenings and the health log

6.1 What is the purpose of health screenings? What is the health log?
- The purposes of health screenings are:
  - **Early recognition of disease** (recognizing diseases that could seriously endanger physical and mental development)
  - Consultation about health matters (for instance, immunization, nutrition, accident prevention)
  - Consideration of social-pediatric aspects (for instance, behavioral problems, prevention of child abuse by recognition of parental stress, signs of abuse, etc.)

- The health log serves to document the early recognition examinations that have been carried out and contains important information about the child's development and illnesses up to the present.

6.2 Explain the usual course of a health screening.
- Taking of body measurements (height/weight, head circumference) and recording them in percentile curves to assess the child's physical development
- See earlier findings to evaluate previous motor, intellectual, and social development

- Attentive observation of the child throughout the screening to determine information about behavioral and motor patterns
- A thorough physical examination of the child, including a neurological examination, to screen for organ diseases
- Age-appropriate vision and hearing tests
- Urine examination (4–5 years)
- Review of immunization status
- Check of Vitamin D/fluoride prophylaxis (up to age 1)

6.3 How would you assess the boy's developmental status?

- There is always assessment of **motor function, social, and play behavior as well as speech development**. At the age of 12 months, a child should be able to do the following:
  - Motor function: Stand while holding on, be able to pull up to standing position alone
  - Social behavior: Show affection to trusted persons
  - Play behavior: Shake, pound, and throw objects
  - Speech development: Imitate speech sounds, form specific double syllables such as "ma-ma," "da-da," directed at a certain person or "um-um" directed at food.
- In part, the boy shows age-appropriate abilities, but there are deficits, especially in motor development. Of particular note is the lack of forearm support that should have been mastered at approximately 6 months. The boy is able to form double syllables, but they are not specific. Evaluation of the developmental stage:
  - Motor function: approx. 9 months
  - Social behavior: approx. 12 months
  - Play behavior: approx. 12 months
  - Speech development: approx. 9 months

6.4 What do you think about the fact that the mother does not perform the physiotherapeutic treatment as you prescribed?

- **Physical therapy according to Vojta:** Stimulation of certain pressure points in certain body positions triggers reflex-like movements of the extremities. These movements present the child with a dilemma: he or she is forced to react actively with a physiological movement that is not natural for a developmentally disturbed child. This causes discomfort, screaming, and resistance. The method is considered very effective for children with spastic paralysis, children with orthopedic problems, or statomotor developmental delay. For parents it is often difficult, due to the child's resistance, to persevere with this treatment
- **Physical therapy by the Bobath method:** Training to normalize the muscle tone and suppress pathological reflex mechanisms, practice of certain motor and postural reflexes. Children usually tolerate this rather passive treatment well. However, the treatment is not quite as effective as the Vojta treatment.
- To be successful, physical therapy requires the parents' collaboration. The best method will have no effect if the treatment is not regularly practiced at home
- With regard to this example, this means that the child needs physical therapy to reverse the motor deficits. Vojta therapy would be more effective but Bobath therapy is better tolerated and therefore would be more regularly administered. The parents' decision can thus be accepted.

Comments

General: The health log serves to document the well-child visits, a voluntary, early disease recognition program for children and adolescents. In Germany, for example, ten visits for early detection of diseases that endanger the normal physical and intellectual development of a child are available to all children and youths up to the age of 13. Health screening programs are also available—according to various periodicity and age schedules—in many countries, including one in the United States that is advocated by the American Academy of Pediatricians (AAP). The information in the following is exemplary for the well-child program in Germany.

The visits take place at suggested intervals. During the visit, there is also a consultation about the child's health, giving an opportunity to ask questions about nutrition, immunizations, etc. This is a way to conduct both secondary prevention—recognition of diseases at the earliest moment possible—and primary prevention—promotion of optimal health and disease prophylaxis. Social pediatric aspects also play an important role in the health screenings.

Public acceptance of the health screenings is good, both because they are covered by health insurance with no additional cost to parents and because most parents have a great interest in their children's best development and want to use all the opportunities that can benefit them.

Practical procedure: Normally, the health screenings take place with the same pediatrician, which means that the child knows the doctor and vice versa. As a result, there is a certain trust between child and doctor. From previous visits, the doctor knows the child's strengths and weaknesses, their preferences and fears. This makes the doctor able to show an interest in the specific qualities of the child and so have a positive influence on the course of the visit. In particular, any abnormalities noticed at the last visit should be compared with the current state of development. The child, on the other hand, knows the office space and the doctor. That leaves them less anxious about being touched, and they know that nothing "bad" will happen to them. The examination usually takes place in a room that is specifically suited to a child, fitted out with appropriate toys and the necessary examining equipment (e.g., wooden blocks with openings to fit geometric shapes, age-appropriate vision charts with animals or symbols, a play mat on which to observe the playing toddler's movements). The mother and child are usually taken into the room 10 or 15 minutes before the doctor comes in, and the age-appropriate toy is handed to the child wherever it is at the moment. The child can get used to the surroundings and the doctor sees them in a relaxed state, which makes it easier to evaluate the developmental stage (ideal case!).

Every health screening proceeds in a standardized order. See answer to question 6.2. In addition to a thorough **physical examination** and **careful observation of the child**, questions are asked about certain symptoms (e.g., seizures, see appendix/examination log). The physical development is evaluated, and body measurements are taken and recorded in percentile curves. The benchmark for normal weight development is that a child's birth weight triples by the end of their first year, increasing by a factor of 6 by the age of 6 and a factor of 12 by the age of 12.

It is often difficult to judge the psychomotor development status of a child. Many factors influence a child's development. A child can develop a different degree in different areas. Therefore, a fairly broad range is given for standard examination values. The importance of individual abnormalities should not be overvalued. Short-term checkups are permitted and useful. Nevertheless, early evidence of disorders must not be overlooked. The developmental status of the boy in the present case is an example of this. Precisely in premature births, developmental delays are to a certain extent physiologically normal. Up to now there are no clear opinions as to the age when the delays must be caught up. In general, it is assumed that by the time the child is of school age, their development should resemble that of children born at term.

Immunizations are not included in the health screenings, but the immunization status is monitored and parents are advised about recommended immunizations as part of the health counseling. Immunization appointments are also often combined with a health screening.

At various points in the child's development, very specific (anamnestic) findings are gathered. Particular attention is paid to these **developmental milestones**. In the following, a description of each health screening in Germany is presented, with the most important findings regarding psychomotor and cognitive development as well as the additional examinations.

1 day of age: This examination is performed a few minutes after birth. Particular attention is given to birth injuries, deformities, and postpartal circulatory and respiratory adaptation.

3 to 10 days of age: In addition to the clinical examination (auscultation, abdominal examination, examination of eyes, auditory canals, and mouth, genitals, skull, motor apparatus), in which particular attention is given to signs of hemodynamically relevant heart defects and signs of heart failure (difficulty drinking, weight gain instead of loss), the so-called newborn screening is performed on a few drops of blood taken from the heel and dropped on a dry blood card. In the United States, newborn blood screening tests are managed by the individual states. The groups from which tests are selected are metabolic, endocrine, hemoglobin, pulmonary, and immune conditions.

Congenital hypothyroidism, which is screened for, is caused by insufficient generation of thyroid hormones (e.g., by agenesis, enzymatic defects, lack of iodine, lack of stimulation by central hormones). Unrecognized and untreated hypothyroidism leads to cognitive defects, short stature, deafness, and neurological disorders. To prevent these serious consequences and ensure normal intellectual development, prompt initiation of treatment (replacement of thyroid hormone) is absolutely necessary.

Phenylketonuria (PKU) is the most frequent autosomal recessively inherited disorder of amino acid metabolism and is caused by a lack of phenylalanine hydroxylase. This disrupts the transformation of phenylalanine to tyrosine. Phenylalanine accumulation in the blood is increased and is excreted in the urine. A mouse-like smell in the urine is typical. Without treatment, PKU leads to psychomotor retardation, cerebral seizures, pigmentation disorders, and skin rashes. If treatment is started early, if possible before the second week of an infant's life, with special diet (low in phenylalanine, enriched with tyrosine), children develop physically and intellectually normal.

In autosomal-recessively inherited **classical galactosemia**, the enzyme galactose-1-phosphate-uridyl-transferase lacks in a galactose degradation pathway. Galactose and galactose-1-phosphate accumulate and damage particularly the liver and brain. Without treatment, the disease is lethal in most cases. The treatment consists of a lifelong lactose-free diet.

Additional recommended tests in the newborn screening that are not universally performed are screening for a lack of biotinidase and adrenogenital syndrome. It has become possible to detect rarer metabolic disorders (e.g., fatty acid oxidation disorders, amino- and organic aciduria) in extended screening with tandem mass spectrometry.

4 to 6 weeks of age: In this examination, the **first behavior patterns** are monitored: social behavior (infant responds to smiles by smiling), play behavior (focus on and follow objects that move in their field of view), and in language (sighing and groaning sounds when content and satisfied). The infant can turn their head to the side in prone position and turn it back and forth in supine position. The primitive reflexes are checked (e.g., Moro response, stepping and placing reactions, palmar and plantar grasp reflexes, see case 80) and Vitamin D and fluoride prophylaxis are administered.

3 to 4 months of age: The infant can control their head in prone position, smile and vocalize spontaneously. They are interested in their hands, clap them together in front of their face, and play with their fingers. In the examination, particular attention must be given to **muscle tone** and the presence of **coordination disorders** so that if there are abnormalities, physiotherapeutic treatment can be initiated in time. In addition, vision (fixation of objects and persons) and hearing (high-pitched rattling [see Fig. Hearing test with a high-pitched rattle], clapping, crumpling paper). There should be nutritional counseling about solid food and solid food combined with breastfeeding.

6 to 7 months of age: Of greatest importance is **screening for cerebral motor disorders** and **evaluation of cognitive development**. The child shows interest in the surroundings (eye contact with mother, reaction to sound stimuli, purposeful reaching for objects and careful examination of them), the child can control head position in every body position, turn from supine to prone position and back again, and prop themselves up with their hands.

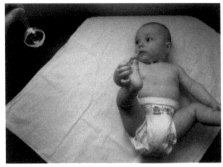

Hearing test with a high-pitched rattle

10 to 12 months of age: In this examination there is a **search for sensory disorders** (e.g., squinting, hearing impairment) and **speech development**. The child must be able to speak in double syllables, react to soft sounds, and examine toys with interest. The child stands, hanging on to something, walks along the furniture, and grasps with a forceps grip (index finger and opposed thumb—see Fig. Forceps grip). During this examination, the doctor also inquires about separation anxiety; this is an important milestone in social development. The immunization status must be checked, and the measles–mumps–rubella–varicella immunization should be discussed.

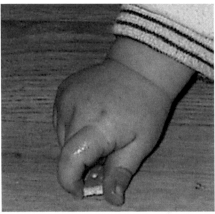

Forceps grip

21 to 24 months of age: In this and the following health screenings, particular attention must be given to **evaluation of sensory and other physical development**. Attention is given to orthopedic problems such as spinal deformities, gait, tipped pelvis, valgus or varus malalignment of the knees, and feet. There must be targeted questioning about behavioral abnormalities (e.g., sleep disorders, tantrums, speech disorders). The child must walk backward and forward freely, walk up and down stairs while holding on, squat and rise, and be able to walk quickly. The child uses at least 20 to 50 words in a meaningful way, can master 2-word sentences such as "Mama come," and understands and carries out simple tasks. He or she imitates simple daily adult actions (see Fig. Imitation of adult actions by a 2-year-old child). The child shares with others and tries to come out on top. The child can build towers of four to six blocks, likes to look at picture books, and exhibits so-called representative play (feeds the doll with a spoon).

→ Cases 6 Page 7

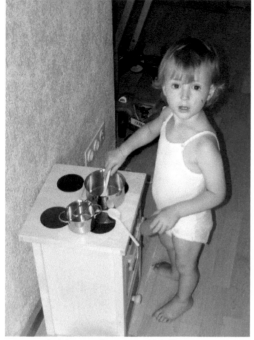

Imitation of adult actions by a 2-year-old child

given particular attention. Hearing and vision tests occupy a good portion of the time. Urinalysis with **urine strips** for glucose, albumin, etc. is a routine part of this health screening.

The child can correctly pronounce all the letters of the alphabet apart from "S," use personal pronouns, singular and plural, correctly, can tell about experiences and chat with others. The child can go up and down stairs without holding on, alternating legs, and stand on one leg for at least 3 seconds. The child concentrates on role and illusion games (make believe), and seeks friendship and cooperation with children of the same age.

The child can cut along lines with a scissors, hold a writing tool that is appropriate for her or his age properly, and create drawings independently.

60 to 64 months of age: This examination resembles the eighth one, especially in determining **whether the child is mature enough to go to school.** Particular importance is given to behavioral disorders or abnormalities. Pronunciation is practically without errors; only small grammatical errors can occur; the child knows their full name. The child can stand on one leg without holding on for at least 5 seconds, hop at least three times on one leg, and draw a circle, a square, and a triangle without error. The child can play persistently and constructively with rules and cooperates with playmates. The child should be able to control stool and urine. The basic program of the ninth visit includes measurement of the blood pressure. The immunization status is checked and completed.

10 to 14 years of age: The E 10/A1 visit includes an extensive medical history with the adolescent (A1). Questions are asked about **chronic and psychological problems,** school developments, family situation, social integration, and sexual hygiene. In this context, there should also be adolescent health counseling (sexual counseling, addiction prevention, offer to talk about problems and conflicts). In the physical examination, special importance is given to the **development of puberty** (see cases 68 and 78). The immunization status is checked; cholesterol and blood pressure are measured.

33 to 36 months of age: In this examination, one is looking for possible deficiencies in social and behavioral skills, the onset of obesity, allergies, and dental or maxillofacial anomalies. In addition, ophthalmological testing is performed in order to detect defective vision, spatial perception, and strabismus and special attention is paid to speech development.

At this age, the child can run confidently, jump from the bottom step of the stairs and land on both feet, use a bobbycar, a tricycle, or a balance bike, draw using the fist grip, and eat with a spoon quite confidently. The child can build sentences with at least three to five words and use their own name.

When playing, the child can take on a role, imitate adult actions, and play "pretend" games (e.g., a stick will become a sword). The child can play with other children for 10 to 15 minutes.

43 to 48 months of age: The examination is similar to the previous one. More importance is given to **evaluation and possibly treatment of behavioral disorders** (e.g., massive acts of defiance, stereotypes, aggressivity). Orthopedic problems (tilted pelvis, valgus and varus legs, abnormal foot arches, scoliosis) are

ADDITIONAL TOPICS FOR STUDY GROUPS
- Immunizations/immunization schedule
- Childhood diseases

7.1   What is the most likely clinical picture here? What is the name of the skin finding shown in the figure?
Lyme borreliosis, rationale: erythema migrans (erythema that spreads in the form of a ring), myalgia, arthralgia, oligoarthritis (joint swelling). The skin changes (here on the ear lobe) appearing in Lyme borreliosis are called cutaneous **lymphoid hyperplasia** (= "lymphocytoma" with circumscribed swelling and redness). Sites of predilection are ears, nipples, and scrotum.

7.2   What further symptoms must be expected with this disease?
The disease has a three-stage course but its first clinical manifestation can also come at an advanced stage.
- **Stage I (early localized stage):** On average, 5 to 12 days (duration: 5–48 days after infection), erythema migrans (ring-shaped erythema with central paleness and centrifugal spread), rarely flu-like symptoms (fever, fatigue, nausea, arthralgia). Spontaneous healing in 99% of cases.
- **Stage II (early generalized stage):** A few weeks after infection, skin changes (cutaneous lymphoid hyperplasia), neurological symptoms (facial nerve paresis, meningitis, or meningoradiculoneuritis), cardiac signs (myocarditis), migrating joint pain and myalgia, oligoarthritis (often gonarthritis) with formation of effusions, eye involvement (chorioretinitis), spontaneous healing in 2/3 of patients.
- **Stage III (chronic stage):** Symptoms persist longer than 6 months after infection, chronic relapsing arthritis, joint complaints and muscle pain, neurological symptoms (chronic encephalomyelitis with para- and tetrapareses, peripheral neuropathy), very rarely (usually not until adult years) acrodermatitis chronica atrophicans (chronic skin inflammation with reddish-livid, initially edematous then atrophically thinned skin, usually starting at extremities, gradually spreading proximally). Chronic inflammatory processes are the most notable; spontaneous healing is no longer possible.

7.3   What treatment do you suggest for the patient?
The patient is in stage II of the disease. Parenteral administration of an antibiotic is indicated. Medications of choice are third-generation cephalosporins, such as ceftriaxone (80 mg/kg body weight/d) or cefotaxime (200 mg/kg body weight/d), or penicillin G (500,000 IU/kg body weight/d, max. 12 million/d) for 14 days.

Comments

Etiopathogenesis: The pathogen of Lyme borreliosis is *Borrelia burgdorferi*, a spirochete primarily transmitted to humans by blacklegged ticks (in the United States, *Ixodes scapularis*). The Borrelia travel through the skin into the lymphatic circulation and from there into regional lymph nodes and blood vessels. They also spread to liver, spleen, joints, CNS, and other organs and can persist there for months to years. **Arthritis** is the **most frequent** form of borreliosis.

Epidemiology: According to the Centers for Disease Control and Prevention, approximately 99% of all reported cases of Lyme disease are confined to five geographic areas: New England, Mid-Atlantic, East-North Central, South Atlantic, and West North-Central). The risk of infection increases with the length of time that the tick is sucking (effective transmission only after > 24 hours). Only about 5% of infected individuals actually become sick.

Clinical aspects: See answer to question 7.2.

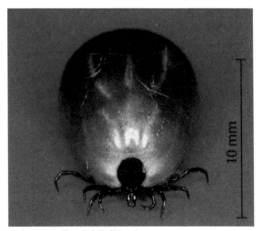

Ixodes ricinus (female full of blood)

Diagnosis: A diagnosis of borreliosis is established on the basis of the **medical history** (tick bites are only remembered in 50% of cases), **clinical symptoms** (see answer to question 7.2), and **serological findings**). In stage I, antibody detection is still frequently negative, so testing is not necessary. However, if symptoms are clinically relevant, serological tests of blood, cerebrospinal fluid, or articular aspirate should be performed 3 to 4 weeks after the start of illness, IgM, and after 6 to 8 weeks, IgG antibodies can be detected. They can persist for months or years after successful treatment. In late forms, high IgG titers can be found. Laboratory results must always be interpreted in the context of the clinical symptoms. *Caution:* Laboratory results can only be compared if they were obtained in the same laboratory. For this reason, always send serum samples to the same laboratory.

Treatment: Treatment depends on the clinical stage. In Stage I, treatment with an oral antibiotic for at least 10 days is sufficient: medication of choice for children < 8-year-old, amoxicillin 50 mg/kg body weight/d; for children > 8-year-old, tetracycline on the first day 4 mg/kg body weight, then 2 mg/kg body weight/d. In advanced stages, parenteral antibiotic treatment is recommended. Medications of choice in this case are ceftriaxone (rocephin) and cefotaxime (claforan).

Prophylaxis: Tick bites are most effectively prevented by skin-covering clothing (long pants, long-sleeved pullovers, firm shoes). Ticks do not fall from trees as generally assumed. Rather, they rest in tall grass and are brushed off in passing. A further recommendation is application of insect repellent with tick repellent (for instance, DEET). A mosquito net should be hung over a baby carriage. After spending time in the woods, children and adults should be searched for ticks naked, over body and hair. After a tick bite, the tick should be removed as quickly as possible. There are special tick tweezers in pharmacies, but the ticks can also be removed with ordinary tweezers. The affected area should *not* be swabbed with alcohol or oil. The tick should be grasped with the tweezers by the head, if possible, held with light pressure, and carefully removed. Sometimes,

parts of the head or mouth may remain in the skin. Although this may scare parents, this is not dangerous. The tick pieces will be expelled from the body in the same way as small wooden splinters, although in rare cases a small blister may appear at the site of the bite, which should then be opened. After the tick has been removed, the site should be disinfected. Prophylactic administration of an antibiotic is not indicated. The parents should be instructed about possible early symptoms of borreliosis (see answer to question 7.2).

Prognosis: The prognosis of Lyme borreliosis is better, the earlier it is diagnosed and treated. Partial recovery is possible. The disease does not generate immunity; reinfections are possible.

Whereas the danger of infection with borreliosis is widespread and worldwide, another tick-borne disease, **early summer meningoencephalitis**, is only transmitted in endemic areas of Europe and Asia. This is an infection of the central nervous system with the tick-borne encephalitis virus (TBE) that belongs to the genus *Flavivirus*. Ticks that transmit the TBE virus are endemic in a large part of East European countries, in Finland and Sweden, as well as in certain regions of Germany. Usually the course of the disease is biphasic: it begins after an incubation period of 7 to 14 days with flu-like symptoms (mild fever, headache, vomiting, and vertigo). After a 1-week symptom-free interval, about 10% of infected individuals develop meningoencephalitis with high fever, headache, and vomiting. Seizures and altered states of consciousness, ranging up to coma, can occur. In children, the disease is usually benign; severe encephalitis with partial recovery and even fatal outcome is extremely rare. Treatment is symptomatic; no causal treatment is available.

But do not spread panic. There is an active TBE vaccine, even for children. However, this vaccine should be limited to children living in endemic areas.

ADDITIONAL TOPICS FOR STUDY GROUPS
- Differential diagnoses
- Tick-borne encephalitis (TBE)

8.1   What is the most likely diagnosis?

Schoenlein–Henoch purpura, rationale: Maculopapulous exanthema with individual petechiae, especially on the extensor side of the lower leg and on the buttocks; abdominal pain; previous respiratory infection

8.2   Which differential diagnoses are you considering? Briefly characterize these diseases.

- **Idiopathic thrombocytopenic purpura** (ITP): Autoimmune thrombocytopenia (thrombocytes < 20,000/μL, often after viral infections, autoantibody against thrombocytes → breakdown of antibody loaded thrombocytes in the RES of the spleen (see case 83)
- **Hereditary purpura simplex**: Autosomal recessive inherited vasculopathy, petechial skin bleeding without therapeutic consequences
- **Seidelmayer cockade purpura**: Vasculitis after mild infections, characterized by target-like, partially raised skin phenomena, especially on the face and extremities. Heals spontaneously after 1 to 2 weeks.
- **Waterhouse–Friderichsen syndrome:** Meningococcal sepsis with a fulminant course with consumption coagulopathy, skin bleeding, microthrombi, and skin necroses (see case 82)

8.3   What treatment do you initiate?

- No causal treatment is possible. High rate of spontaneous healing. With a mild course, bed rest is no longer recommended.
- If the clinical course is severe: Bed rest; analgesics (for instance, paracetamol); in joint involvement antiphlogistics (for instance, ibuprofen)
- For abdominal symptoms (for instance, bloody stools, colic): Prednisolone 1 to 3 mg/kg body weight/d p.o. until symptoms are gone
- For nephritis, see Comments

Comments

Definition and epidemiology: Schoenlein–Henoch purpura is a **generalized allergic vasculitis** of the small vessels Toddlers and school children are most frequently affected.

Etiopathogenesis: The disease often occurs after viral infections. There is a type III immune reaction (Arthus reaction) with subendothelial deposit of IgA-containing immune complexes in the small vessels and activation of the complement system.

Clinical aspects: The disease progresses in bursts, often over the course of weeks. **Maculopapulous exanthema with petechiae and ecchymoses**, especially on the **extensor side of the lower leg and on the buttocks**. If the gastrointestinal tract is infected, mucosal edema and bleeding lead to colic-like abdominal pain. Tarry stools and invagination frequently occur in this case. If the joints are involved, painful periarticular swelling and limitation of motion occur. In a third of cases, the renal blood vessels are also infected. However, development of nephritic syndrome (micro- or macrohematuria, proteinuria, edema, arterial hypertonia) as a result of glomerulonephritis is rare. Seizures and altered states of consciousness are symptoms of a (rare) involvement of cerebral vessels.

Diagnosis: The diagnosis can be established on the basis of the **medical history** (prior infection) and clinical aspects (purpura with normal coagulation and thrombocyte values, joint involvement, abdominal symptoms, occult blood in the stool, etc.). If the kidneys are involved, micro- or macrohematuria and proteinuria are observed.

Treatment: See answer to question 8.3. No causal treatment is known. The disease usually heals spontaneously within a few weeks.

Suspicious findings resulting from renal involvement are quite frequent. If the course is uncomplicated, no treatment is necessary. There is no advantage to using steroids.

Very rarely, glomerulonephritis ends in terminal renal failure. In that case, there is no ensured treatment protocol. Care should be taken that the diet is carbohydrate rich, low in protein and salt, and fluid intake should be balanced. Edema and high blood pressure are treated with diuretics and antihypertensives. Because of the role of the autoimmune process, the best procedure is collaboration with a pediatric nephrological center to administer glucocorticoids and immunosuppressive agents (chlorambucil, azathioprine, or rifampicin).

Prognosis: The prognosis is usually very good except in rapidly progressive glomerulonephritis (terminal renal failure). Very rarely, the cause of death is acute gastrointestinal complications or acute renal failure.

Case

8

ADDITIONAL TOPICS FOR STUDY GROUPS
- Other vasculitides
- Immunological reaction types according to Coombs and Gell
- Invagination

9.1   Describe what you see on the ultrasound image in the figure.

In cross section, the image shows a thickened muscle diameter and in longitudinal section, a lengthened pyloric canal (see Fig. Sonography).

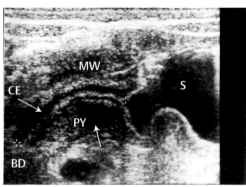

Sonography in hypertrophic pyloric stenosis (imaging of the distinctly thickened muscle wall [MW], the severely narrowed canalis egestorius [CE], with elongated pylorus [PY, ++] as expression of high-grade pyloric stenosis with enlarged overall diameter [→]; fluid in stomach [S], duodenal bulb [DB])

9.2   Explain the pathogenesis.

This is a muscular hypertrophy of the pylorus and neighboring portions of the antrum causing a disorder of stomach emptying.

9.3   List the typical symptoms

- Projectile vomiting after every meal
- Visible stomach peristalsis ("peristaltic wave")
- Failure to thrive: Weight loss, "senile" appearance
- Dehydration, electrolyte shift; laboratory: hypokalemic, hypochloremic alkalosis
- Restlessness, possible altered state of consciousness
- Pseudo-constipation
- Upper abdominal meteorism

9.4   What treatment do you suggest?

- Compensation for dehydration and electrolyte shift
- Weber–Ramstedt pyloromyotomy (see Comments)

Comments

Definition and epidemiology: Postnatal hypertrophy of the circular pyloric muscles and neighboring portions of the stomach causes obstruction of the pyloric canal, leading to emptying disorders of the stomach. Hypertrophic pyloric stenosis occurs with a frequency of 1:500. Boys are affected approximately five times more frequently than girls. The diagnosis is usually established between the 3rd and 12th week of an infant's life.

Clinical aspects: See answer to question 9.3. Infants are hungry, restless, drink greedily, appear distressed and "senile" (see Fig. Typical facial expression...). After the meal, painful gastric hyperperistalsis—usually visible as a peristaltic wave in the upper abdomen—leads to projectile vomiting that never contains bile. In the course of this vomiting, the child can spit as far as 2 meters!

Diagnosis: The diagnosis is confirmed by sonography, with **the typical medical history and clinical factors.** The pylorus appears thickened and elongated; the stomach is well filled, even hours after the meal.

The laboratory results show electrolyte shift and characteristically, hypochloremic, metabolic alkalosis. If the findings are ambiguous, other obstructions in the gastrointestinal tract (for instance, polyps, annular pancreas) must be ruled out radiologically with an upper gastrointestinal passage examination using water-soluble contrast medium.

In the outpatient department, a provocation test can be performed with 50 mL of tea. In palpating the abdomen, you feel an olive-shaped structure in the right upper abdomen. This is the pylorus.

Differential diagnoses: Systemic infection (for instance, urosepsis), gastroenteritis, symptoms of cerebral pressure, duodenal or jejunal atresia, gastroesophageal reflux, adrenogenital syndrome with loss of salt, intolerance of cow milk protein.

Treatment: After compensation for dehydration and electrolyte shift by infusion therapy, the treatment of choice is **Weber–Ramstedt pyloromyotomy.** The pyloric muscles are completely severed except for the mucosa. The operation is associated with low risk and a high success rate.

In very rare cases, the pyloric obstruction disappears spontaneously, usually after the 12th week. In mildly progressing cases, an attempt can be made to avoid surgery with conservative treatment (spasmolytics before meals, elevating the upper body, sedation, infusion therapy, frequent, small meals).

Prognosis: After postoperative nutritional buildup, the infant will do well with a normal diet.

ADDITIONAL TOPICS FOR STUDY GROUPS
- Clinical aspects, diagnosis, and treatment for the differential diagnoses

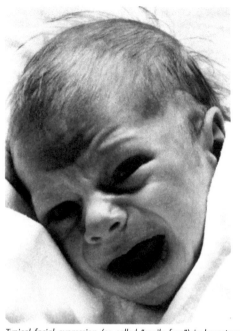

Typical facial expression (so-called "senile face") in hypertrophic pyloric stenosis (4-week-old boy who has been vomiting for 10 days and is losing weight. He always has a sour, dissatisfied expression, often frowns and screams.)

10   Bronchial asthma

10.1   Describe the thoracic X-ray result. What do you notice? What is your diagnosis?
- **Thoracic X-ray:** Massive overinflation of the lungs with increased transparency; low, flattened diaphragm between the 10th and 11th rib; narrow heart silhouette; slightly increased streaking in the right pulmonary hilum (= prominent hilum but no pneumonic infiltrate, so-called infection hilum; indication of possible infection-triggered [infection-exacerbated] asthma]
- **Diagnosis: Acute asthma attack with probable allergic bronchial asthma**; rationale: history of allergy, increasing shortness of breath, dry cough, wheezing, massive thoracic retractions, "silent chest"; for thoracic X-ray results, see above.

10.2   Explain the pathogenesis of this disease.
- Bronchial asthma is characterized by **spasmodic occurrence, obstructions of the respiratory pathways** reversible spontaneously or by treatment resulting from **hypersensitivity of the bronchial mucosa.** The cause of the bronchial hyperreactivity is a chronic inflammation of the bronchi. The triggers are usually allergens, but other irritants, such as infections, gastroesophageal reflux, cigarette smoke, chemical irritants, cold air, emotional stress, also act as triggers.
- Contact with the trigger is via an IgE-mediated degranulation of mast cells to **release histamine** (early reaction). The consequences are smooth muscle spasms, mucosal swelling, and dyscrinia that lead to narrowing of the respiratory pathways, especially in the middle-sized and smaller bronchi.

→ Cases 10   Page 11

- 12 to 24 hours after the start of the early reaction, inflammatory cells enter the tissue (T lymphocytes and eosinophils) and release inflammation mediators. This late reaction plays a significant role in maintaining the inflammation.
- Chronic inflammation is not only involved in the development of hyperreactivity; it can also induce so-called airway remodeling, which is a permanent modification of the respiratory pathways.

10.3 What acute treatment do you initiate?
- **Elevate upper body**, calm the patient
- Pulse oximetry
- **Administration of oxygen** (2 L/min) through a nasal cannula or mask, only at O_2 saturation < 90% (*Caution:* hypoxemia may be the only stimulus for breathing; uncontrolled administration of oxygen can inactivate this, and cause breathing cessation)
- **Inhalation of a β_2-sympathomimetic such as salbutamol**, one drop per birth year ([max. 8] diluted with 0.9% saline) possibly in combination with an anticholinergic such as ipratropium bromide, two drops per birth year, most effectively by moist inhalation (for instance, with a Pari-Boy device). In case of severe obstruction, undiluted salbutamol can be used for constant inhalation with monitoring of the pulse rate.
- Placement of an indwelling catheter for infusion therapy (fluid replacement, secretolysis) with blood draw (blood gas analysis, inflammation parameters [CRP, sedimentation rate, leukocytes])
- **Glucocorticoids** i.v., such as methylprednisolone as bolus (2–5 mg/kg body weight), then every 6 hours, 1 to 2 mg/kg body weight. Duration of steroid therapy depends on the clinical symptoms. Usually it can be discontinued after a few days. If the therapy lasts for more than 7 days, the steroid must be tapered off. Inhaled glucocorticoids have no effect in acute cases.
- Possibly **theophylline** i.v.: initial brief infusion over 20 minutes (with pre-treatment 2–3 mg/kg body weight, without pre-treatment 5–6 mg/kg body weight), then prolonged infusion with a perfusor with 1 mg/kg body weight/h.
- Possibly **sedation** with ketamine (for instance, ketanest S 0.5 mg/kg body weight gradually, up to 2.5 mg/kg body weight with monitor oversight; ketanest also has a strong bronchodilator effect); *caution:* respiratory depression. Always be prepared for intubation in the intensive care ward.
- Administration of **antibiotics** (for instance, cefuroxime, 30–100 mg/kg body weight/d or amoxicillin

50–100 mg/kg body weight/d) only when there are signs of a bacterial infection.
- In case of worsening, **intensive care**, possibly ventilation

10.4 What long-term treatment would you consider useful?
- **Allergen avoidance**
- Individual treatment planning is more important than any stepwise schema; the following points must be taken into account:
  - What can child and family really accomplish in addition to kindergarten, school, and daily stress? It is better to have less treatment, but systematically administered, than a great deal of treatment that is seldom performed.
  - In every long-term therapy, there must first be **asthma education**—outpatient or inpatient—for both patient and family. The objectives are information and counseling (What is asthma? How should I react in an emergency? What can I do to prevent an attack? How can I evaluate my breathing [peak flow, asthma journal?] etc.) to reduce fear of the disease, learn the right way to deal with the disease, and thus achieve the best possible long-term treatment. In this process, close collaboration of physicians, nurses, physiotherapists, psychologists, etc. with the family is very important; depending on the patient's situation, a suitable treatment must be found, with information about the purpose, the effect, and side effects of the treatment.
  - *In general the following applies:* reduce complications as much as possible; keep things as normal as you can.
- **Stepwise long-term medical treatment**: see Tab. Stepwise long-term medical treatment, for individual drugs, see Comments
- Always keep emergency medications at hand
- Sport and physical activity are a significant basis for asthma therapy. Targeted breathing exercises and exercises to make breathing easier (use of auxiliary breathing muscles, pursed lip breathing) for emergencies should be learned and regularly practiced.
- If necessary, hyposensitization, if not too many allergies are evident and patient is > 6 years: every 1 to 2 weeks subcutaneous injection or sublingual application of specific antigen solutions in increasing doses. *Caution:* Must only be done by trained allergologists under careful monitoring.
- Choice of occupation: Avoidance of occupations that favor hyperirritability of the bronchial system (for instance, baker, hairdresser)

Comments

Definition: Bronchial asthma is a chronic inflammatory disease of the airways with bronchial hyperreactivity and variable airway obstruction. It is usually associated with an atopic disposition. Narrowing of the airways is usually spontaneous or reversible after treatment.

Etiopathogenesis: See answer to question 10.2. Like allergic rhinitis and neurodermitis, bronchial asthma is on the spectrum of atopic diseases. In more than 90% of cases, asthma is associated with allergies. In children, only 15% of asthma cases is exclusively allergic in origin. Usually, the disease is **mixed asthma**, triggered by allergens, infections, and non-specific irritants. Many allergens are pollen, animal epithelial cells, and house dust mites. In addition to numerous non-specific irritants (for instance, cold air, dust, ozone), bronchial hyperreaction can be triggered by psychological (for instance, school, family, friends) and physical stress (= exercise-induced asthma in sport, climbing stairs) as well as endocrine causes (for instance, hyperthyroidism, menstruation) and medications such as analgesics.

Clinical aspects and classification: **Cardinal symptoms** are attacks of shortness of breath with expiratory wheezing that in part can even be heard at a distance without a stethoscope (distance wheezing, see case) as well as cough and dyscrinia. In an acute asthma attack, the patient sits upright, uses auxiliary breathing muscles, is anxious and produces cold sweat. Different degrees of severity are distinguished on the basis of the number of symptoms and limitations of pulmonary function (in the symptom-free interval) (see answer to question 10.4).

Diagnosis: Diagnosis of an acute asthma attack is always established clinically (shortness of breath, prolonged expiratory phase, dry cough, use of auxiliary respiratory muscles, massive expiratory wheezing, buzzing and whistling over the lungs, tachycardia, cyanosis, in severe cases weakened respiratory sounds [= "silent chest"]). At the start, the **blood gas analysis** often shows hypercapnia and progressively increasing hypoxia. When the progress is severe, global respiratory failure with hypoxia and hypercapnia can occur in the advanced stage. After the patient has been stabilized, a thoracic X-ray is made. It is particularly necessary if the medical history or the clinical picture creates suspicion of comorbidity such as pneumonia, atelectasis, or pneumothorax. The following abnormalities are seen in thoracic X-ray results in an acute asthma attack: pulmonary overinflation, that is, increased transparency, flat diaphragm, narrow heart silhouette, increased perihilar streaking (see Fig. Thoracic X-ray in Cases).

The typical history (for instance, family history, seasonal occurrence of symptoms) and examination findings lead to a diagnosis of bronchial asthma.

The examination findings include **prolonged expiratory phase, expiratory wheezing, whistling, and thrill**; alveolar overinflation causes a **hyperresonant percussion sound**. In severe obstruction, the respiratory sound can be so soft that it can hardly be heard ("silent lung"). **Pulmonary function tests** (spirometry, full-body plethysmography) make it possible to objectivize increased airway resistance or overinflation of the lungs as well as the reversibility of an obstruction. With latent symptoms, a non-specific bronchial provocation can be helpful (methacholine [MCH] provocation test, running stress). The prick test can give a suggestion about the pathogenetic significance of an allergen, and allergen-specific IgE antibodies can be detected in the RAST test. Elevated values for total IgE can be found in the laboratory and eosinophilia can be detected in the differential count. Other pulmonary diseases should be ruled out with a thoracic radiograph.

Treatment: For acute treatment, see answer to question 10.3. For stepwise treatment, see answer to question 10.4. The objective of the treatment is to reduce the frequency of attacks, moderate bronchial hyperreactivity, and to protect the patient from late damage (for instance, development and growth disorders, cor pulmonale). The most important treatment principle is to avoid asthma triggers: Allergen avoidance (for instance, mattress slip covers impermeable to mites, no wall to wall carpeting in cases of dust mites, no pets in cases of animal allergy, etc.), avoidance of non-specific irritants such as active and passive smoking. Parents and patients should learn how to deal with the disease through so-called asthma training. Physical training (asthma sport) is another important pillar of asthma therapy for maintaining and improving pulmonary function.

The objective of drug therapy is the reduction of inflammation, and thus the sensitivity of the bronchial mucosa. Anti-inflammatory drugs include first and foremost inhaled glucocorticoids (for instance, budesonide, beclomethasone, fluticasone), oral glucocorticoids (and glucocorticoids, prednisolone) as well as oral leukotriene receptor antagonists (LTRA, antileukotrienes such as montelukast). There are short-acting and long-acting β_2 sympathomimetics. Anti-IgE antibodies (omalizumab) are restricted to patients with IgE-proven pathogens. Treatment is designed according to a monitoring schema adjusted to the severity of the asthma (see Tab.). For this treatment, only as many drugs should be prescribed as needed for optimal asthma control (see Tab.).

→ Cases 10 Page 11

	Controlled bronchial asthma (fulfills all criteria)	Partially controlled bronchial asthma (fulfills 1–2 of the criteria within a week)	Uncontrolled bronchial asthma (fulfills ≥3 of the criteria within a week)
Daytime symptoms	no	> 2 times per week	
Nighttime symptoms /Awakening from sleep	no	yes	
Restriction of everyday activities	no	yes	
Administration of medication, as needed/ Emergency care	no	> 2 times per week	
Pulmonary function (FEV1 or PEF)	normal range	< 80% of the reference value of FEV1 or optimal personal value of PEF	
Exacerbation[a]	no	at least one time per year	at least one time per week

Abbreviations: FEV1, forced expiratory volume in 1 second; PEF, peak expiratory flow.

Source: Deutsche Atemwegsliga und Deutsche Gesellschaft für Pneumologie und Beatmungsmedizin (DGP). Kurzfassung der Asthma-Leitlinie 2017. Stuttgart: Thieme 2018; *German Respiratory League and German Society for Pulmonology and Respiratory Medicine. Abridged Edition of the Asthma Guidelines 2017.*

Note: The level of bronchial asthma control should be monitored at regular intervals and treatment should be adjusted, i.e., reduced or intensified, accordingly.

[a] Each weekly exacerbation is per definition "uncontrolled asthma." Exacerbation: Episodes with increasing shortness of breath, coughing, wheezing, and/or tightness in the chest, which are proceeded by an attack of FEV1 or PEF.

Stepwise long-term medical treatment for bronchial asthma of children and adolescents

Step	Treatment	Supplementary treatment
Step 1		Salbutamol or ipratropium bromide as needed
Step 2	Inhaled corticosteroids (ICS) at low doses **Alternatively:** montelukast	Salbutamol or ipratropium bromide, as needed
Step 3	ICS at medium doses	Salbutamol or ipratropium bromide
Step 4	ICS at medium doses +/− long-acting β₂ mimetic +/− montelukast **Alternatively**: ICS at high doses +/− long-acting β₂ mimetic **+/−** montelukast	or ICS/formoterol (at low doses, only in adolescents > 12), as needed

Inhalation is an important building block of the therapy. Correct technique is particularly important, so that the active agents are deposited intrabronchially and not only in the nose and throat. The highest concentration of active agents in the lungs is obtained with moist inhalation but powder and aerosol inhalation are also possible. Ideally, this should be done with devices such as Aerochamber or Babyhaler. After inhalation of inhaled glucocorticoids, patients should rinse their mouth or eat or drink something, in order to avoid thrush.

Prognosis: Asthma is not curable, but (long-term) therapy adapted to the severity of the condition can make life with the disease easier. There will be a lifelong atopic disposition and a tendency to asthma. Remission in or around puberty occurs in less than 50% of cases. There is often a residual airway hyperreactivity and asthma symptoms occur again later. Transition to adult chronic-obstructive pulmonary disease is possible.

 ADDITIONAL TOPICS FOR STUDY GROUPS
- Immunological reaction types according to Coombs and Gell
- Additional causes of eosinophilia
- Side effects of treating asthma with drugs
- Allergic rhinitis, neurodermitis
- Principle of desensitization

11.1 Describe the otoscopic finding. What is your diagnosis?
- **Otoscopic findings:** Eardrum with perforation and inflammatory secretion
- **Diagnosis: Otitis media right**; rationale: disturbed sleep (child brought to the emergency department at night), restless child, purulent secretion in auditory canal, the frequent touching of the ear is taken as indication of pain, pain on pressure to tragus, swollen lymph node in right jaw angle (for otoscopic findings, see above) with infection of upper airways (serous rhinitis, fever, reddened tonsillar ring)

11.2 List the most frequent causes of this disease.
- Usually viral infection, possibly a bacterial superinfection
- Frequent pathogens for superinfections: *Streptococcus pneumoniae, Haemophilus influenzae, Moraxella catarrhalis*
- Rare pathogens for superinfections: *Streptococcus pyogenes, Staphylococcus aureus, Pseudomonas aeruginosa, Escherichia coli*

11.3 What possible serious complications do you know of?
Hearing impairment in cases of middle ear effusion that results in delayed speech development, inner ear involvement (for instance, labyrinthitis with vertigo), mastoiditis, chronic-relapsing otitis, facial nerve paralysis, spread of infection from skull bone to meninges, intracranial abscesses, sinus venous thrombosis.

11.4 What therapeutic procedure would you consider useful here?
- The toddler has a bacterial infection (purulent secretion, high fever) that should be treated with **antibiotics**. Drugs of first choice: amoxicillin (50–100 mg/kg body weight/d in three separate doses p.o.), alternative in case of allergy/intolerance macrolide (for instance, clarithromycin 15 mg/kg body weight/d in two separate doses) or oral cephalosporins (for instance, cefixime 8 mg/kg body weight in one single dose) for 5 to 7 days
- In case of nasal congestion, nose drops three to four times daily to reduce mucosal swelling, especially at bedtime
- Sufficient fluid for secretolysis
- Analgesia/Fever reduction with ibuprofen (10 mg/kg body weight p.o., max. 3 × daily) or paracetamol supp. (10–20 mg/kg body weight, max. 3 × daily)

111

Case

11

Comments

Definition: Acute otitis media is a one- or both-sided **serous to purulent inflammation of the middle ear**. Usually there is an accompanying upper airway (rhinopharyngitis) infection (see case description).

Epidemiology and etiopathogenesis: Especially infants and toddlers frequently contract otitis media, due to the immunologically determined, elevated susceptibility to infection in this age group, as well as anatomical characteristics. The short and usually wide Eustachian tube facilitates migration of germs from the nasopharyngeal space into the middle ear. Moreover, enlarged adenoids are often present.

Airway infections accompany mucosal edema of the Eustachian tube. This results in a disorder of the tubal function (so-called tubal catarrh) with insufficient ventilation of the middle ear. This facilitates secondary bacterial infection of a primary otitis media that is usually viral. For pathogens, see answer to question 11.2.

Clinical aspects: See case and answer to question 9.3. For complications, see answer to question 11.3.

Diagnosis: The taking of the medical history is followed by a physical examination with checking, among other things, **for tragus pain on pressure and the meningism sign** as well as palpation of **the lymph nodes and mastoids. Otoscopy** shows a red ear drum, swollen, possibly bulging or retracted, or perforated with secretion. Otoscopy is usually quite difficult because most children are uncooperative due to the pain. An attempt at distracting the child with something like "Do you think there's a mouse in your ear?" sometimes helps. It can also be useful to inspect the healthy ear first so that the child notices that the examination is not as terrible as she thinks. In practice, however, the situation often ends with the mother and the nurse holding the child still for otoscopy. For this reason, auscultation and other examinations should always come first, since after otoscopy, another physical examination is no longer possible, due to lack of cooperation. In otoscopy, it is important to hold the otoscope in the right hand (for left-handed people, in the left hand), to grasp it with the thumb and index finger, and support it with the middle finger at the zygomatic arch while gently pulling the outer ear upward and outward in order to straighten the auditory canal and obtain a better

→ Cases 11 Page 12

view of the eardrum (see Fig. Otoscopy in a child). For the sitting position of the child during otoscopy, see case 80.

Further examinations, such as a smear or laboratory work, are not necessary if the clinical examination and the otoscopic findings are unambiguous. If there are additional symptoms, such as dehydration and meningism, hospital admission with extensive diagnosis and appropriate therapy should follow.

Treatment: See answer to question 11.4. Decongestant nose drops relieve cold symptoms and regulate the ventilation problem. Since middle ear inflammation is often very painful, systemic analgesics should be administered. Paracetamol is usually well tolerated and with the appropriate dose has relatively minor side effects. Ibuprofen has both analgesic and anti-inflammatory properties. Anesthetizing ear drops are not efficacious in acute middle ear inflammation. They are used in otitis externa.

It is not possible to make a general recommendation for antibiotic administration because of the high rate of spontaneous healing with symptomatic treatment and the mostly viral cause of the disease. As long as there are no unambiguous signs (fever, purulent effusion, and swollen lymph nodes) of a bacterial (secondary) infection, the course of the disease is continuously controlled, with symptomatic treatment. Antibiotic treatment should not be given unless the patient's condition deteriorates or there is unambiguous proof of a bacterial infection. In children under the age of 2, however, the risk of complications is higher, thus leading to a more frequent indication for antibiotic therapy in this age group. Amoxicillin is the agent of choice, because of the pathogenic spectrum, but cephalosporins or macrolides are efficacious too. Treatment lasts for 7 to 10 days.

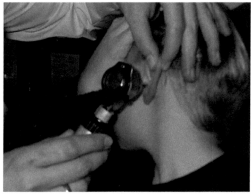
Otoscopy in a child

In relapsing otitides, possible causes, such as adenoid vegetations, should be eliminated. Persistent middle ear effusion is treated by paracentesis (incision of the tympanic membrane in the posterior or anterior lower quadrant) and, if necessary, by placement of a tympanostomy tube.

Prognosis: Healing is usually uncomplicated within 10 to 14 days. If the tympanic membrane is perforated, the defect closes by itself.

 ADDITIONAL TOPICS FOR STUDY GROUPS
- Differential diagnoses with criteria for differentiation of acute otitis media
- Anatomy and physiology of the ear, nose, and sinuses
- Additional ENT diseases such as acute sinusitis, rhinopharyngitis, tonsillitis, and adenoids

12 Varicella (chicken pox)

12.1 Explain the typical symptoms of the disease to the parents.
- Rarely prodromes (fever, fatigue, headache)
- Within a few hours, changes in skin (also skin of head) and mucosa (especially oral cavity, conjunctiva, genitals); palms of hands and soles of feet are usually not affected.
- These efflorescences are simultaneously present in various developmental stages (so-called **starry sky**, see Fig. Varicella exanthema), that is, red spots, papules, little blisters, and pustules.
- Little blisters and pustules tear open, dry, crust over, and the scabs fall off after approximately 2 weeks.

- Frequently concomitant catarrhal symptoms with and without fever

12.2 In your opinion, how could the boy have become infected? When would you expect to see the first symptoms?
- **Droplet infection** from contact with sick persons, possibly also airborne transmission; contagious 1–2 days before outbreak of rash until fifth to seventh day after occurrence of rash
- **Incubation time:** Approximately 2 weeks (8–21 days)

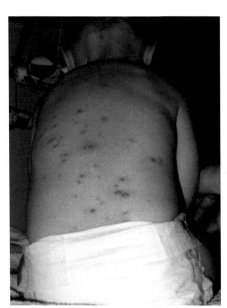

Varicella exanthema (back with efflorescences at various stages of development—"starry sky")

12.3 **Are there any dangers to mother and child at this stage of pregnancy? Would you have to expect complications if the mother were in another stage of pregnancy?**
- **General:** With existing immunity (mother has been infected) → no danger
- **In first infection:**
  - **In the third trimester up to 5 days before birth:** Intrauterine infection usually also leads to infection of the fetus; the disease is benign in the unborn and newborn, thanks to the mother's acutely produced antibodies. This means that in the example case there is a danger that the mother will contract chickenpox if she has no immunity. With the mother infected, it is likely that the unborn child will be infected, but not with serious effects.

- **In the first and second trimester:** Varicella embryopathy is very rare (connatal varicella syndrome) possibly with skin defects (scars), skeletal and muscular hypoplasia, deformities in eyes (chorioretinitis, microphthalmus, cataract, and anisocoria), CNS (cortical atrophy, ventricular dilatation, cerebellar hypoplasia). The course is asymptomatic in 75 to 97% of cases; interruption of pregnancy is not indicated for this low fetal risk. The pregnant woman receives *Varicella zoster* immunoglobulin, careful surveillance of the pregnancy (repeated ultrasound examinations).
- **Peripartal, that is 5 days before the birth until 2 days after the birth**, danger of connatal varicella (mother's antibodies can no longer be transmitted to the child), course and degree of severity are very variable (isolated efflorescences to severe organic manifestations such as pneumonia, encephalitis), outbreak between the ages of 10 and 12 days, lethality up to 30%; therefore with suspicion of peripartal infection, the newborn should always be admitted to the hospital with monitoring, possibly i.v. administration of acyclovir or passive immunization.

12.4 **Is there any possibility of inoculation?**
- **Passive immunization within 72 hours of exposure:** Varicella zoster immunoglobulin (indications: seronegative pregnant woman in case of Varicella contact; newborns whose mothers became ill with varicella 4–7 days before or 2 days after delivery or had varicella contact; newborn in the first days after birth with varicella contact; immunodeficient patients)
- **Active immunization:** Live vaccines, immunization recommended by the Center for Disease Control and Prevention (CDC) for children 12 months old, with a booster dose between 4 and 6 years old The chicken pox shot can be given in a single vaccine together with a measles–mumps–rubella shot (MMRV) or separately, up to 4 weeks later at the soonest. This immunization is also recommended for all children from 9 to 17 years old who have neither had chicken pox nor been immunized against it.

Comments

Definition and epidemiology: Varicella is an **acute, highly contagious viral disease.** A generalized, vesicular exanthema appears in bursts. Ninety percent of all children up to the age of 14 years are infected (so-called childhood disease). Infants in the first six months usually do not become ill because of maternal passive immunity. Exception: peripheral infection (see answer to question 12.3).

Etiopathogenesis: The pathogen for chickenpox is the **Varicella zoster virus** that belongs to the *Herpes* virus group of human pathogens. Human beings are the exclusive pathogen reservoir. For transmission

path/contagiousness/incubation time, see answer to question 12.2. The virus enters the body through the airway mucosa. This results in viremia with hematogenous distribution in skin and mucosa, giving the clinical picture of chickenpox. Subsequently the virus persists in the cells of the sensory ganglia and can be reactivated, for instance, in case of immune system weakness, stress, advanced age, malignant diseases—but usually not in childhood. This results in shingles, a very painful neuritis with little groups of blisters in one or more dermatomes. It rarely appears all over the body.

Clinical aspects: See answer to question 12.1. **Complications** of the disease are bacterial superinfections, usually with *Staphylococci* or *Streptococci*. Possible sequelae are impetigo, abscesses, phlegmones, necrotizing fasciitis. Cerebellitis, pneumonia, and keratitis have been observed as further complications. In immunodeficient patients, some occasionally life-threatening courses have been observed, with encephalitis, severe pneumonia, hepatitis, and pancreatitis.

Diagnosis: The diagnosis is clinical. In case of doubt it is possible to detect specific antibodies or the pathogen.

Differential diagnoses: Disseminated *Herpes simplex*, insect sting, strophulus infantum (prurigo simplex), urticaria, erythema exsudativum multiforme.

Treatment: In uncomplicated courses, local anti-itch suspensions such as anaesthesulf lotion. These suspensions promote the drying of the rash and by cooling (for this reason, they should be stored in the refrigerator) they relieve the pain and itch, thus preventing a bacterial superinfection caused by scratching. If there is a fever, **antipyretics** such as paracetamol may be used, but not ASA, because of the danger of Reye syndrome. In patients with risk factors such as immunodeficient patients, a severe course, newborns with connatal varicella infection or infected premature babies, antiviral treatment

with acyclovir is indicated (250–500 mg/m² body surface over 1 hour every 8 hours for 10 days). This treatment should be started within the first 4 days after exposure or immediately upon appearance of the first rash. Bacterial superinfections must be treated with antibiotics, for instance, erythromycin or cephalosporins, for at least 7 days.

Prophylaxis: A child with varicella, presumed to have varicella, or varicella contact must be admitted to the hospital and isolated. This also applies to babies newly born to mothers with varicella. On the other hand, newborns with connatal varicella syndrome do not need to be isolated.

Children with uncomplicated chickenpox may return to kindergarten when the contagious stage is over. A doctor's clearance certificate is required for the return.

For active and passive immunization, see answer to question 12.4.

Prognosis: Varicella usually heals well. However, there are often scars because blisters are scratched open. Complications such as CNS involvement and varicella pneumonia also have a good prognosis if treatment is begun early.

ADDITIONAL TOPICS FOR STUDY GROUPS
- Other viral infectious diseases (rubella, measles, mumps, etc.)

13 Lymphadenitis colli

13.1 Name the possible causes of swollen neck lymph nodes.
- Often a concomitant disease with mild infections of the upper airways
- Local infections, for instance, in oral mucosa/teeth, in ENT region, at skin and head skin, (usually) one-sided lymph node swelling with streptococcal or staphylococcal infections
- Generalized infections such as cat scratch disease, toxoplasmosis, infections with EBV, CMV, measles, rubella, atypical mycobacteria among others, with generalized lymph node swelling
- Mucocutaneous lymph node syndrome (Kawasaki syndrome)
- Lymphoma, malignant neoplasm
- Lymph node tuberculosis (rare)

13.2 What other studies do you order for this girl?
- **Laboratory:** (differential) Blood count, inflammation parameters (CRP, sedimentation rate)

- **Throat smear:** Diagnosis of pathogen
- **Sonography of the swollen lymph nodes:** Size, extent, necrolysis

13.3 What treatment do you initiate?
- Antibiotic treatment (active against Staphylococci/Streptococci) see Comments
- Possibly hospital admission: Depending on the form of the lymphadenitis colli and changes in laboratory parameters, preferably a generous indication since oral administration of antibiotics is not as effective and an abscess can often develop rapidly
- In case of abscess, incision

13.4 What pathological finding can you determine? What treatments does this require?
- **Microbiological findings:** Acid-fast bacilli
- **Most likely diagnosis: Lymphadenitis colli caused by atypical mycobacteria**; rationale: in spite of appropriate treatment, continuing lymphadenitis

colli, one-sided involvement, general condition not impaired; for microbiological finding, see above
- **Differential diagnoses:** Lymph node tuberculosis (very rare in children)
- **Treatment of atypical mycobacteriosis:**
  - Order an antibiogram

- Surgical removal of the lymph node and all fistular channels
- In complete removal: Treatment with clarithromycin (15–30 mg/kg body weight/d) or azithromycin (10–12 mg/kg body weight/d) in combination with rifampicin (350 mg/m² body surface) for 6 months, possibly modification after receipt of antibiogram.

Comments

Definition: An **inflammatory** swelling of the regional neck lymph nodes is called lymphadenitis colli. Non-inflammatory swellings are called lymphadenopathies.

Etiopathogenesis: See answer to question 13.1. In many healthy children, neck lymph nodes up to the size of beans are palpable; these swell up as a result of frequent infections in the ears, nose, and throat. Thus, not every palpable lymph node is pathological.

Lymph node swelling also occurs in malignant diseases (leukemia, solid tumors) as well as generalized infections (lymphotropic viruses such as EBV or CMV, in toxoplasmosis [*Toxoplasma gondii*] or cat scratch fever [*Bartonella henselae*]), but they are usually generalized.

One-sided lymph node swelling with abscesses is usually lymphogenic in origin. The pathogens are often *Staphylococci* or *Streptococci*, in infections of the ENT region, the teeth, or the skin. Sometimes a one-sided lymphadenitis colli is caused by atypical *Mycobacteria* (Mycobacteria other than tuberculosis [MOTT]). *Mycobacterium avium* can be detected in 80% of cases. The infectious pathway has not yet been found, but transmission from human to human is ruled out. The pathogen can be found in tap water, soil, wild animals, and pets.

Clinical aspects: Swelling of the neck lymph nodes can be one- or two-sided, painful and movable. If the inflammation extends into the surrounding area, the node can be firmly attached to it. Redness and infiltration into the skin can occur. The general condition can be significantly impaired. Lymphadenitis colli caused by atypical *Mycobacteria* usually develops slowly and only on one side; this does not impair the patients' general condition.

Diagnosis and Treatment: A thorough physical **examination with assessment of all lymph node stations** and the size of liver and spleen (hepatosplenomegaly chiefly in EBV infection). The ENT area and the teeth should be examined with particular care.

If there is a suspicion of tuberculosis (see case 72), in addition to a thorough medical history with particular inquiry about contact with persons suffering from tuberculosis or with persons at risk, a tuberculin test should be performed. In addition, a thoracic X-ray should be made.

In case of a local infection, an attempt should be made **to identify the pathogen** (for instance, by means of smears), since a specifically targeted **antibiotic treatment** must be administered. The efficacy spectrum of the antibiotic must include Staphylococci. This means that penicillin alone is not sufficient. Specific findings are treated with intravenous antibiotics (for instance, with cephazoline 50 mg/kg body weight in three individual doses or cefuroxime 100 mg/kg body weight/d in three individual doses) to achieve a sufficiently high tissue concentration of the active agent.

A surgical intervention cannot be avoided always in this way. If the infection produces abscesses, the abscesses should be lanced. If there is a suspicion of a mycobacterial origin, the abscess, with all fistular tubes, should be removed completely. The resected tissue must be worked up histologically and bacteriologically. If MOTT infection is verified and the abscess cannot be completely removed, tuberculostatic treatment is administered for 6 months (see answer to question 13.4).

Surgical therapy is also necessary to rule out a malignant growth if in spite of treatment, the lymph node does not shrink in a period of 2 to 4 weeks or even grows larger.

ADDITIONAL TOPICS FOR STUDY GROUPS
- Complications of acute Lymphadenitis colli
- Differential diagnoses
- Tuberculosis, other MOTT infections

14.1 What do you think causes these symptoms? What are your next steps?

- **Possible diseases:** Bronchiolitis, pneumonia, severe bronchitis, foreign body aspiration
- **What are your next steps?**
  - Upset the child as little as possible! If necessary, sedation (diazepam 0.5 mg/kg body weight i.v., *caution:* respiratory depression)
  - Pulse oximetry: if pO_2 < 90%, administer oxygen (enrichment of the air child is breathing with oxygen, using nasal cannula/mask/funnel or introduction into warming bed)
  - BGA: hypoxia, hypercapnia
  - Placement of i.v. port, blood draw for determination of inflammation parameters (blood picture with differential blood count, CRP, sedimentation rate)
  - Thoracic X-ray: infiltrates, shadows

14.2 What is your diagnosis on the basis of the thoracic X-ray and the medical history? Describe the radiological changes typical for this clinical picture.

- **Diagnosis: Bronchiolitis**; rationale: onset of the disease with non-specific airway infection, tachypnea, dyspnea, nostril flaring, weakened breath sounds, isolated fine crackles
- **Typical radiological changes (see Fig. Thoracic X-ray in Cases):**
  - **Significant overinflation** of both pulmonary lobes (flat diaphragm, increased transparency)
  - Increased bronchial visibility in the perihilar area
  - Possibly small poorly aerated regions (atelectasis)

14.3 List the most frequent pathogens of this disease.

Respiratory syncytial virus in 80% of cases (Syn.: **RS virus**, RSV)

14.4 What therapeutic possibilities are available?

- **Hospital admission:** Every infant with bronchiolitis should be monitored as an inpatient. The breathing situation deteriorates dramatically in the early morning hours (minimal body-intrinsic glucocorticoid production); often nutrient, at least fluid replacement via feeding tube, is essential, since every additional stress endangers the infant significantly. In young infants with bronchiolitis, there is an elevated risk of apnea.
- **Symptomatic treatment:** Minimal handling, oxygen administration, for instance, via nasal cannula or funnel, dampening the air with a cold air nebulizer, sedation, fluid administration (stomach tube or i.v.), monitor surveillance, decongestant nose drops.
- **Inhalation therapy:** Attempt at treatment by inhalation of bronchodilators such as salbutamol (0.1–0.5 mg/kg body weight in 2 mL physiological NaCl solution) or epinephrine (1 mL of the 1:1,000 diluted solution in 1 mL physiological NaCl solution) with careful pulse oximeter monitoring. If the situation shows no clinical improvement or even deterioration, the inhalation therapy is discontinued.
- **Glucocorticoids:** Systemic administration only if the course is severe (initial bolus 1–3 mg/kg body weight, then 2 mg/kg body weight/d).
- Only if there is a suspicion of a bacterial superinfection (blood picture, CRP), **antibiotic treatment** with cephalosporins (for instance, cefuroxime 30–100 mg/kg body weight in three individual doses i.v. for at least 8 days) should be conducted.
- If there are signs of respiratory failure (rising pCO_2 values, marked tachypnea [> 100/min] or apnea), pharyngeal CPAP should be attempted. If this fails, intubation and ventilation should be considered.
- **Ribavirin:** The virostatic ribavirin is potentially mutagenic; subsequently, its use necessitates adherence to strict clinical practice guidelines for best safety of the patient and the nurses. This treatment should only be used if the course of the disease is severe.

Comments

Definition and epidemiology: Bronchiolitis is an acute viral, obstructive inflammation of the bronchioles that occurs almost exclusively in the first year of a child's life. Children contract it most frequently in the winter months.

Etiopathogenesis, clinical aspects and diagnosis: RS viruses, and less frequently parainfluenza, influenza, rhino-, and adenoviruses attack the entire respiratory tract and lead to a severe inflammation of the lower airways. After **3 to 5 days with symptoms of a**

cold (prodromal stage), children increasingly develop tachypnea, inspiratory and expiratory dyspnea, cough, circulatory centralization and weakness in drinking.

Bad general condition; on auscultation, "soundless" tachypnea (silent chest), and dyspnea with unambiguous radiological signs of pulmonary overinflation indicate bronchiolitis.

The clinical symptoms in the case example could also suggest severe pneumonia. But in that case, the X-ray would show pneumonic infiltrates.

→ Cases 14 Page 15

Treatment: No causal treatment is known. There-fore, the treatment is exclusively symptomatic (see answer to question 14.4).

Prophylaxis: Endangered children (for instance, infants with heart defects, bronchopulmonary dys-plasia, immunodeficiency, premature birth) should be protected in the winter months of the first year of the child's life by means of passive immunization with monoclonal antibodies (palivizumab). At pres-ent, an active vaccine is not available.

Prognosis: In the first months or years after an RSV infection there is increased susceptibility to bron-chopulmonary infection, especially with obstruc-tive symptoms. The prevalence of asthma after RSV infection also increases.

ADDITIONAL TOPICS FOR STUDY GROUPS
- Foreign body aspiration
- Pneumonia
- Bronchial asthma
- Pulmonary deformities

15   Infectious mononucleosis

15.1   What is your suspected diagnosis?
Infectious mononucleosis, rationale: Patient's age (so-called kissing disease in adolescents); high fever, tiredness, fatigue, sore throat, difficulty swallow-ing, feeling of pressure in upper abdomen, transient exanthema

15.2   With your suspected diagnosis, what exam-ination findings do you expect?
- Pharyngitis and tonsillitis with extensive, smudgy coating (angina lacunaris) and possibly unpleasant breath
- Largely symmetrical, often multifocal lymph node swelling, most intense in the neck
- Hepato- and splenomegaly
- Possibly icterus, livid, fine to moderately spotty exanthema

15.3   List the most frequent causes of this dis-ease.
- **Tonsils:** Secondary bacterial tonsil infection, usually with Streptococci; distinctive tonsillar hyperplasia ("kissing tonsils") → obstructive apnea possible
- **Immune system:** Hepatitis, ruptured spleen, lym-phoma, hypo-/hypergammaglobulinemia, formation of autoantibodies
- **Hematopoietic system:** Thrombocytopenia, anemia, granulocytopenia; in immunodeficiency often

severe, even lethal lymphoproliferative clinical picture
- **Heart:** Myocarditis, pericarditis
- **Central nervous system:** Meningoencephalitis, Guil-lain–Barré syndrome
- **Skin:** Slight, transient maculopapular exanthema, urticaria, vasculitis, ampicillin exanthema (resulting from ampicillin administration→ itching, mea-sles-like exanthema)
- **Other organ involvements**: Pneumonia, nephritis
- **EBV-associated malignant tumors:** Burkitt lym-phoma, Hodgkin disease, T-cell lymphoma, naso-pharyngeal carcinoma

15.4   What advice do you give the patient? When will the symptoms improve?
- There is no causal treatment. Virostatics and antibi-otics are without effect.
- **Symptomatic treatment:** Bed rest, antipyretics (paracetamol), soft (or liquid) diet, if necessary infu-sion therapy for fluid replacement
- High doses of glucocorticoids (for instance, one-time prednisolone 12–53 mg/kg body weight i.v. bolus; possibly repeat 1–2 times) only in case of airway obstruction, hemolytic anemia, thrombocytopenia
- Antibiotic therapy in case of superinfection (mac-rolide), ampicillin contraindicated (see answer to question 15.3)
- **Improvement of symptoms:** Symptoms up to 4 weeks; fatigue, easy tiring up to 1 year

117

Case

15

Comments

Etiopathogenesis and epidemiology: Infectious mononucleosis (Syn.: Pfeiffer glandular fever) is trig-gered by the Epstein–Barr virus (EBV) in the group of herpes viruses. Transmission is by infected saliva. For this reason, it is also called the kissing disease. Adolescents are most frequently affected. The level of endemic infection after the age of 30 is over 80%.

Clinical aspects: After an incubation period of 10 to 50 days, a first infection with EBV in immuno-competent older children, adolescents, and adults exhibits the clinical picture of infectious mono-nucleosis with fever, lymph node swelling, severe angina, hepatosplenomegaly, and exanthema (see case). Sometimes there is also icterus. In children,

→ Cases 15 Page 16

the course is mostly asymptomatic or atypical (slight influenza-like symptoms). In immunodeficient patients, there can be severe lymphoproliferative clinical pictures (for instance, malignant B-cell lymphomas). For complications, see answer to question 15.3.

Diagnosis: The diagnosis is based on typical clinical symptoms (see case and answer to question 15.2) as well as characteristic changes in the blood picture (see Fig.). Because of the associated hepatitis the transaminases are almost always elevated.

The **Paul–Bunnell test** (Syn.: Monospot, mononucleosis quick test) that verifies the presence of heterophilic antibodies, typical of infection, can facilitate diagnosis in older children and adolescents. In children under 5 years, the test usually gives a false negative because antibody formation is still insufficient. A positive EBV antibody test is definitive proof. In a recently acquired infection, antibodies against the virus capsid (anti-VCA [virus capsid antigen]-IgM) and anti-EA (early antigen)-IgG are found. Subsiding infections can be confirmed by anti-EBNA (nucleus-associated antigens).

Treatment: See answer to question 15.4.

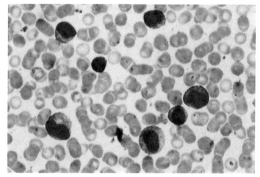

Blood picture in infectious mononucleosis (atypical lymphocytes with oval or bean-shaped nucleus and fine vacuoles in cytoplasm, partially reminiscent of monocytes, so-called Pfeiffer cells)

Prognosis: The prognosis is usually good. In immunocompetent patients, this is a self-limiting disease. EBV persists lifelong in B lymphocytes and can, especially in immunodeficiency or on immunosuppressive therapy, be reactivated. Various lymphomas, for instance, Burkitt lymphoma, are associated with EBV.

ADDITIONAL TOPICS FOR STUDY GROUPS
- Further causes of tonsillopharyngitides
- Differential diagnoses of hepatitis

16 Foreign body aspiration

16.1 **What typical clinical symptoms and examination results do you expect if this is really a foreign body aspiration?**
- Typical history: Cough attack
- Usually shortness of breath, followed by tachypnea; possibly cyanosis
- Auscultation: Weakened breath sounds on the affected side, sometimes bizarre secondary sounds, inspiratory and/or expiratory stridor, possibly moist crackles
- Percussion (reliable findings only in children 5 years and older): Hyperresonant percussion sounds

16.2 **You order a thoracic X-ray (see Fig.). Describe the abnormalities.**
- Distinct overinflation of the left lung (increased transparency and low diaphragm left)
- Mediastinal displacement right
- No foreign body visible

16.3 **What treatment do you initiate if this is really an aspiration?**
Bronchoscopic foreign body removal

Comments

Definition and etiopathogenesis: Aspiration of foreign bodies is an accident frequently affecting toddlers. In addition to small objects made of the most varied materials (for instance, a toy) solid bits of food such as peanuts, apple or carrot pieces are often aspirated.

In newborns and infants, in cases of gastroesophageal reflux, (relapsing) aspirations of milk must also be considered.

The valve mechanism arises through a valve stenosis in bronchial shift. In this process, air passes into deeper sections of the lung during inspiration and can no longer escape during expiration. As a result, there is overinflation and mediastinal shift to the opposite side.

The right main bronchus is more often affected than the left one because of its steeper branching.

Clinical aspects: The symptoms described in the case are typical for foreign body aspiration. Aspiration is not always followed by shortness of breath; often the coughing attack is the only indication that aspiration has occurred. If the aspirated foreign body is not removed, the area behind the aspirated object, which receives less air, can become inflamed. Chronic bronchitis or pneumonia can develop and bronchiectasis can be formed. For this reason, in case of long-lasting coughing, a possible foreign body aspiration should be considered and specific questions about it should be asked while taking the medical history.

Diagnosis: In auscultation, an asymmetrical breath sound can be heard. Usually it is weaker on the aspiration side. On percussion, the sound is hyperresonant because of overinflation caused by the valve mechanism.

The aspirated foreign body is only radiopaque in about 10% of cases, so indirect signs, such as valve mechanism (80%) and atelectasis (20%), principally indicate aspiration. The valve mechanism causes overinflation of the affected lung (increased transparency, low diaphragm) in some cases with mediastinal shift (see answer to question 16.2). Fluoroscopy of the thorax visualizes the decreased mobility of the diaphragm on the affected side.

Foreign bodies can be so small that they do not cause obstruction to either inspiration or expiration and thus cannot be found with the usual roentgen diagnostics. If the suspicion is supported by medical history and clinical findings, bronchoscopy is required. This is always done under anesthesia.

Treatment: In principle, pounding the child on the back, Heimlich maneuver, raising up the child by the legs, etc. are not wrong, but usually do not have the desired result. In case of acute choking, one should try to calm the child and notify the emergency physician **immediately**. Foreign bodies should be removed **bronchoscopically** as promptly as possible, in order to prevent atelectasis and inflammatory tissue reactions.

Prophylaxis: In principle, toddlers should not eat small, solid pieces of food such as nuts, apple slices, raw carrots, nor play with very small objects such as little buttons, peas, little toys. But even with great care and a maximum of monitoring, it is not always possible to prevent an aspiration accident.

Prognosis: Bronchoscopic removal of foreign bodies in children is almost always successful. Complications can arise if, for instance, a peanut crumbles during removal and secondary pneumonia develops. However, this is very rare. Children can usually be discharged from the hospital on the day after the intervention.

ADDITIONAL TOPICS FOR STUDY GROUPS
- Differential diagnoses of chronic cough

---

17 Testicular torsion

17.1 What is your suspected diagnosis? What differential diagnoses can be considered?
- **Suspected diagnosis: Testicular torsion**; rationale: patient's age, testicles painful, reddish-livid color, coarsely swollen
- **Differential diagnoses:** Orchitis, hydatid torsion, epididymitis, direct trauma, incarcerated inguinal hernia, testicular tumors

17.2 How do you confirm the diagnosis?
Duplex ultrasonography: Confirmation of absent or insufficient perfusion of the testicle, *caution:* at the slightest suspicion of testicular torsion, **operate immediately** (there is only a max. of 6-hour time from the start of pain to infarction of the seminiferous tubules, 12 hours until infarction of the Leydig cells. However,

this clearly depends on the remaining residual perfusion). Duplex ultrasonography is not definitive, since if perfusion is found to be present, there could still be a hydatid torsion or incomplete torsion endangering the testicle. Therefore, the indication for diagnostic surgery is broadly defined.

17.3 What are your next steps?
- Laboratory: blood picture, differential blood count, CRP, sedimentation rate (inflammatory parameters to rule out the differential diagnoses of orchitis, epididymitis). Detailed medical history regarding coagulation disorders, tendency to bleeding, to prevent perioperative complications of hemorrhaging
- Inform Pediatric Surgery/Pediatric Urology or Urology
- Inform Anesthesia (premedication)

→ Cases 17 Page 18

- Surgical exposure of the testicle, untwisting and orchidopexy (attachment of the testicle to the scrotum)
- If this does not result in reperfusion (livid discoloration does not disappear): semicastration

- Always perform prophylactic orchidopexy of the contralateral testicle, but usually in a later second surgery

Comments

Definition and etiopathogenesis: The turning of the testicle around its longitudinal axis and the ductus deferens interrupts the circulation of the testicle. The result is a hemorrhagic infarction. The cause of testicular torsion is often abnormal motility of the testicle in its sheaths because of an abnormality in the tunica vaginalis testis or the mesorchium. This abnormality is usually bilateral.

Clinical aspects: Testicular torsion occurs chiefly in infants and in puberty. Extremely intense pain in the testicle and the groin sets in while the patient is in a state of complete wellbeing. The infant usually screams out of a state of complete wellbeing, makes a distressed impression, and cannot be soothed by the usual means. He no longer wants to breastfeed at the breast. Sometimes there is nausea and vomiting because of peritoneal irritation.

The scrotal skin is discolored reddish-livid, the testicle is swollen.

(Differential) diagnostics: Establishing a differential diagnosis of orchitis is achieved by a detailed medical history, and the clinical course and duplex ultrasonography of the testicle. A **sudden onset of symptoms** is typical for testicular torsion. Parents usually come to the Emergency Department shortly after the start because they cannot interpret the child's screaming and cannot soothe him.

Orchitis, which usually occurs in adolescence and young adulthood, is often associated with a mumps infection. In this case there is a prodromal stage with fatigue and tiredness, followed by the typical mumps symptoms with swelling of one or both parotid glands and fever. In sonography, it may be possible to see enlargement of the affected testicle. It appears hypoechoic, homogeneous, with smooth borders. In addition, there is thickening of the scrotal mass and an associated hydrocele. Duplex ultrasonography shows increased circulation of blood with hyperemic flow profile. In orchitis, the serological inflammatory parameters (CRP, sedimentation rate) are elevated.

The so-called **Prehn sign** in the clinical examination can give an additional indication. Intensification of pain when the testicle is raised points to testicular torsion; decrease of pain suggests orchitis.

Treatment: See answer to question 17.3. Testicular torsion is a urological emergency. The diagnosis must be established quickly because the ischemic time of the testicle is only 4 to 6 hours. If this time is exceeded, the germ cells die, with subsequent testicular atrophy and loss of ability to father a child (infertility).

Spontaneous untwisting is rare. The risk of a relapse is very high, so that in this case as well, an operation for fixation should be scheduled.

Prognosis: The prognosis depends on the time of the operation. If it is done on time and if the other testicle is fixated in a second operation, there will be no residual damage.

ADDITIONAL TOPICS FOR STUDY GROUPS
- Anatomy of the testicle
- Cardinal symptom inguinal and testicular pain
- Epididymitis, Orchitis

18 Post-streptococcal glomerulonephritis

18.1 What causes of macrohematuria do you know? What other causes are there for "red urine"?
Macrohematuria is the visible red coloring of the urine caused by excretion of erythrocytes. As little as 0.5 mL blood in 500 mL of urine color the urine red. A distinction is made between:
- **Glomerular hematuria** in glomerulonephritis (GN), for instance, post-streptococcal GN, systemic GN (Schoenlein–Henoch purpura, lupus erythematosus, etc.), familial GN

- **Non-glomerular hematuria,** for instance, in concretions, urinary tract infections, trauma, foreign body, tumor, hemorrhagic diathesis (thrombocytopenia, hemolytic anemia, etc.)

Further causes of "red urine" are, for instance,
- Foods such as red beets, blackberries, rhubarb, food dyes (aniline)
- Medications such as rifampicin, metronidazole, phenytoin

- So-called brick dust deposit (yellow-red sodium urate occurring in acid urine)
- Hemoglobinuria in hemolysis (for instance, march hemoglobinuria [walking for a long time, which challenges the feet] leads to microtraumatization and destruction of erythrocytes], hemolytic crises in hemolytic anemia, incompatible blood transfusion)
- Myoglobinuria (destruction of muscle tissue, for instance, after severe muscle injury)

18.2 What is your suspected diagnosis?

Poststreptococcal glomerulonephritis, rationale: prior purulent angina, macrohematuria, arterial hypertension

18.3 What is your diagnostic procedure?

- **Laboratory** (pathological findings in poststreptococcal GN expanded):
  - Blood/serum: Sedimentation rate ↑, blood picture, urea, creatinine ↑, electrolytes, ASL ↑ (antistreptolysin), complement (chiefly C3) ↓, immune complexes, possibly ANA, immunoglobulins, albumin
  - Urine: Erythrocyturia (micro- and macroscopic), red blood cell casts, leukocyturia, proteinuria,

specific weight, urine culture, amount of urine, GFR ↓.
  - Throat smear: Streptococci
- **Sonography of kidneys:** Enlarged kidneys, blurred parenchyma–pyelon border, echogenicity resembles liver

18.4 How do you treat the boy?

- There is no causal treatment.
- **Symptomatic treatment**: Fluid restriction (700–1,000 mL/1.7 m² and day), bed rest
- In verified infection, antibiotic treatment after antibiogram; if *Streptococci* are detected, penicillin 50,000–100,000 IU/kg body weight/d p.o. for 10 days
- Control: Daily weight control, pathological laboratory results, blood pressure
- Treatment of possible complications:
  - Severe arterial hypertension: antihypertensives, for instance, with calcium channel blockers (nifedipin) and ACE inhibitors (captopril)
  - Oliguria and edema: Diuretics, such as furosemide
  - Anuria: Dialysis, hemofiltration
  - Heart failure: digoxin
  - Encephalopathy: If there are seizures, diazepam or long-term sedation with phenobarbital

Comments

Definition and forms: **Glomerulonephritis** (GN) is an inflammation of the glomeruli caused by deposit of immune complexes or autoantibody formation as well as complement activation. A distinction is made between acute poststreptococcal GN and chronic GN (for instance, in autoimmune diseases).

Nephritic syndrome is characterized by hematuria, mild proteinuria (1.5–3 g/d), limited kidney function with formation of edema, and arterial hypertension. If, in addition, large-scale proteinuria develops (> 3 g/d), the condition is called nephrotic syndrome (see case 47).

Etiopathogenesis: One to two weeks after tonsillitis or skin infection by β-hemolyzing group A *Streptococci* (so-called nephrogenic *Streptococci*), an inflammatory reaction in the glomeruli can occur. This is possible in spite of a previously adequately treated Streptococcal infection. Bacterial antigens use complement C_3 to form immune complexes (immune complex nephritis) that deposit on the mesangium. Microscopic accumulations of subepithelial immune aggregates ("humps") are typical. Approximately 80% of patients exhibit symptoms of GN; approximately 20%–50% remain asymptomatic and only exhibit microhematuria. Poststreptococcal GN is the most frequent cause of nephritic syndrome. No prophylaxis is possible.

Clinical aspects: In addition to general symptoms like paleness, loss of appetite, vomiting, and headache,

there are typical symptoms such as macrohematuria, oliguria, proteinuria, and edema (only with severely limited kidney function, especially around the eyelids and pretibially). Possible complications (approximately 5% of cases) include elevated blood pressure up to hypertensive crises with cerebral seizures, acute renal failure, encephalopathy, and heart failure.

Diagnosis: See answer to question 18.3.

Treatment and prognosis: In 95% of cases, with symptomatic treatment (see answer to question 18.4), the symptoms regress in a few days or weeks. Microhematuria can persist for weeks to months and increase in febrile infection or with stress, without expectation of an unfavorable prognosis.

In 5% of cases, patients develop kidney failure and require dialysis. Encephalopathy and heart failure can be avoided through appropriate therapy (see answer to question 18.4).

Tonsillectomy is only indicated in relapsing tonsillitides requiring antibiotics; poststreptococcal GN is not an indication.

ADDITIONAL TOPICS FOR STUDY GROUPS
- Nephrotic syndrome
- Hemolytic–uremic syndrome

19.1   What is the purpose of percentile curves? What are somatograms? What important information do they provide?

- **Percentile curve:** The measurements of body height, weight, and head circumference are entered in the screening documentation at every health examination (E1–10). This gives an overview of the child's development and a comparison to the "average child." Measurements that lie between the 3rd and 97th percentile are normal; if the results fall above or below these two percentiles, it must be assumed that there is some illness, even if only one of the measurements is not normal in comparison with the others. There is a characteristic percentile curve for each nationality.
- **Somatogram:** The child's current age, height, and weight are entered next to each other in the curve provided and this should yield a horizontal line. This is done as soon as the child arrives, to provide a quick impression of his physical development.

19.2   What information do you derive from the percentile curves of the 11-month-old boy?

- Height and weight development up to approximately the age of 6 months normal (running approximately to the 50th percentile).
- From the sixth month, development (height/weight) remains static and is now under the 10th percentile; no growth/no weight gain since the sixth month is a **failure to thrive**.

19.3   What is your suspected diagnosis on the basis of the medical history, the growth and weight development, and the external appearance of the boy? What differential diagnosis must you consider?

- **Suspected diagnosis: Celiac disease**; rationale: failure to thrive, small amount of subcutaneous fat tissue, sour, voluminous stools several times a day, swollen abdomen, loss of appetite, bad mood (see answer to question 19.2; Interpretation: probably until the age

of 6 months, the boy was fed entirely on mother's milk. Since the mother's milk contains no gluten, development has been normal; with the addition of porridge and similar foods [containing gluten] from the sixth month, development has stalled).
- **Differential diagnoses:**
  - Other malabsorption or maldigestion syndromes: cystic fibrosis, cow milk protein intolerance/allergy, malnutrition, congenital intestinal enzymatic defects
  - Chronic diseases: HIV (HIV enteropathy), heart failure, kidney disease, ulcerative colitis, Crohn disease, tuberculosis, malignant tumor, etc.
  - Disruptions in the social environment/psychiatric disorders: neglect, child abuse, eating disorder, etc.

19.4   With your suspected diagnosis on physical examination, what further findings do you expect?

- Skin folds on buttocks caused by lack of fatty tissue
- Meteorism and many fluid-filled intestinal loops
- Muscle hypotonia, muscle weakness
- Pallor caused by anemia
- Possibly edema caused by lack of protein

19.5   How do you confirm your suspected diagnosis?

- Typical medical history and examination findings (see answers to questions 19.3 and 19.4)
- Symptoms beginning with consumption of grain-containing foods
- **Laboratory:** Hypochromic anemia due to lack of iron, electrolyte shift (Ca ↓), extended prothrombin time, lack of protein, **anti-gluten antibodies** (IgA and IgG), **anti-endomysium antibodies** (IgA), **anti-tissue transglutaminase antibodies** (IgA), **total IgA** (in selective IgA deficiency, the tests can give a false-negative response)
- **Small intestine biopsy:** Required for establishing diagnosis; total villous atrophy, flat small intestine mucosa, hyperplastic and deep crypts, lymphocyte infiltration

Comments

Definition and pathogenesis: Celiac disease (syn.: gluten-sensitive enteropathy) is a chronic malabsorption disorder caused by intolerance of the protein-containing elements (gliadin fraction of the cereal seed storage protein) of native grains. Gliadin triggers an immune reaction (delayed-type [type IV] hypersensitivity reaction). Autoantibodies against the endomysium (the autoantigen is the enzyme tissue transglutaminase) are formed.

The chronic inflammatory process leads to total villous atrophy in the small intestine. The results are

malabsorption with disordered absorption of all nutrients (loss of digestive enzymes) and failure to thrive. The full-blown disease does not always occur in toddlers. Sometimes it is only diagnosed in adulthood. The disease is then called "native sprue."

Epidemiology and etiology: The incidence of the disease in average, healthy people in the United States is approximately 1:133. The etiology is not yet completely understood. There is a genetic predisposition (association with HLA antigens DQ2 and DQ8).

Clinical aspects: Most children fall ill between 8 months and 2 years of age, that is, the symptoms begin with the start of a grain-containing diet. Retrospectively, a "percentile kink" is often found. For typical clinical examination findings, see case and answers to questions 19.3 and 19.4.

Diagnosis: See answer to question 19.5. Information leading to a diagnosis includes detection of anti-gliadin and more-specific anti-endomysium and anti-tissue transglutaminase antibodies and the obligatory histological examination of the small intestine mucosa. This is usually obtained endoscopically in a gastroduodenoscopy as a forceps biopsy at the duodenojejunal flexure. The Watson capsule formerly used for a biopsy is virtually never used today because endoscopes have become steadily finer and better.

In addition to total villous atrophy (see Fig.), the histological examination shows hyperplasia of the crypts with lymphoplasmocytic infiltration of the lamina propria and the epithelium.

Treatment: Celiac disease is incurable but it can easily be treated. Therapy consists of a systematic, lifelong gluten-free diet. This means that gluten-containing foods such as wheat, rye, oats, barley, spelt, green spelt, einkorn wheat, and malt are forbidden. Even the slightest amounts of gluten-containing foods must be avoided. *Caution:* Prepared foods can contain hidden gluten. On the other hand, rice, corn, millet, buckwheat, soy, and potatoes are allowed. With this treatment, the mucosa is regenerated within 6 to 12 months. The success of the treatment can be seen in improvement of the child's mood, rapid gain in height and weight, as well as disappearance of the diarrhea. At the start of the therapy, vitamin and iron replacement should be initiated.

Prognosis: With a consistent diet, the prognosis is good and a healthy life is possible.

👪 ADDITIONAL TOPICS FOR STUDY GROUPS
- Symptoms, diagnosis, and treatment of other malabsorption disorders (for instance, cow's milk intolerance)
- Chronic inflammatory intestinal diseases
- Development of height and weight in childhood

123

Case

19

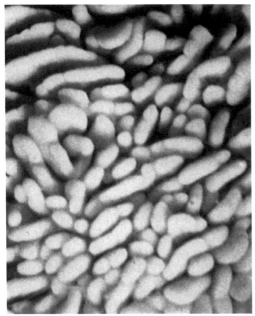

Normal small intestine mucosa obtained by suction biopsy, seen under a loupe

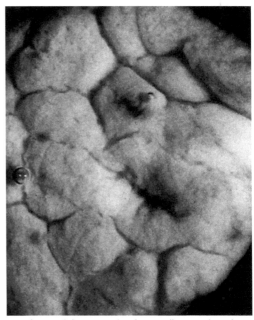

Typical mucosal changes in celiac disease: Villous atrophy and cerebral cortex-like changes

→ Cases 19 Page 20

20.1 **What could the soft swelling on the head be? Name a typical differential diagnosis and distinguish the two clinical pictures from each other.**
The soft swelling on the head, high parietal right, could be a **caput succedaneum** (birth swelling) that often occurs after a protracted birth. It arises at the leading point of the child's head as a result of pressure and congestion of blood and lymph vessels. An important

differential diagnosis is **cephalhematoma** (head blood swelling). The tangential forces acting on the head during birth cause a shearing off of periosteum from the bone. Small vessels are torn, causing subperiostal bleeding. Sometimes there is an associated skull fracture. Especially where there are coagulation disorders, the hematoma can result in copious blood loss with anemia or hyperbilirubinemia requiring treatment.

Swelling	Caput succedaneum	Cephalhematoma
Consistency	soft, doughy-edematous, not fluctuating	firmly elastic, fluctuating
Location	between the galea aponeurotica and the skull cap (subcutaneous)	usually parietal, subperiostal bleeding
Limited to skull seams	no	yes
Prognosis	no treatment, regression within a few days	usually no treatment, regression within a few days to weeks, calcification is possible, children often develop hyperbilirubinemia (breakdown of hematoma → hemoglobin ↑ → breakdown in liver → liver "over-challenged" because of immaturity → bilirubin ↑); regular bilirubin check and if necessary, phototherapy

The caput succedaneum is distinguished from the cephalhematoma clinically and sonographically (see Tab. Fig. caput succedaneum and cephalhematoma).

20.2 **What is the most probable cause of the position of this newborn's arm?**
The newborn's arm position is most probably caused by an **upper plexus paralysis** (Erb–Duchenne). This is caused by a birth trauma to the nerve fibers of segments C5 and C6 with paralysis of the corresponding muscles as well as sensory and sweat-secretion damage of the affected region. The strength and sensory function of the hand are not impaired. It is typical of upper plexus paralysis that the arm hangs by the body limp, adduced, pronated, and internally rotated ("Waiter's hand"). These symptoms are particularly noticeable when the Moro reflexes and the intrinsic muscle reflexes of the arm (biceps tendon reflex and radius-periosteum reflex) are being tested. These cannot be elicited. If the phrenic nerve is also affected (this is rare), the diaphragm is paralyzed with dyspnea.

20.3 **List additional birth injuries.**
Clavicular fracture, lower plexus paralysis (Klumpke's palsy), facialis paralysis, torticollis (wry neck), epiphysiolysis, and/or diaphyseal fracture of the humerus, very

rarely injury of the internal organs (for instance, adrenal gland hemorrhage, liver capsule, or spleen rupture)

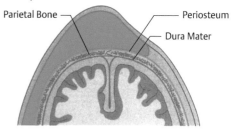

a Caput Succedaneum

Parietal Bone — Periosteum

Dura Mater

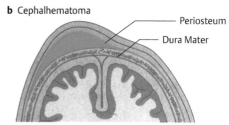

b Cephalhematoma

Periosteum

Dura Mater

Caput succedaneum and cephalhematoma

Comments

General: Birth injuries are observed after (traumatizing surgical) delivery in both protracted and normal deliveries. The most important ones are presented below.

Caput succedaneum (birth swelling): See answer to question 20.1.

Cephalhematoma (blood swelling of the head): See answer to question 20.1.

124

Case

20

Damage to the brachial plexus: These can be caused by pulling on the arm or the head. Depending on which segments are affected, a distinction is made between an upper and a lower plexus paralysis.

For **upper plexus paralysis** (Erb–Duchenne paralysis), see answer to question 20.2.

The less frequent **lower plexus paralysis** (Klumpke's palsy) affects segments **C7**, **C8**, and **Th1**. Paralysis of the hand and finger muscles (the so-called Trousseau sign) is characteristic. If the sympathetic fibers of the Th1 segment are affected, an ipsilateral Horner syndrome appears (miosis, ptosis, enophthalmus). **Treatment of the plexus paralysis** consists of positioning arm and hand in the middle position to avoid excessive stretching of the muscle and joint capsule, as well as physio- and motion therapy (start after 2–3 weeks). Most cases can be well treated with this method. If the paralysis persists longer than 3 to 6 months (very rare), the nerve plexus must be reconstructed with neurosurgical techniques.

Clavicle fracture: Clavicle fracture is a birth injury because in development of the shoulder, even in a normal birth, strong forces are acting on the clavicle. The injury occurs chiefly in macrosomal children. In newborns, there is a protective position of the arm on the affected side; the Moro reflex is lacking or weakened. Palpation of the clavicle is painful; sometimes a crepitation or a step can be felt. However, the fracture is often only recognized after 2 to 3 weeks due to callus formation with thickening. The prognosis is good; usually no special treatment is needed.

Torticollis: Torticollis (wry neck) is caused by an injury of the sternocleidomastoid muscle during birth, with hematoma formation. Healing of this hematoma leads to a scarred shortening of the muscle. The head is tipped to the injured side and turned to the healthy side. A therapy with physical therapy and corrective positioning is indicated. Surgical correction is only rarely necessary.

Facial nerve palsy and asymmetrical screaming face: Facial nerve palsy is the most frequent birth injury of peripheral nerves. It is caused by compression of the facial nerve, for instance, by the mother's promontorium or the forceps in a forceps birth, and is characterized by a lack of lid closure and a missing nasolabial fold on the affected side as well as a pulling of the mouth (for instance, when screaming) toward the healthy side. With incomplete eyelid closure, the eye must be protected from drying out with salves (for instance, dexpanthenol salve) or eye drops. The prognosis is good; in 90% of cases, symptoms regress in a few days or weeks.

In paralysis of the facial nerve, differential diagnosis must consider the benign "asymmetrical screaming face" which is caused not by a paralysis but by a unilateral aplasia of the depressor anguli oris. The differentiation is clinical, by observing the child while it is screaming and at rest. In facial nerve paresis, the paralysis is also present when the child is not screaming and the eyelid is not completely closed. In the "asymmetrical screaming face" the eyelid closure is unremarkable, and the nasolabial fold during screaming does not disappear (see Fig. "Asymmetrical screaming face").

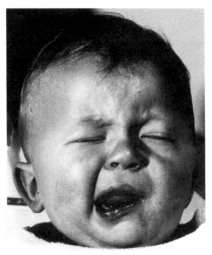

"Asymmetrical screaming face" (At rest, normal appearance. While the child is screaming or crying, the right corner of the mouth is pulled down and the relevant half of the lower lip is turned outward. The nasolabial fold on the side that is not distorted is clearly emphasized. This is not a facial nerve palsy. The cause is a missing M. depressor anguli oris left.)

👪 ADDITIONAL TOPICS FOR STUDY GROUPS
- Normal and pathological development birth process
- Newborn reflexes

21.1 What is your suspected diagnosis?

Acute sinusitis; rationale: rhinitis, cough, secondary high fever, intense frontal headache, worse when bending forward

21.2 What additional symptoms found on physical examination would confirm your suspected diagnosis?

- Impaired nasal breathing
- Purulent or bloody nasal secretion
- Postnasal drip at the rear wall of the throat
- Headache over the frontal and/or maxillary sinus
- Painful nerve exits (supraorbital, infraorbital nerves)
- Possibly lymph node swelling in the jaw angle and jugular
- Possibly swollen cheeks and bridge of the nose
- Lower lid edema

21.3 List the most frequent causes of this disease.

Often the sinusitis is accompanying a viral rhinitis. The pathogen of bacterial superinfection is chiefly Pneumococcus, *Haemophilus influenzae*, or *Moraxella catarrhalis*.

21.4 What do you do next?

- Antibiotic treatment (for instance, amoxicillin or cephalosporins)
- Muco- and secretolysis, with drugs (ambroxol), with adequate liquid consumption, inhalation, infrared therapy, humidifier
- Decongestant nose drops (3 × daily) oxymetazolin 0.025% or 0.05% improve air flow and elimination of secretions, but not longer than 7 days because of rebound effect with mucosal edema
- Antipyretics/analgesics (paracetamol, ibuprofen)

126

Case 21

Comments

Definition and epidemiology: Sinusitis is an inflammatory reaction of the mucosa in the paranasal sinuses (paranasal sinuses [ethmoidal cells, maxillary sinus, frontal sinus, sphenoid sinus]) to infectious, allergic, or toxic irritants. A sinusitis lasting more than 3 months is called chronic sinusitis. Even younger children can contract acute sinusitis.

Etiopathogenesis: Inflammation of the ethmoid cells (ethmoid labyrinth) is already possible in infants since these paranasal sinuses are pneumatized from birth. The maxillary sinuses are formed at approximately the age of 3 years (inflammation of the maxillary sinuses from the age of 3 years), the sphenoidal sinuses at approximately the age of 6 years (sphenoidal sinus inflammation from the age of 6 years), and the frontal sinuses around the age of 8 years (frontal sinus inflammation from the age of 8 years). Usually, in cases of viral rhinitis, there is an accompanying inflammation of the sinus mucosa. Impaired aeration of the sinuses and backup of secretions due to impaired outflow (adenoids) prepare the way for bacterial superinfection that then, as in the reported case, lead to fever and worsening of the general condition. Typical bacteria participating in acute sinusitis are *Pneumococci*, *Haemophilus influenzae*, and *Moraxella catarrhalis*. In chronic sinusitis, the most frequently found pathogen is *Staphylococcus aureus*, but *Streptococci* and anaerobes can also be involved.

In relapsing sinusitis, hypertrophic adenoids and allergies should be considered, as well as ostia displaced by foreign bodies. Immune deficiency and cystic fibrosis are additional important but rare causes.

Clinical aspects and complications: See answers to questions 21.1 and 21.2. There are catarrhal symptoms such **as cough, cold, and sore throat**, but also **intense (head-) aches** and **fever**.

Complications arise from intracranial transmission of the inflammation. Rare, but dreaded, are orbital phlegmones, frontal bone osteomyelitis, meningitis, and cavernous sinus thrombosis.

Relapsing sinusitis can also lead to sinobronchial syndrome in childhood and thus be the cause of chronic bronchitis and bronchiectasis.

Diagnosis: The diagnosis is usually established **clinically**. Collections of secretion in the frontal and maxillary sinuses can easily be seen sonographically. Thus an X-ray can usually be avoided.

Therapy and prognosis: See answer to question 21.4. The rate of spontaneous healing of acute sinusitis is high. However, intense bacterial colonization, recognizable by purulent rhinitis, fever, and lymph node enlargement after a catarrhal onset, requires antibiotic treatment with amoxicillin (50–100 mg/kg body weight in 3–4 divided doses) or cephalosporins (cefpodoxime 5–12 mg/kg body weight in two divided doses) over a period of 7 days.

ADDITIONAL TOPICS FOR STUDY GROUPS
- Adenoids
- Cystic fibrosis
- Anatomy of the facial bones

22.1 **What is your suspected diagnosis? What are the grounds for this? Describe typical symptoms, incubation period, and treatment of the disease.**
- **Suspected diagnosis: Scarlet fever**; rationale: onset with sudden high fever; sore throat, small-spotted, slightly raised, pale red rash, especially in the inguinal folds and inner thighs, with no rash around the mouth; red oral mucosa and tonsils.
- **Symptoms:**
    - Prodromal stage: high fever, sore throat, tonsillo-pharyngitis, impaired general condition
    - After 2 to 3 days: maculopapulous rash (beginning in the groin, no rash around mouth), enanthem, "raspberry tongue," submandibular lymph node swelling
    - After 1 to 3 weeks: lamellar skin flaking on palms and soles
- **Incubation time:** 2 to 5 days
- **Treatment:** Antibiotics
    - Medication of choice Penicillin V (50,000 IU/kg body weight/d in 2–3 divided doses for 7 days; in case of vomiting or difficulty swallowing, penicillin G i.v.
    - In case of penicillin allergy: Macrolide, such as erythromycin (50 mg/kg body weight) for 7 days or cephalosporins of second (for instance, cefuroxime 30–100 mg/kg body weight/d) and third (for instance, cefpodoxime 8 mg/kg body weight/d) generations over a period of 5 to 7 days (*Caution:* Cross-allergies)

22.2 **The aunt suspects "measles." What are the characteristic symptoms of measles?**
Typical 2-phase (febrile) course:
- *Prodromal stage (2 days):* catarrhal symptoms such as conjunctivitis, cold, sore throat; enanthem on gums and Koplik spots (like grains of salt on a wet background) on the buccal mucosa; fever

- *After 3 to 4 days:* fever elevated again with outbreak of rash (maculopapulous, onset behind ears and in the face); rash pales again after 7 days

22.3 **Why can the disease not be mumps? Name the most important symptoms, incubation period, and treatment of mumps.**
- Mumps is not an **exanthemic children's disease**.
- **Symptoms:** Subfebrile temperatures, usually (painful) swelling of the parotid gland on one or both sides, possibly with involvement of pancreas, testicles, ovaries, CNS, no sore throat
- Incubation time: 12 to 25 days
- **Treatment:** No causal treatment is known. Symptomatic analgesics/antipyretics (for instance, paracetamol), possibly warm or cold compresses for pain relief, pureed diet, oral hygiene

22.4 **An additional children's disease is whooping cough. What are the clinical symptoms of whooping cough? How long is the incubation time? How would you proceed with treatment?**
- **Symptoms:** Three-stage course
    - Catarrhal or incremental stage (lasts 1–2 weeks): flu-like symptoms such as cough, cold, slight fever
    - Paroxysmal stage (lasts 4–6 weeks): typical attacks of staccato coughing, especially at night, inspiratory whooping, cyanosis, expectoration and vomiting of tough, colorless slime, frequently subconjunctival hemorrhages; in newborns, instead of coughing, menacing apnea attacks with risk of sudden death
    - *Decremental stage:* Fading away of symptoms (duration, untreated 6–10 weeks)
- **Incubation time:** 7 to 14 (20) days
- **Treatment:** Erythromycin p.o. (50–60 mg/kg body weight for 14 days); shortens duration of the illness only in the prodromal stage; in all stages interrupts contagiosity; antitussives are ineffectual

127

Case

22

Childhood diseases: Childhood diseases are contagious diseases that produce long-lasting immunity and that most people have already had as children. The typical exanthemic childhood diseases include varicella, measles, rubella, scarlet fever, fifth disease (infectious exanthema), and roseola (exanthema subitum). Mumps and pertussis are typical non-exanthemic childhood diseases. For an overview table, see appendix.

Note: Parents should be informed about the following points if their child is sick with a childhood disease:
- Danger of contagion (for how long)

- Taking of prescribed medications (how? when?)
- Attending kindergarten/school or other facility for children possible or when is it possible again?
- Contact with siblings
- Danger of contact for a pregnant person
- Possibility of immunization (for instance, mumps, measles, rubella, pertussis)
- Possible complications/problems (for instance, dehydration with high fever), so that the parents can consult a doctor in case of the corresponding symptoms

Scarlet fever: See answer to question 22.1. The clinical picture described in the example case best corresponds to scarlet fever. The pathogens are various exotoxin-forming β-hemolyzing group A *Streptococci*. It is always possible to create immunity to a single toxin, so that infections with other exotoxin-forming *Streptococci* can lead to a repeated scarlet fever infection. The disease is spread by droplet transmission; contagiosity is very high. The disease usually begins with a purulent angina tonsillaris, but wound infections are possible as the origin of scarlet fever (so-called wound scarlet fever). The rash is also described as "sand paper-like" since it feels like fine sandpaper when it is brushed with the hand.

Scarlet fever is a diagnosis at a glance; a smear or a rapid test for *Streptococcus* is not absolutely necessary. Treatment is with penicillin or in case of penicillin allergy with macrolides or cephalosporins of the second or third generation. (*Caution:* Cross-allergies.) The disease is no longer contagious 24 hours after the start of antibiotic treatment. There is no inoculation against the disease.

Possible **secondary diseases** are rheumatic fever (see case 61), which occurs much less frequently in recent years, thanks to systematic antibiotic treatment, and acute poststreptococcal glomerulonephritis (see case 18).

Measles: See answer to question 22.2. Measles is caused by paramyxoviruses and characterized by a 2-phase disease course. The incubation time is 8 to 12 days. Measles is highly infectious. Infected persons are contagious for 3 to 5 days before onset of the rash and for 4 days afterwards. The patient is left with lifelong immunity. No causal treatment is known. Antibiotics are indicated in case of bacterial superinfection. Particularly dreaded are complications of the disease, such as otitis media (a frequent bacterial superinfection), measles pneumonia, laryngotracheitis with croup, and measles encephalitis. The last-mentioned disease has a high lethality (30%). A very rare late complication is subacute sclerosing panencephalitis (SSPE) that manifests some 6 to 8 years after the measles infection. It begins with psychological and intellectual changes and has a progressive course. Neurological disorders ranging up to loss of cerebral functions follow. The prognosis is unfavorable. It is possible to inoculate against measles.

Mumps: See answer to question 22.3. Mumps is a systemic infectious disease caused by the mumps virus (an RNA virus in the group of paramyxoviruses), usually with a benign course. The patient is left with lifelong immunity. The disease is spread by droplet transmission; contagiosity is very high. It is not associated with a rash but attacks the parotids and other salivary glands. An associated pancreatitis is often observed. Contagiosity begins 7 days before and ends 9 days after the parotid swelling. Complications are mumps meningitis (usually with a good prognosis) as well as ovarian or testicular inflammation. For this reason, especially in adolescence or adulthood, mumps is a dreaded disease since it can result in infertility. It is possible to inoculate against mumps.

Pertussis: See answer to question 22.4. Pertussis (Syn.: Whooping cough) is caused by the bacterium *Bordetella* pertussis. Especially young infants are endangered by the highly contagious disease, because at this stage, they do not have adequate immunity. The immunity borrowed from the mother (so-called passive immunity) after she has had pertussis, or has been previously inoculated against it, does not provide sufficient protection to an infant infected with pertussis. Consequently, it is recommended for women to receive the Tdap vaccine (Tetanus–diphtheria–acellular pertussis vaccine) in the third trimester, even if they have previously received Tdap vaccine in order to protect the newborn against pertussis during the first weeks after birth.

Because of the particular danger of apnea, infants with pertussis, or suspicion of pertussis, should always be admitted to a hospital for surveillance with a breathing monitor. Persons with the disease are infectious in all three stages, but most intensely in the catarrhal stage. Other frequent complications of whooping cough are pneumonia and otitis media, through secondary infection with *Haemophilus influenzae* or *Pneumococci*. Cerebral seizures and hypoxic encephalopathy are described as very rare complications. Patients recover from the disease with long-lasting but not lifelong immunity, so that adults can contract the disease again. Inoculation is possible. Because of the severity of whooping cough in infants, the CDC recommends checking the pertussis immunization status of the family and updating it if necessary.

👪 ADDITIONAL TOPICS FOR STUDY GROUPS
- Further typical infectious childhood diseases (for instance, rubella, varicella, fifth disease)
- Krupp syndrome
- Immunization (see case 35)

23.1 What is your diagnosis? What are the grounds for your decision?

Grade I traumatic brain injury or cerebral concussion (Syn.: Mild traumatic brain injury); rationale: short period of unconsciousness, relapsing vomiting, retrograde amnesia, normal neurological examination

23.2 What further measures do you undertake?

■ If necessary Skull X-ray: see Comments

■ Care of the laceration
■ In-patient observation for 24 to 48 hours depending on the symptoms, monitoring of blood pressure, pulse, pupillary reaction, respiration
■ Reassure parents: No reproaches! No blanket assignment of blame. Point out the frequency of this kind of event. Good chance of recovery

23.3 List possible complications.

Traumatic cerebral bleeding, cerebral edema

Comments

Definition and clinical aspects: Cerebral concussion denotes an acute neuronal functional disruption of the brain caused by a mechanical trauma. It is characterized by a brief (< 1 hour), acute disruption of vigilance, retro- and/or anterograde amnesia, headache, nausea, and vomiting, as well as other associated vegetative symptoms, such as transitory psychomotor restlessness but no neurological loss.

Diagnosis: In the physical examination—with particular attention to neurological losses and vital signs—fractures, spinal, thoracic, and soft tissue injuries must be ruled out. In the differential diagnosis, the possibility of child abuse must always be kept in mind (see case 75).

Recent flow of secretion from the nose can be a symptom of a CSF fistula in fracture of the base of the skull that can manifest clinically as a "simple" cerebral concussion. To differentiate between CSF and nasal secretion, the glucose content in the secretion is determined with a test strip. The glucose test is positive for CSF and negative for nasal secretion.

An X-ray of the skull is not vitally necessary; however, in strong suspicion of skull fracture it can be helpful. The indication criteria for an X-ray must be strict, in order to avoid an unnecessary radiation load for the child. In suspicion of cerebral bleeding or pressure on the brain, a CT scan should be performed. EEG examinations are not vitally necessary, but they are a good method for monitoring progress without subjecting the child to a radiation load. Neurological function disruptions can appear in the EEG as unspecific dysrhythmias.

Treatment and prognosis: All children with cerebral concussions must be admitted to the hospital. If parents do not understand this, one must explain that at home, in the absence of adequate monitoring and treatment that might be necessary, the outcome could be lethal. One should also document that this has been done.

Circulatory function and pupillary reaction should be constantly monitored for at least 24 hours, for prompt recognition of cerebral pressure symptoms. Even after 24 hours, bleeding can set in on the following days. The parents should be informed that if their child's behavior changes or other abnormalities are noted, they should immediately consult their pediatrician or the emergency service. No special treatment is required for uncomplicated cerebral concussion; healing takes place without sequelae.

👫👤 ADDITIONAL TOPICS FOR STUDY GROUPS
 ■ Cerebral contusion and compression
 ■ Skull fractures
 ■ Intracranial hemorrhage
 ■ Glasgow-Coma-Scale
 ■ Neurological examination (reflexes, motor function, paralysis, tone, sensory perception, cerebral nerves, meningism)

129

Case

23

24 Urosepsis/Urinary tract infection

24.1 Give the grounds for your decision to admit the child. What do you suspect?

■ Clinical aspects (high fever, circulatory centralization, sensitivity to touch) and diagnostics (CRP ↑

sedimentation rate, ↑) suggest **sepsis** (for instance, meningitis, urosepsis) → indication for admission.
■ **Suspected diagnosis: Urosepsis**; rationale: severely ill infant with high fever, sucking weakness,

→ Cases 24 Page 25

relapsing vomiting, inflammation parameters/urea/creatinine elevated, leukocyturia, proteinuria, erythrocyturia, nitrite detected in urine, leukocyte casts in urine sediment (see Fig. example case).

24.2 **How do you confirm the diagnosis?**
- **Confirm urinary tract infection:** see Comments
- **Urine culture, blood culture:** Determination of pathogen, antibiogram
- **Lumbar puncture:** to rule out the differential diagnosis of meningitis (poor general condition, sensitivity to touch, vomiting); *Note:* in infants, broad indication in fever of unknown origin
- **Sonography of the kidneys:** Congestion in the renal pelvis, rule out malformations

24.3 **List the most frequent causes of this disease.**
- *Escherichia coli* (80%)
- *Proteus* species (10%) *Enterococci, Klebsiella, Pseudomonas*, fungi, etc.

24.4 **What treatment do you initiate? Are any additional measures required?**
- **Treatment:** Antibiotics for 10 to 14 days (initial i.v. administration; if inflammation parameters decrease, possible change to oral from the seventh day), for instance, ampicillin + gentamicin or ceftazidime + gentamicin
- **Other measures:** Analgesics/antipyretics (for instance, paracetamol), increased fluids, search for congenital malformations of the urinary tract in the free interval (see Comments)

Comments

Definition: A urinary tract infection is characterized by colonization or invasion of the urinary tract and kidneys by bacteria and subsequent significant bacteriuria. This results in local or generalized signs of inflammation (for instance, leukocyturia, fever). In urosepsis, the septic event proceeds from the urinary passages.

Epidemiology: Urinary tract infection is one of the most frequent bacterial infections in children. Approximately 3% of all girls and 1% of all boys have such an infection at least once. Girls are more frequently affected than boys because of the short urethra.

Etiopathogenesis: For pathogens, see answer to question 24.3. In infants, the infection is predominantly hematogenous; later it is an ascending infection over the urethra and bladder. In every child with a confirmed febrile urinary tract infection, especially if the child is younger than 1 year, it is necessary to look for malformations of the urinary tract (obstructions/outflow impediments, vesicoureteral reflux, etc.) as the cause of the infection.

Clinical aspects and diagnostics: The fever of unknown origin of the infant described in the case, as well as his poor general condition, high inflammation parameter values, and abnormal urine findings raise a high suspicion of urosepsis.

However, the urine findings should be cautiously evaluated because the tests were conducted on urine collected in a bag. Bag urine has a high rate of contamination with germs occurring everywhere in the environment and is therefore not suitable for establishing a diagnosis. A pathological finding on fresh urine with little or no contamination confirms the diagnosis. Ideally it is collected from the midstream, or even better, by means of bladder catheterization or puncture.

The latter method should always be used for infants. More than 10^4/mL organisms in the midstream, 10^3/mL organisms in catheter urine and any organisms in bladder puncture urine confirm the infection. Other definitely pathological values are the detection in the urine of leukocytes > 50/µL, erythrocytes (> 20/µL in bladder puncture urine because of puncture trauma), nitrite (bacterial metabolic product), and protein (participation of kidney parenchyma).

Various malformations and urine transport disruptions should be ruled out sonographically (see etiopathogenesis). Micturating cystourethrography (MCU) is used to rule out vesicoureteral reflux. This examination is only useful after healing of the urinary tract infection and with antibiotic prophylaxis because otherwise, the finding can be distorted by functional disorders due to infection. Other examinations, such as renal scintigraphy, i.v. pyelography, can be conducted, depending on the finding.

Treatment: See answer to question 24.4. If abnormalities are found in the urinary tract, thought must be given to long-term antibiotic prophylaxis and/or surgical correction of the malformation.

Prognosis: Usually the disease heals well with promptly started, adequate treatment. Where there are malformations of the urinary tract, there is a high risk of relapsing urinary tract infections. Delayed renal growth or parenchymal scars can be observed after relapsing pyelonephritis in 5% of cases. These can lead to limited kidney function and arterial hypertension.

ADDITIONAL TOPICS FOR STUDY GROUPS
- Malformations of the urinary tract
- Pyelonephritis

→ Cases 24 Page 25

25.1 **What should the mother have done imme-diately? What are the first aid measures?**
- **First aid** (at the accident site, this is what the mother should have done at once): Remove the child from the source of heat. Remove clothing only if it is not stuck to the burned area; in that case, cut around the clothing leaving the burn intact. Cool the burned area with cool water for no more than 30 minutes or until the pain is reduced or alleviated without inducing hypothermia. Cooling also reduces the risk of shock, if applied up to 45 minutes after heat exposure. In the case of young children, infants, and newborns, with burns extending over more than 15% of the body surface, cooling treatment should be waived altogether, as the resulting hypothermia will have a negative effect on the prognosis.
- Analgesia, for instance, with paracetamol supp., ibuprofen.
- If there are wounds, cover them with the best sterile materials possible, for instance, with metalline sterile compress, sterile sponges from the automobile/home first aid kit.
- Call emergency doctor/go to pediatric clinic.

25.2 **Determine the extent of the burns this child has suffered. Why is it important to determine the extent?**
- Rule of Nines: Gives an approximate idea of the extent of the burns (see Fig.)
  - **Children/Youths > 9 years of age:** Head 9%, trunk 4 × 9%, upper extremity 9%, lower extremity 2 × 9%
  - **Children < 9 years of age:** Per birth year, add 1% to head and subtract 0.5% from the legs
- **Hand surface rule:** The patient's hand surface, incl. fingers, corresponds to 1% of the body surface area (BSA)
- This means that in the 2-year-old girl, the burns encompass: Left arm 9% + left half of thorax 9% + 1% of the thigh = 19% of the BSA
- Determination of the extent of burns is important for:
  - Decision about in-patient treatment and/or transfer to a special burn hospital
  - Further treatment planning (for instance, infusion plan)
  - Estimation of possible complications, such as danger of shock due to fluid shift from intra- to extracellular because of increased capillary permeability, starting at burns on 10% of BSA

131

Case

25

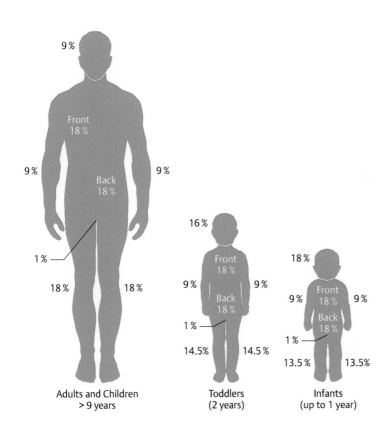

| Adults and Children > 9 years | Toddlers (2 years) | Infants (up to 1 year) |

Rule of Nines according to Wallace (modified for children)

→ Cases 25 Page 26

- For first measures, see answer to question 25.1
- **Pain therapy**, for instance, pethidine (1–2 mg/kg body weight, s.c. or i.v.)
- **Stabilization of circulation with** 0.9% NaCl solution (10–20 mL/kg body weight for 1 hour, if necessary, repeat)
- **Hospital admission** (always from burns > 15% of BSA) for fluid replacement, prevention of infection, monitoring the status of consciousness/circulatory parameters
- **Infusion therapy** to compensate for losses and stabilize circulation, according to the following schedule:
  - In addition to maintenance requirement (for calculation, see case 4)
  - In the **first 24 hours**: 4 mL × kg body weight× % burned BSA, 50% in the first 8 hours, 50% in the following 16 hours, after start of diuresis add potassium (1–2 mmol/kg body weight/d) (electrolyte control)
  - **On the second day**: 3 mL × kg body weight× % burned BSA
  - *Caution:* Infusion amount must be adjusted to diuresis, blood pressure, central nervous pressure. Oliguria generally means a lack of fluid. Avoid over-infusion
- **Wound care:** Clean with sterile saline and remove necrotic tissue, if necessary under short-term anesthesia; depending on extent of the burns
  - First-degree burns require treatment with lotions and ointments; first-degree burns are usually not bandaged.
    - Second-degree burns require disinfecting wound management systems such as Suprasorb, bandaging, antibiotic ointments, and daily cleaning of the wound to remove dead skin or ointment.
  - Grade III burns (see question 25.4): Treatment will most likely include most of the following, namely, cleaning and debriding, IV fluids and/or antibiotics, pain medications, tetanus shot, synthetic or biological skin grafting.
- **Check tetanus protection status**! If protection lacking, simultaneous vaccination
- **Reassure parents:** No blanket assignment of blame! Point out the frequency of this kind of event; emphasize good chance of recovery, for instance, when dressings are changed show the parents the progress that has been made or even include them in the wound care. Active participation in recovery can often compensate for feelings of guilt.

25.4 What degrees of burn severity do you know?

- **Grade I:** Redness, mild swelling, painful, no blisters, affects only the epidermis
- **Grade II:** Deep redness, may be white in an irregular pattern, may appear shiny and wet, swelling, painful, surface blistering, affects epidermis and part of the dermis layer
- **Grade III:** White or charred, black, brown, or yellow, swelling, necrosis of epidermis and entire layer beneath the dermis, lack of pain sensation due to destruction of nerve endings
- **Grade IV:** Damage extends to underlying bones, muscles, and tendons, lack of pain sensation due to destruction of nerve endings

Comments

Definition: Burns involve thermal damage of the skin caused either by the direct effect of heat or by contact with hot liquids (scalding), heated objects (contact burn), chemicals (chemical burn), electric current (electric burn), or radiation.

Classification: The severity of the damage and thus the effect on the whole body is determined by the depth (degree of severity) and the surface extent (Rule of Nines or modified form according to Wallace) (see answers to questions 25.2 and 25.4).

Etiopathogenesis and clinical aspects: Burns and scalding are among the most frequent childhood accidents. Scalding (80%) usually occur when the child pulls down vessels containing hot liquids (see case) or fall into hot liquids. But touching hot objects, such as a stove burner or iron, or flame burns (playing with fire, grills) is often what causes the accident.

The possibility of child abuse must always be kept in mind!

In children, a grade II burn or a burn of 10% of the BSA is enough to trigger shock symptoms. Intense pain causes neurogenic shock, and loss of water, electrolytes, and protein (exudate, loss through edema formation when capillary permeability is increased, imperceptible perspiration, loss as urine) cause hypovolemic shock (burn shock). Complications that can be expected are respiratory failure due to formation of pulmonary edema (ARDS), renal failure due to prolonged hypovolemia, hepatic dysfunction, ulcer formation (stress ulcers), and paralytic ileus. In case of larger skin defects the infection risk is elevated because the natural barrier is lacking; wound healing can be impaired by bacterial superinfection. From grade IIb burns and up, there is scar formation, and in children there is a particular tendency to cheloid formation.

Diagnosis: The diagnosis is established on the basis of the medical history and the clinical examination. Often the entire extent of the burn cannot be clearly determined because there can be so-called after-burning. In this process the tissue slowly releases the stored heat and this leads to further damage.

Treatment: See answers to questions 25.1 and 25.3.

Small superficial scalding/burns can be treated on an outpatient basis.

Patients should be admitted to the hospital for grade I burns of more than 15% of the body surface, grade II burns/scalds of more than 5%, especially if the face, hands, feet, genitals, and joints, and all grade III burns. Depending on the extent and severity of the burns, a decision must be made as to whether transfer of the patient to a burn center is indicated. The indication should be broadly established, especially for children. There are currently 139 self-designated burn centers in the United States; 70 of these have been designated burn centers by the American Burn Association and the American College of Surgeons.

For head and neck burns, associated inhalation trauma with formation of laryngeal edema requiring intubation must be expected.

Because of the high risk of infection, wound care should be performed under the most sterile conditions possible. If wounds are not infected, antibiotic prophylaxis is not necessary, but in the presence of infection, targeted (after antibiogram) antibiotic treatment is required.

Scar formation can be avoided by means of compression, for instance, with compression garments that must be worn constantly for 1–2 years, daily massage with moisturizing creams or oils, and protection against sunlight. Active physiotherapy is indicated for prevention of contractures; corrective surgery may become necessary.

Prophylaxis: Most accidents occur at home, so the best preventive measure is comprehensive parent education regarding avoidance of burn/scalding injuries.

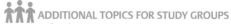 ADDITIONAL TOPICS FOR STUDY GROUPS
- Shock
- Heat exhaustion/Heat stroke
- Overcooling and frostbite

26   Oxyuriasis

26.1   What is your suspected diagnosis?
Oxyuriasis; rationale: child's age, abdominal pain, itching with traces of anal scratching, disturbed sleep (visiting emergency department during the night), no other pathological findings

26.2   How do you confirm the diagnosis?
Microscopic confirmation of eggs laid in the anal region with the sticky tape method (pasting a strip of transparent tape on the skin in the anal region [ideally not until the child is asleep], remove the tape and paste it to a slide (see Fig.); for diagnosis (and later to monitor treatment), tape preparation from **three successive days** are needed, since the females do not lay eggs every day.
In strong infestations, living pinworms, which can be seen as moving threads on the surface of stools, are often excreted.

26.3   Explain the path of infection to the parents.
Oxyuriasis is often contracted by fecal–oral **autoinfection**. This means that the females wander to the anal region at night and lay their eggs there. This leads to itching. By scratching in the anal region, the eggs are transferred to the fingers, from where they are taken up into the mouth and return to the intestine. The eggs can also adhere to the pajamas, underwear, or bed linens and be inhaled.

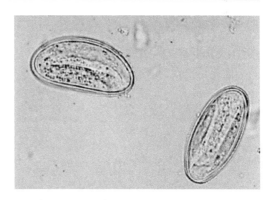

Eggs of Oxyuris vermicularis

26.4   What treatment do you initiate?
- Interrupt the infectious pathway by **hygienic measures** (wash hands, cut fingernails short, change linens, and boil them)
- **Medicamentous treatment**, for instance, with pyrantel embonate, one-time administration of 10 mg/ kg body weight, repeat after 14 days, since the drugs are only efficacious against the adult worms, and not against larvae and eggs
- Concomitant treatment of family members to prevent re-infection, since other family members are often infected through smear and dust infection (asymptomatic infections are also possible)

→ Cases 26 Page 27

Definition and epidemiology: Oxyuriasis (Syn.: Enterobiasis) is an intestinal infection with *Oxyuris vermicularis* (pinworm). It is the most common worm infection in the United States and affects primarily kindergarten- and school-age children.

Etiology: *Oxyuris vermicularis* is a small, maggot-like threadworm that belongs to the class of nematodes. Human beings are the only host. The worm lives in the lower small intestine, colon, and the vermiform appendix. It grows to about 12 mm in length. The female lays 10,000 eggs in its lifetime of an average of 40 to 90 days. For the path of infection, see answer to question 26.3.

Clinical aspects: The symptoms are chiefly nighttime itching and the resulting disrupted sleep. Children often complain of abdominal pain. Superinfection of the excoriations and vulvovaginitis by worm immigration into the female genital tract is possible. Presumably appendicitis can be caused by Oxyuridae, since Oxyuridae are found in excised appendices fairly often.

Diagnostics: The diagnosis is established **clinically**. Often the pinworms can be seen macroscopically when the anus is spread open. In suspicion of oxyuriasis, the presence of eggs can often be confirmed by means of cellotape (see answer to question 26.2; Fig.). When the stool is examined, worms or eggs are only seen by chance.

Treatment: See answer to question 26.4. In re-infection, a therapy attempt with mebendazole (1 × 100 mg/week) for 8 weeks is recommended. A face mask should be worn when working with contaminated linens to avoid the inhalation of worms.

Prognosis: The prognosis is good and the disease is easily treatable. Re-infection is possible.

 ADDITIONAL TOPICS FOR STUDY GROUPS
- Ascaridiasis
- Tapeworms
- Acute appendicitis

134

Case

27

27   Anorexia nervosa

27.1   What is your suspected diagnosis?

Anorexia nervosa; rationale: patient's age, extreme, voluntary weight loss, excessive physical activity, suspicion of self-induced vomiting, social withdrawal, body image disorder (distorted perception of body: at 40 kg, still thinks she is too fat), conspicuous eating behavior

27.2   List the most important diagnostic criteria.

- Body weight at least 15% below the norm (Body mass Index [BMI body weight in kg/height in m²] < 17.5)
- Caused the weight loss herself
- Disturbed body image (afraid of "getting fat," although she is underweight)
- Endocrine disorder along the hypothalamic–hypophyseal–gonadal axis (the extreme weight loss and resulting underweight cause a shift of releasing hormones of the hypothalamus, the hormones of the hypophysis, or the hormones that act on the end organs, especially the gonads; the results are amenorrhea and hair loss). If the disease begins before puberty, delayed or lacking sequence of pubertal developmental steps

27.3   List causes of this disease.

The causes of eating disorders like anorexia nervosa are multifactorial. A role is played by:
- **biological factors:** Physical changes at the start of puberty; vulnerability of the serotonergic system
- **sociocultural causes:** For instance, the ideal disseminated throughout Western countries of thinness, and consumer and achievement orientation
- **individual factors:** Typical personal characteristics (depressive alienation, orientation toward achievement, ambition, anxiety and compulsion disorders, tenacity to the point of rigidity, introversion, need for harmony, good intelligence), disturbed search for identity, authority, and autonomy conflicts, psychosexual development, and role finding disorder
- **genetic factors:** Familial predisposition

27.4   What do you do next?

- **Physical examination:** Typical examination findings are restless patient, little or no subcutaneous fat tissue, cool extremities, signs of dehydration (dry, coated tongue, dry mucosa, skin turgor ↓), bad breath (acetone is a sign of hunger metabolism), dry, scaly skin, blotchy skin, acrocyanosis, lanugo, brittle/dull hair, hair loss, short stature, possibly delayed development of puberty, body temperature between 36°C and 37°C, bradycardia, hypotension, decreased capacity.

- **Hospital admission:** Search for somatic complications or elimination of organic / psychiatric diseases that could have led to extreme weight loss:
  - Laboratory, abdominal sonography, blood pressure / heart rate checks, ECG
  - Consultation with a child or youth psychologist or psychiatrist: Decision about further procedure (outpatient treatment or referral to a facility for child or youth psychiatric facility). This depends on the general/nutritional condition and the patient's compliance; the patient can also be admitted against her will. In the present case, the parents, as entitled to custody, made the decision.
- Nutritional therapy and weight gain measures depend on the patient's compliance / general and nutritional condition
  - outpatient treatment or non-parenteral nutritional buildup: adequate amounts of a balanced, mixed diet
  - inpatient treatment/low compliance: administration of high-caloric nutrition via gastric tube, possibly in an induced coma, by means of a central venous catheter
- If necessary treat somatic complications, for instance, correction of the electrolyte and water balance
- **Behavioral therapy:** Written agreement regarding weight gain and target weight
- One-on-one psychotherapeutic conversations and family therapy
- Supplemental measures such as occupational and music therapy

Comments

Definition and epidemiology: Anorexia nervosa is a frequently occurring, severe eating disorder in children and youth. It is characterized by an extreme effort to be thin, in which underweight and danger to one's own weight are denied for a long time. It typically occurs between 12 and 25 years of age, with a peak age between 14 and 15 years of age (prevalence rate 0.3–1%). Girls are affected in 95% of cases, but boys are affected with increasing frequency.

Etiopathogenesis: See answer to question 27.3.

Clinical aspects: Onset of the disease is insidious. Because patients want to "watch their figure," they avoid high-calorie foods and limit themselves to a "healthy" diet. Typically, they also increase their physical activity. In some of the patients, the trigger is a (supposedly) negative remark about their body weight by someone in their social circle.

Intense concern about appearance, body weight, and calorie and fat content of food is characteristic of anorexia nervosa. "Weight phobia" leads to an extremely low desired weight and increasingly restrictive eating behavior, combined with weight-loss measures (e.g., appetite depressants, laxatives, diuretics, self-induced vomiting, and excessive physical activity).

Finally, food is only consumed to prove to others that the patient is eating ("look here, I am eating, even though you think I'm not." Most patients actually believe that they are eating enough. They know precisely how many calories there are in the food they have consumed, and they only drink water (usually without carbonation). But they can also have binge attacks. The extreme weight loss, going as far as cachexia, lead to primary or secondary amenorrhea, constipation, hair loss, hypothermia, changes in the blood picture (leukopenia, anemia),

hypoglycemia, hypotension, bradycardia, osteoporosis (sometimes life-threatening), electrolyte shifts, and ECG changes.

The patients' failure to understand that they are sick is typical. They suffer from an inaccurate body image with overestimation of their physical proportions.

Diagnostics: The **clinical picture** of anorexia nervosa is generally so **typical** that the diagnosis can be established without difficulty. In differential diagnosis, somatic and psychiatric diseases associated with weight loss should always be ruled out (e.g., neoplasms, diabetes mellitus, celiac disease, severe depression). For diagnostic criteria, see answer to question 27.2.

Treatment: The treatment of anorexia nervosa rests on three pillars: treatment of somatic complications, nutritional therapy, and psychotherapy. The decision as to whether the patient should be treated as an outpatient or inpatient depends on the extent of the symptoms and the patient's compliance. Weight loss of more than 25% of the original body weight or underweight with physical complications, frequent appearance of a voracious appetite, complete refusal to eat or drink, life-threatening physical or emotional changes (e.g., abnormal electrolyte levels, danger of suicide), progressive weight loss in spite of outpatient treatment, a gridlocked family situation, and social isolation are indications for hospital admission, usually long-term.

A prerequisite for successful psychotherapeutic work is attainment of an adequate body weight. For this reason, the most important part of treatment is weight normalization. Girls have achieved an adequate weight when menstruation reappears. It is recommended to set the 25th percentile of the Body mass-Index, in writing, as the target weight.

→ Cases 27 Page 28

A motivation during weight rehabilitation can be expansion of the range of activity, which had been restricted at the beginning of treatment. In the course of treatment, **normalization of eating behavior** should be achieved (e.g., balancing nutrients, a planned diet, addition of "forbidden" foods, regular meals). Adequate Vitamin D and calcium replacement is recommended as osteoporosis prophylaxis. Individual psychotherapy is provided as support, possibly also family therapy to overcome intrafamily conflicts. Supplementary occupational and music therapy are also added. So far, drug therapy of anorexia nervosa has not been successful.

Prognosis: In about half of patients, the eating disorder disappears completely, in 30% there is residual disease, and in 20%, the disease becomes chronic. Five percent of affected persons die as a result of anorexia nervosa.

 ADDITIONAL TOPICS FOR STUDY GROUPS
- Bulimia nervosa
- Obesity

28 Diabetic (embryo-) fetopathy

28.1 What clinical picture are you considering? Explain the pathogenesis of the child's clinical picture.
- **Suspected diagnosis: Diabetic Fetopathy**
- **Rationale:** Macrosomal newborn, hypoglycemia, hypocalcemia, incipient respiratory distress syndrome (tachypnea, expiratory sighing, acrocyanosis, BGA: respiratory acidosis)
- **Pathogenesis:** Mother's poorly managed diabetes mellitus during pregnancy with hyperglycemia that passes through the placenta to the fetus (fetal blood sugar is 70% of the mother's concentration). This leads to hyperplasia of the fetal pancreatic β cells with resulting hyperinsulinism. The insulin stimulates the fetal glycogen storage, fat and protein synthesis, and inhibits pulmonary surfactant formation. Postpartum, the hyperinsulinemia leads to hypoglycemia in the newborn, resulting in the clinical picture described above.

28.2 What symptoms can generally be expected in newborns with this clinical picture?
- Macrosomia, birth weight > 4,000 g with mechanical complications of birth (e.g., protracted course of parturition, arrested parturition, clavicular fracture, central obesity)
- Organomegaly with organ immaturity
- Tendency to hypokalemia; clinical aspects: hyperexcitability, tremors, sweating, sucking weakness, apnea, seizures, frequent but also asymptomatic
- Tendency to hypocalcemia, hypomagnesemia; clinical aspects: hyperexcitability, irritability, tremor, seizures, apnea, relapsing vomiting, tachycardia, tachypnea, tetany
- Frequent lack of surfactant with resulting respiratory distress syndrome
- Increased risk of deformity, e.g., heart (hypertrophic cardiomyopathy, hypertrophic subaortal stenosis, aortic isthmus stenosis, septal defects, etc.), CNS (neural tube defects, e.g., meningomyelocele), caudal regression syndrome (malformation complex with agenesis or hypoplastic lower extremities), gastrointestinal

tract (atresia, colon hypoplasia), urogenital tract (renal agenesis, ureteral duplications), situs inversus
- Polyglobulia (insulin leads to elevation of erythropoietin) with risk of renal vein thrombosis
- Severe, prolonged neonatal jaundice (see case 38): hemoglobin breakdown in polycythemia, hepatic immaturity

28.3 What measures do you undertake? As consultant, what do you recommend to your colleague in gynecology?
- **Therapeutic and diagnostic measures:**
  - Transfer of the child to a **neonatology unit** for intensive monitoring (pulse oximetry, monitoring)
  - Place child in incubator; if pulse oximetric oxygen saturation < 90% feed oxygen into the incubator; if oxygen requirement > 40% or hypercapnia, CPAP; if this treatment fails, intubation and ventilation (see case 55)
  - Pre-prandial blood sugar (BS) checks in the first 3 days of an infant's life (target BS value: > 45 mg/dL [2.5 mmol/L])
  - **Controlled (early) feeding** with 15% maltodextrin solution (5–10 mL/kg body weight every 3 hours); feed infant diet as early as possible; if the infant wants to breastfeed, offer the breast frequently; consider supplementary feeding until nursing is successful
  - BS ↓ in spite of controlled feeding: 10% glucose as continuous infusion (4 mL/kg body weight/h); if blood sugar < 25 mg/dL (1.4 mmol/L) or < 40 mg/dL) with symptoms, 10% glucose i.v. bolus (2.5 mL/kg body weight over a period of 10 minutes)
  - Calcium replacement in case of hypocalcemia (e.g., 10% calcium gluconate 2 mL/kg body weight every 8 hours oral; only with severe symptoms of calcium lack (clinical aspects: seizures, tetany, laryngospasm, tachycardia, apnea) 10% calcium gluconate 1–2 mL/kg body weight slowly i.v. with monitor control (*caution:* bradycardia, heart rhythm disturbance, asystole)

– Rule out childhood malformations (e.g., echo-cardiography, ECG, thoracic X-ray, abdominal sonography)

! 28.4 What prophylactic measures are recommended to women with Type 1 diabetes during pregnancy? What are the grounds for this?

- Early instruction to type 1 diabetics so that they can achieve good blood sugar values for planned pregnancies. The frequency of cardiac malformations and caudal regression syndrome as well as perinatal mortality depends significantly on the quality of the blood sugar adjustment.
- Intensive supervision of the pregnant woman by a diabetologist and a gynecologist experienced in diabetology.
- The goal is a **normoglycemic metabolism**:
  - **First trimester**: The insulin requirement falls (to approximately the 16th week of pregnancy)
  - In the **second and third trimester**: From the 16th week of pregnancy continual **increase of insulin requirement** (in the 28th to 32nd week of pregnancy, adjustment to the requirement before pregnancy) until 36th week of pregnancy, and then, insulin requirement is stable
- Prenatal care **every 2 weeks**, more frequent ultrasound examinations, Doppler sonography, regular CTG checks to diagnose fetal condition
- Broad indication for hospital admission in case of pregnancy complications (e.g., inclination to premature contractions because of elevated vulnerability to infection and over-expansion of the uterus in polyhydramnion; elevated risk of a hypertensive disease / (pre-) eclampsia; placental insufficiency because of diabetic microangiopathy)
- Delivery in a perinatal center
- No post-term pregnancy (placental insufficiency, macrosomy of the child)

Comments

Epidemiology: In approximately 0.3% of pregnancies, there was a type 1 diabetes mellitus before the pregnancy. Gestational diabetes develops in 1% to 5% of all pregnancies. For every subsequent pregnancy, there is a high chance (66%) of another gestational diabetes.

Etiopathogenesis: As a result of a poorly managed maternal diabetes mellitus during pregnancy, the clinical picture of diabetic (embryonic) fetopathy (see answer to question 28.1).

Clinical aspects: See answer to question 28.2.

Diagnostics: In principle, newborns of diabetic mothers should be carefully watched during the first few days from birth, particularly with continual blood sugar checks. In the first 3 days, the blood sugar should be checked immediately postpartum, at the age of 30 minutes, 1, and 3 hours, as well as always preprandially (normoglycemic blood sugar values: Premature babies > 25 mg/dL [1.4 mmol/L] in the first 24 hours, > 35 mg/dL [1.9 mmol/L] from the second day; Newborns > 35 mg/dL [1.9 mmol/L] in the first 24 hours, > 45 mg/dL [2.5 mmol/L] from the second day). If the blood sugar values remain stable above 45 mg/dL (2.5 mmol/L), the checks can be reduced and finally discontinued. With polycythemia, the hematocrit and with symptoms of hypocalcemia, the serum calcium should be regularly checked. Because of the inclination to hyperbilirubinemia, the bilirubin concentration must also be carefully monitored.

The application of further diagnostic measures depends on clinical symptoms (e.g., thoracic X-ray for respiratory symptoms and oxygen need). Sonography of heart and kidneys are performed to rule out organ malformation.

Treatment: See answer to question 28.3. In addition to treatment of respiratory symptoms, polyglobulia (dilution of the blood by infusion therapy) and hyperbilirubinemia (see case 38) as well as balancing hypocalcemia, stabilization of blood sugar values is of great importance. In hypoglycemia that is not stabilized on oral maltodextrin solutions and early feeding of infant nutrients (already at the age of 3–4 hours), 10% glucose infusions are required. During this treatment, the blood sugar values must be checked at 30-minute intervals. Administration of more concentrated glucose solutions may be necessary. These infusions must be administered through a central venous catheter because of the poor tolerance of the veins. If possible, bolus administration should be avoided because this triggers a rebound effect through insulin release.

Prophylaxis: See answer to question 28.4. In all pregnant women, diabetes screening (oral glucose tolerance test [oGTT]) should be performed in the 24th to 28th week of pregnancy. The urine is tested for glucose at every prenatal care visit. If there is glucose in the urine, an oGTT must be performed.

Prognosis: The prognosis is closely dependent on the presence of accompanying malformations. It is usually good if there are no complications.

ADDITIONAL TOPICS FOR STUDY GROUPS
- Surfactant
- Respiratory distress syndrome
- Hyperbilirubinemia

→ Cases 28 Page 29

29.1 **Describe the sonography result. What is your suspected diagnosis? What differential diagnosis must you consider?**

- **Sonographic diagnosis:** Tumor in the right kidney (see Fig.)
- **Suspected diagnosis: Nephroblastoma**; rationale: patient's age, macroscopic hematuria, convex abdomen, resistance in the right upper abdomen, pale skin as a sign of anemia, tiredness and fatigue, laboratory results (anemia, sedimentation rate ↑, leukocyte / erythrocyte / proteinuria)
- **Differential diagnoses:** Neuroblastoma, teratoma, adrenal cortex tumor

29.2 **How do you proceed?**

- **Hospital admission**, preferably contact with a pediatric oncology center, university hospital, or children's hospital with an oncology unit, to discuss further procedures with this suspected diagnosis, so as to spare the child repeated examinations
- **Radiological diagnosis:**
  - Abdominal MRI or CT scan: Precise location and delineation of the tumor, search for metastases (so-called staging); in children, usually MRI (no radiation load)
  - i.v. urogram: Visualization of the urinary tract, extent of the tumor (ureters cannot be visualized in abdominal CT or MRI)
  - Thoracic X-ray: With a confirmed tumor, to rule out pulmonary metastasis
  - Thoracic CT: For further differentiation of suspected metastases in the thoracic X-ray
  - Skeletal and hepatic scintigraphy: With a confirmed tumor, to rule out intra-abdominal metastasis or skeletal metastases

- For distinction from the differential diagnosis of neuroblastoma, determination of vanillic and homo-vanillylmandelic acid in (24 hours) urine collection (in neuroblastoma ↑)
- For evidence of a neuroblastoma: see Comments/Treatment

29.3 **What do you know about the prognosis for the disease you suspect?**

The prognosis depends decisively on the tumor stage (see Comments). Whereas in stage I the healing rate is 95%, by stage III–IV the healing rate falls to approximately 50%. The survival rate in primary lung metastases is higher than for metastases or relapses that develop after the start of treatment. Pulmonary relapses have a better outcome than abdominal relapses.

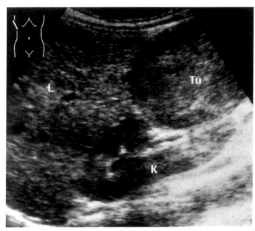

Tumor (Tu) in the right kidney (K); liver (L)

Definition: The nephroblastoma (Syn.: Wilms tumor) is a **malignant embryonic mixed kidney tumor** with epithelioid, fibroblastic, and myogenic sarcomatous portions.

Epidemiology: The incidence is 1:10,000, the peak frequency is between 2 and 5 years of age. Girls develop the tumor slightly more frequently than boys.

Classification and prognosis: There are five stages (see Tab. Tumor stages).

Etiopathogenesis: The etiology is not known. In 5% to 10% of cases, bilateral tumors are found. These are often associated with other abnormalities (aniridia, hemihypertrophy, Beckwith–Wiedemann

syndrome). The origin is a defective differentiation of the embryonic kidney tissue. The tumor arises in the kidney parenchyma. It grows expansively, compressing and distorting the system of hollow spaces in the kidney. Neighboring organs are infiltrated early. The metastasis is lymphogenic (pararenal and paraaortic lymph nodes) as well as hematogenous (lungs, liver, brain). Rarely, tumor thrombi are found in the Vena cava and the right atrium.

Clinical aspects: The clinical symptoms are very unspecific. Children are often—even in advanced stages—only slightly impaired, so that the tumor is discovered by chance, e.g., during a health screening. Often the first clinical indication is the abdomen distended by the tumor. Only approximately every third patient shows symptoms such as abdominal pain, hematuria, vomiting, fever, arterial hypertension, loss of weight, or constipation.

Diagnosis: See answer to question 29.2. *Caution:* Take great care in palpation and sonography of the abdomen because the risk of tumor rupture is very high. **No tumor biopsy before the start of treatment**, because of the danger of hematogenous dissemination of the tumor This means that the diagnosis is established only on the basis of imaging and confirmed histologically after surgical resection.

Treatment: Treatment depends on the stage of the tumor and patient's age and should only take place as part of clinical studies. The usual sequence is preoperative polychemotherapy (vincristin, prednisone, adriamycin, cyclophosphamide, and etoposide in several cycles), tumor nephrectomy, and postoperative chemotherapy, with radiation (from stage II with lymph node involvement). Preoperative chemotherapy can reduce the size of the tumor before it is removed. In over 50% of cases, it is possible to achieve a return to prognostically more favorable

tumor stages (I or II). Moreover, the intraoperative risk of tumor rupture and thus the danger of tumor dissemination can be reduced and postoperatively treated less aggressively (possibly no radiation, shorter courses of chemotherapy).

In patients under 6 months, a primary operation without preoperative chemotherapy is possible, since at this age, the occurring variants are almost exclusively of low malignancy and progress of the tumor during preoperative chemotherapy is very likely.

Prognosis: See answer to question 29.3 and Tab. Tumor stages and prognosis of nephroblastoma according to the National Wilms Tumor Study (NWTS).

👫👫 ADDITIONAL TOPICS FOR STUDY GROUPS
- Distinction criteria for differential diagnoses of nephroblastoma
- Complications of chemo- and radiation therapy
- Other pediatric tumors (e.g., bone tumors)

Tumor stages and prognosis of nephroblastoma according to the National Wilms Tumor Study (NWTS)

Stage	Extent	Healing rate
I	Tumor limited to one kidney	95%
II	Tumor extends past the renal capsule, surgically completely resectable; lymph node involvement possible	90%
III	Tumor extends past the renal capsule, no complete surgical removal possible; no hematogenous metastases	70%
IV	Hematogenous distant metastases (lung [80%], liver [20%], bone, CNS)	50%
V	Bilateral tumor	< 50%

30 Neurofibromatosis (von Recklinghausen disease)

30.1 What is your suspected diagnosis regarding the skin changes?
Neurofibromatosis (von Recklinghausen disease); rationale: cafe au lait spots (not raised, light brown, sharp, irregular borders, usually pigment spots several centimeters in size, see Fig. example case), prepubertal > 5 (size > 0.5 cm) are confirmatory.

30.2 What further clinical abnormalities/changes can be associated with this disease?
- Axillary/inguinal small spots of hyperpigmentation (usually not until adolescence)
- Neurinoma, neurofibroma along peripheral nerves, possibly with sarcomatous degeneration, epileptic attacks, mental retardation

- Iris harmatoma (Lisch nodules)
- Vision disorder caused by optic nerve glioma
- Possibly skeletal changes (e.g., scoliosis, skull asymmetry, tibial pseudoarthrosis)
- Frequent occurrence of pheochromocytomas, cerebellar astrocytomas
- Frequent hydrocephalus
- Underachievement, concentration disorders

30.3 Which classification of this disease do you know of?
- **Neurofibromatosis type I:** Peripheral form, 90% of cases; cafe au lait spots from birth; clinical aspects: see answer to question 30.2

- **Neurofibromatosis type II:** Central form, 10% of cases. Clinical: manifestation age around 20 years, bilateral acoustic neurinoma with resulting auditory deficit, tinnitus, vertigo, meningioma, schwannoma, rare skin manifestations, and neurinomas

! 30.4 List other diseases in the same spectrum and give their characteristic symptoms.
- **Tuberous cerebral sclerosis (Bourneville–Pringle disease):** Sebaceous adenoma (multiple reddish brown butterfly-shaped nodules around the cheeks), amelanotic naevi (white spots), epilepsy (Blitz–Nick–Salaam spasms), intellectual impairment, polycystic renal degeneration
- **Ataxia telangiectasia (Louis–Bar syndrome):** Ataxia, oculocutaneous telangiectasia, pigment spots, polyneuropathy
- **Encephalotrigeminal angiomatosis (Sturge–Weber syndrome):** Nevus flammeus of the facial skin, usually one-sided, in the supply area of the first trigeminal branch, angiomatosis of vessels of the pia mater, choroid, facial asymmetry frequently with glaucoma, epilepsy with focal attacks, frequent hemiparesis, and homonymous hemianopia
- **Hippel–Lindau syndrome:** Angiomatosis retinae, cerebellar hemangioblastoma, visceral cystic changes

! 30.5 The boy was brought in because of a blow to the head. What diagnostic and therapeutic procedures do you initiate?
- Medical history and clinical details do not indicate a cerebral concussion.
- The child need not be admitted to the hospital, but the parents must be told to observe him.
- Inform the parents that in case of vomiting, headache, or the loss of consciousness, the child must be brought back immediately.
- For cerebral concussion, see case 23.

Comments

Case 30

Definition and etiopathogenesis: The clinical pictures described above are part of the spectrum of **phacomatoses** or neurocutaneous syndrome. They arise as the result of ectodermal tissue dysplasias of the skin and CNS with some tumor-like proliferation (hamartomas), but mesodermal abnormalities can also occur.

Usually this is an autosomal-dominant hereditary gene mutation that can occur spontaneously in 50% of cases. They have high penetrance with variable expressivity, i.e., within one family the severity of the disease can differ.

The cause of type I neurofibromatosis is mutations of the NF gene on the long arm of chromosome 17. It is one of the most frequent genetically caused diseases. The disease occurs with a frequency of 1:4,000.

Clinical aspects: See answers to questions 30.2, 30.3, and 30.4.

Diagnostics: The diagnosis of type I neurofibromatosis can be clinically confirmed if at least two of the following seven criteria are met:
- 5 cafe au lait spots (prepubertally > 5 mm, postpubertally > 15 mm); possibly visible under Wood light
- Proof of at least two neurofibromas located in the skin or deeper or a plexiform neurofibroma (often does not occur until puberty)
- Sprinkles of freckles in the axillary hollows or the groin
- At least two Lisch nodules in the iris
- Proof of an optic nerve glioma (frequent in childhood)
- Specific skeletal dysplasias (e.g., sphenoid bone dysplasia, bending of long bones, pseudoarthroses of the tibia)
- First-degree relatives with type I neurofibromatosis

The symptoms develop over the course of years. For this reason, it can be difficult to establish a diagnosis in children.

If neurological symptoms are present, a skull MRI should be performed to rule out hydrocephalus or intracerebral space-occupying lesions (e.g., cerebellar astrocytoma). Regular ophthalmological examinations should be performed yearly to rule out optic nerve gliomas.

A prepartum diagnosis is possible, based on examination of chorion cells.

Treatment: Treatment is limited to **symptomatic measures** (e.g., anticonvulsive therapy in epilepsy, support in cases of mental retardation). Removal of peripheral tumors is indicated in case of pain and excessive growth. If possible, intracranial tumors are resected early. This should be followed by genetic counseling.

Prognosis: The prognosis depends on the form of the disease. In 60% of cases, the course of the disease is mild. The risk of developing malignant tumors (nephroblastoma, neurofibrosarcoma, etc.) is increased.

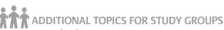 ADDITIONAL TOPICS FOR STUDY GROUPS
- Cerebral seizures
- Cerebral concussion

→ Cases 30 Page 31

31.1 What is your suspected diagnosis?

Contagious impetigo in atopic dermatitis; rationale: pustulous-crusty skin changes with honey yellow crust; previously existing itchy skin disease (here: atopic dermatitis) favors manifestation and spread.

31.2 What triggers the disease?

There are two forms of the disease:

- **Small-blister form**, chiefly triggered by β-hemolyzing group A Streptococci (*Streptococcus pyogenes*)
- **Large-blister form** (more frequent), chiefly triggered by *Staphylococcus aureus*
- Sources of infection are nose and throat infections or impetigo foci in contact persons

31.3 List one complication of the disease.

- **Lymphadenitis colli** caused by transmission of the infection into the local lymph nodes (see case 13)

- **Post-infectious glomerulonephritis:** Infection with group A β-hemolyzing *Streptococci* can lead to formation of immune complexes that are deposited in the mesangium and lead to inflammatory reactions and glomerulonephritis (see case 18)
- **Staphylogenic Lyell syndrome** in infection with exfoliatin-forming *Staphylococcus* strains (see Comments)

31.4 What treatment do you initiate?

- Indication for systemic antibiotic treatment because of marked skin findings and fever, e.g., with cephalosporins (e.g., cephalexin 60–100 mg/kg body weight p.o. in three individual doses) or erythromycin (40–60 mg/kg body weight p.o. in two individual doses) for 7–10 days
- Local disinfection, e.g., moist compresses with chinosol
- Simultaneous treatment of the brother, also with systemic antibiotic therapy, to prevent reinfection

141

Case

31

Comments

Definition and etiopathogenesis: Contagious impetigo is a frequent, contagious, superficial infection of the skin in children, which manifests preferentially periorally and on the hands. For pathogens, see answer to question 31.2. Itching skin diseases, such as neurodermitis, favor development of the disease.

Forms and clinical aspects: A distinction is made between a large-blister and a small-blister form. The **small-blister form** is characterized by short-lived, thin-walled blisters on erythema that become pustules with honey yellow crusts. In the **large-blister form**, the blisters are more stable and up to several centimeters in size. The skin manifestations can be associated with painful lymph node swelling.

For complications: See answer to question 31.3. **Staphylogenic Lyell syndrome** (Syn.: bullous impetigo, staphylococcal-scaled-skin- (SSS-) syndrome, Ritter dermatitis) is characterized by extensive bullous detachment of the skin that is caused by epidermolytic toxins (exfoliatin A and B) of certain *Staphylococcus* strains. It occurs chiefly in infants and toddlers a few days after a *Staphylococcus* infection (contagious impetigo, otitis media, pharyngitis). The onset of the disease is acute with high fever, and at first, a scarlet fever-like rash. After 1 to 2 days, flaccid blisters are formed that tear quickly and lead to extensive erosion (scalded skin). The blisters can be provoked by slight rubbing (positive

Nikolsky sign). The course can be severe, and pneumonia or sepsis can occur. The treatment consists of maximal doses of intravenous antibiotics (penicillinase-resistant penicillin, e.g., flucloxacillin [100 mg/kg body weight in three individual doses] or cephalosporins [e.g., cefuroxime 75–150 mg/kg body weight in three individual doses]) and local antiseptic application.

Differential diagnoses: Superinfected *Herpes simplex* infection, acrodermatitis enteropathica (autosomal-recessively inherited zinc malabsorption with bullous skin changes, chiefly perioral, on hands and feet, as well as the anogenital area, and chronic diarrhea.

Diagnostics: The diagnosis is by visual examination. A pathogen smear and determination of the ASL titer are not necessary. Urine examination to rule out post-infectious glomerulonephritis should be performed up to 3 weeks after healing, by the private pediatrician.

Treatment: Local anesthetic application (e.g., compresses with chinosol) is usually sufficient. Local antibiotic treatment should no longer be administered because this can elicit an allergy that might later complicate necessary oral antibiotic treatment. Moreover, local antibiotic treatment contributes significantly to development of resistance. For

→ Cases 31 Page 32

treatment when the course is severe, see answer to question 31.4. For treatment of post-infectious glomerulonephritis, see case 18.

Prognosis: The disease usually heals without scarring, often spontaneously, but it can also last for weeks with significant spread through reinfection.

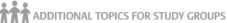

ADDITIONAL TOPICS FOR STUDY GROUPS
- Other *Staphylococcus* or *Streptococcus* infections
- Atopia
- Neurodermitis
- Enteropathic acrodermatitis and celiac disease
- Staphylogenic Lyell syndrome

32 Ullrich–Turner syndrome

32.1 Which clinical picture do these symptoms suggest?

Ullrich–Turner syndrome; rationale: intrauterine growth retardation (→ hypotrophic newborn), dwarfism, signs of dysmorphia (pterygium colli, high palate, nipples far apart, low hairline on neck), lymphedema on backs of hands are pathognomic at birth (see Fig. example case)

32.2 What other abnormalities do you expect?

- Cubitus valgus (hyperextensible elbow joints)
- Shortened metacarpal IV
- Frequently melanocytic pigmented naevi
- Various malformations of internal organs (e.g., cardiac defects, renal malformations, rudimentary ovaries)
- Lymphedema on foot dorsum
- Flat chest
- Hypoplastic nails

32.3 How do you confirm the diagnosis?

Chromosomal analysis: Chromosome set 45 X0 (about 55% of cases), but also mosaics (45 X0/XX, 45 X0/XY among others) or X-structural disorders (deletion of the short arm, Ring-X among others) are possible.

32.4 What do you tell the parents about the course and prognosis of the disease? What therapy does the diagnosis call for?

Information and counseling for parents: Explain to the parents that there is a suspicion of Ullrich–Turner syndrome, a chromosomal disorder in which the second X-chromosome has been lost. The Ullrich–Turner syndrome is not inherited and has a good prognosis. Briefly list the child's symptoms that led to the suspected diagnosis and explain that further diagnostics (see Comments) are necessary. The life expectancy is normal. Physical and mental developments are almost always normal, but heart and kidney defects that might occur must be corrected. In comparison to the average population, affected girls are below normal in stature (final height without treatment: 114–147 cm) and are infertile. For this reason, children must receive treatment with estrogen and growth hormones (see below) and receive psychosocial support from their parents (because of the possible stigma of dwarfism and infertility). There is no restriction of possible career.

Therapeutic consequences:
- With growth hormone treatment from toddler age until puberty, the patient can reach a final height in the lower normal range for women.
- Hormone therapy with estrogen for development of secondary sexual traits/menstruation (even for psychological reasons) and prevention of osteoporosis from a bone age of 12 to 13 years, possibly with a shift to a pill form, but this cannot affect fertility.
- Possible surgical correction of the pterygium colli, heart defects, kidney malformations, etc.

Comments

Definition and etiopathogenesis: The abnormalities described in the sample case are characteristic for Ullrich–Turner syndrome (Syn.: Monosomy X. In English-speaking countries the condition is simply called Turner syndrome, although the first description was made by the German physician Ullrich). This is a **numerical chromosomal aberration of the gonosomes** in which the X or Y chromosome is lost after fertilization. Often there are also mosaics, or disorders of the X structure (see answer to question 32.3).

Epidemiology: The syndrome occurs with a frequency of about 1:2,500 in females. The mother's age is not a factor. There is no increased risk of repetition.

Clinical aspects: In addition to **morphological abnormalities** (see Fig. and answers to questions 32.1 and 32.2) there are often malformations of internal organs. There is sterility with primary amenorrhea. The ovaries are only rudimentary (connective tissue strands or "streak gonads"). Intelligence is normal.

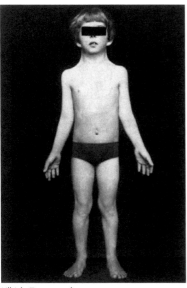

Ullrich–Turner syndrome

physician because she feels she is too short or she is not experiencing puberty.

The lymphedema in hands and foot dorsa are pathognomic for the disease. The diagnosis is confirmed by chromosome analysis (see answer to question 32.3). Hypergonadotrophic hypogonadism can be confirmed in the laboratory (FSH and LH ↑, estrogens and progesterone ↓).

In particular, it is important to search for renal abnormalities with sonography and for heart defects (primarily aortic isthmus stenosis, aberrant large vessels) with echocardiography.

Differential diagnosis: **Noonan syndrome** (Ullrich–Turner stigmata in girls or boys with normal female or male chromosome sets without verifiable chromosomal aberrations)

For treatment: **See answer to question 32.4.**

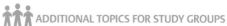

ADDITIONAL TOPICS FOR STUDY GROUPS
- Additional chromosomal aberrations (e.g., Klinefelter syndrome, Down syndrome)
- Mechanism of origin of numerical and structural chromosomal aberrations (non-disjunction, erroneous distribution of gonosomes and autosomes)

Diagnostics: The phenotype of the Ullrich–Turner syndrome is not always as characteristic as described in the sample case. When the abnormalities are less clearly visible, the syndrome is first discovered when the girl or adolescent visits a

---

33 Hip diseases in childhood

33.1 What is your diagnosis? Justify your decision.

Coxitis fugax; rationale: previous airway infection, patient's age, protective limping, painful limitation of movement in right hip joint, sonographically, hip joint effusion (see Fig. Coxitis fugax)

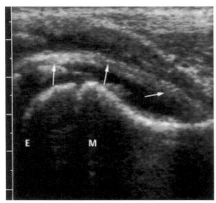

Coxitis fugax. Sonographic longitudinal section of the proximal femur in the area of the femoral neck 5-mm wide hip joint effusion, barely 4 mm thick, sharply definable joint capsule (arrows); E = epiphysis, M = metaphysis

33.2 Explain the clinical picture of Perthes disease

- **Definition:** Aseptic femoral head necrosis of unclear etiology
- **Epidemiology:** Peak age between 5 and 7 years
- **Pathogenesis:** Disruption of blood flow to the femoral head leads to disrupted growth of the ossification center (widened intra-articular space in X-ray), later necrosis of the ossification center, break down of the necrotic trabeculae and regeneration of the ossification center (see Fig. Perthes disease)
- **Clinical aspects:** Protective limping, load-dependent hip and knee pain
- **Diagnostics:** Clinical examination (limited movement, especially in abduction and rotational movements [positive Patrick's test]), MRI (verification of the early stage), X-ray (establishing diagnosis), sonography (verification of the joint effusion)
- **Treatment:** Unloading the affected leg (no sports, crutches, etc.), therapeutic exercises to avoid deformation of the femoral head; where deformation has begun, surgical restoration of joint congruence (e.g., realignment osteotomy)
- **Prognosis:** Depending on the start of the disease, usually good, but also possible subluxation with

permanent limitation of movement and later hip joint arthrosis

33.3 What do you know about slipped capital femoral epiphysis?

- **Definition and pathogenesis:** Loosening and (usually slow) slipping of the epiphysis of the femoral head (see Fig. epiphysiolysis of the femoral head), but also acute slipping off is possible; this disrupts blood flow to the femoral head with danger of femoral head necrosis, malpositioning and shortening of the affected leg

- **Epidemiology:** During the pubertal growth spurt, especially in boys
- **Etiology:** Speed of growth, hormonally predisposing factors (adiposogenital dystrophy, eunuchoid gigantism)
- **Clinical aspects and diagnosis:** Constitution type, knee and hip pain, in dislocation, the hip joint shifts into outward rotation and abduction on hip flexion (positive Drehmann sign), diagnosis of acute slipping corresponds to the finding of a femoral neck fracture (acute inability of the hip to bear a load, running no longer possible); dislocation often only recognizable in axial beam path (so-called Lauenstein imaging).
- **Treatment:** Immediate load relief of the hip joint, surgical repositioning and fixation (wire nail, corrective osteotomy)
- **Prognosis:** Usually good, early coxarthrosis is rare

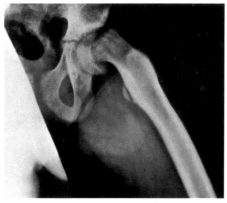

Epiphysiolysis of the femoral head (Lauenstein imaging hip joint)

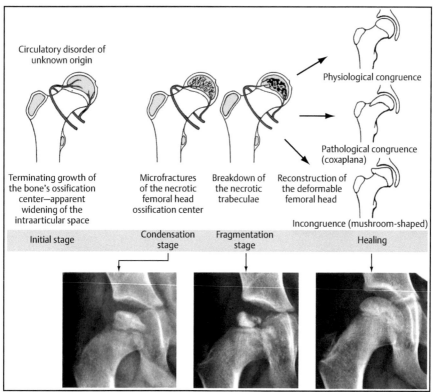

Circulatory disorder of unknown origin

Physiological congruence

Pathological congruence (coxaplana)

Terminating growth of the bone's ossification center—apparent widening of the intraarticular space

Microfractures of the necrotic femoral head ossification center

Breakdown of the necrotic trabeculae

Reconstruction of the deformable femoral head

Incongruence (mushroom-shaped)

Initial stage | Condensation stage | Fragmentation stage | Healing

Perthes disease (pathogenesis and course)

General: Knee pain in childhood must be considered to be a symptom of hip disease until there is proof to the contrary. The most important ones are presented below.

Transient synovitis: In the sample case, the medical history and clinical aspects suggest **transient synovitis** (see answer to question 33.1). The so-called irritable hip frequently occurs in association with a respiratory infection. An accompanying inflammation of the hip joint capsule (synovialitis) produces pain and limitation of movement in the hip joint. A hip joint effusion can be verified sonographically. It usually recedes within a few days. In differential diagnosis, bacterial coxitis must be ruled out (fever, elevated serological inflammatory parameters). Transient synovitis is treated purely symptomatically with analgesics and antiphlogistics (e.g., ibuprofen, diclofenac) and, if necessary, with rest.

Perthes disease: See answer to question 33.2. This is an ischemic femoral head necrosis with an etiology that is presently unclear. It is assumed that the cause is malformation of the femoral head blood vessels. The age of onset lies between 3 and 12 years, with a peak age of 5 to 7 years. Boys have the disease more frequently than girls. In one-quarter of the cases, both femoral heads are affected. Knee pain and protective limping are early symptoms. The clinical examination can be unremarkable; limitations of motion (abduction, rotation) do not set in until the involvement is extensive. The course of the disease has four stages (see Fig. Perthes disease) that are classified according to radiological criteria (pelvic overview and axial Lauenstein imaging). *Caution:* The Roentgen diagnosis is often far behind the clinical course. It is increasingly being replaced by MRI, since the latter does not impose a radiation load on the patient and the diagnosis can be established much earlier.

Epiphysiolysis of the femoral head: See answer to question 33.3. In this condition, loosening of the epiphyseal seam of the femoral head leads to a slipped epiphysis with a risk of femoral head necrosis. Youths in puberty are affected, boys more often than girls. The disease often lasts for several weeks (slow slipped capital femoral epiphysis), but acute events are possible (acute slipped capital femoral epiphysis). The latter always constitute an orthopedic emergency. In the slow form, the usual symptoms are discrete with pain in knees and hips, later increasing outward rotation and shortening of the affected leg. In the acute form, the hip immediately becomes unable to bear a load, as in a femoral neck fracture.

Treatment is always operative. Usually, the prognosis is good; rarely, an early coxarthrosis develops.

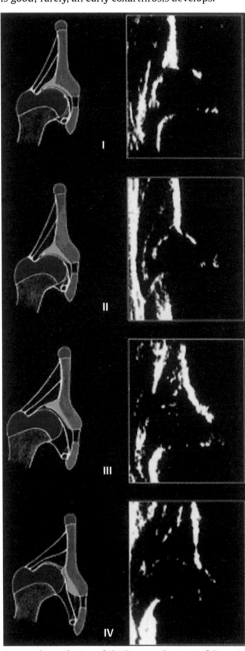

Sonographic evaluation of the hip according to Graf (Type 1 = mature hip joint, type II = hip is (still) physiologically immature, type III = decentered hip, type IV = luxated hip)

145

Case
33

→ Cases 33 Page 34

Congenital hip joint luxation and dysplasia: In congenital hip joint luxation (incidence 2:1,000) there is a disruption of the joint closure with subluxation or luxation of the femoral head out of the acetabulum. Hip dysplasia (incidence 2–4:100) is malformation of the hip shape, especially around the acetabulum. Risk factors for occurrence of hip dysplasia are prepartal anomalies of position (e.g., breech presentation), multiple pregnancy, and female sex of the baby. Familial clustering has been observed. In 40% of cases both hips are affected. In infants, there is limited abduction of the affected hip and asymmetry of the gluteal folds, occasional instability of the joint, and leg shortening with complete dislocation of the hip joint. The Ortolani sign (= "clunk" phenomenon), which was formerly tested in well-baby screening, is currently no longer checked. There is a danger of injuring the blood vessels that supply the femoral head. In any case, the test is not very sensitive; abnormalities are only found in 50% of patients with hip dysplasia. The diagnosis is established on the basis of the ultrasound findings. In Germany, the standardized sonographic hip examination (according to Graf, see Fig. Sonographic assessment of the

hip according to Graf) is regularly performed on all infants during the third initial examination. Treatment depends on the severity. Centered, stable, or mildly unstable hip joints are treated by wearing a pediatric hip abduction orthosis for 6 weeks up to 6 months. Severely unstable hip joints are immobilized with splints or plaster cast for several weeks if there is danger of luxation. Luxated hip joints are repositioned slowly and gently with bandages (Pavlick bandage); in the presence of severe contractures, by overhead extension. After successful repositioning, a splint or plaster cast is applied for several weeks to normalize the acetabulum, thus stabilizing the hip joint. The prognosis depends on when treatment was started. With early diagnosis and treatment, the child can be restored to a normal condition.

ADDITIONAL TOPICS FOR STUDY GROUPS
- Other aseptic bone necroses (e.g., Scheuermann disease, Osgood–Schlatter disease, Osteochondrosis dissecans)
- Foot deformities

34 Hepatitis A

34.1 What diseases can be considered? What is the most likely diagnosis?
- **Differential diagnoses:** Hepatitis A, Meulengracht disease, hepatitis with mononucleosis, cytomegaly
- **Suspected diagnosis: hepatitis A**; rationale: The child's visit to a camping spot where there is a risk of hepatitis A; start of the disease about 3 weeks after his visit there (incubation time of hepatitis A 14–48 days), upper abdominal pain, nausea, loss of appetite, tiredness, fatigue, slight fever, scleral icterus

34.2 What diagnostic procedures do you order to confirm your suspected diagnosis? What findings would you expect?
- **Laboratory:** Serum transaminases ↑ (already in the pre-icteric phase), bilirubin (direct and indirect) ↑, alkaline phosphatase (↑), anti-HAV-IgM (shortly after start of illness; for a total of about 3 months), anti-HAV-IgG (for years to lifelong, expression of immunity)
- **Abdominal ultrasound**: hepato(spleno)megaly

34.3 Name additional clinical signs you would find if your suspected diagnosis is confirmed.
- Hepatomegaly with pain on pressure

- Dark ("beer brown") urine and bleaching of stool ("acholic") (see Comments)
- Itching
- Possibly splenomegaly

34.4 What do you know about the infectious pathway and incubation time of the disease? When may the boy return to school?
- **Infectious pathway:** Fecal-oral via smear infection or ingestion of contaminated food (e.g., shellfish)
- **Incubation time:** 25–30 days (15–50 days)
- **Infectiousness:** 1–2 weeks before to 1 week after onset of the disease. This corresponds to excretion of the hepatitis A virus (HAV) in the stool; i.e., return to school is possible 1 week after the start of the disease

34.5 Do cases of this disease have to be reported?
- **Endangered persons:** Personnel of infectious units, children, staff in facilities for children and handicapped persons, workers in waste water treatment plants
- Obligation to report suspicion, illness, and death

→ Cases 34 Page 35

Epidemiology: In the past, the level of endemic infection of hepatitis A in the United States was high. The disease was counted as a childhood disease. Today, because of good hygienic conditions and because of universal infant vaccination since 2006, there is increasing evidence of vaccine-induced immunity in young patients.

Infections are mainly acquired in the course of travel. Hepatitis A is endemic in tropical and subtropical countries. For the pathway of transmission, see answer to question 34.3.

Pathogenesis of the icterus: In viral hepatitis, there is **intrahepatic cholestasis**, i.e., secretion of bile from the hepatic cell into the bile canaliculi is disrupted. The result is congestion of the entire biliary tree. As a result, the concentration of conjugated (water soluble) and later unconjugated (water insoluble) bilirubin, bile acids, cholesterol, alkaline phosphatase, and phospholipids is elevated in the blood. Bilirubin is deposited in the tissues, causing yellow coloration (icterus) of skin, mucosa, and sclera. Generalized itching (pruritus) is caused by the increased concentration of bile salts in the skin. More conjugated (water soluble) bilirubin is excreted by the kidneys, giving a beer-brown color to the urine. Normally, bilirubin is discharged into the intestinal lumen in the form of bilirubin glucouronide, where it is transformed into urobilinogen and stercobilinogen by bacterial action. Oxidation produces urobilin and stercobilin that give the stool its dark color. In cholestasis, bilirubin is not discharged into the intestine and therefore cannot be transformed. The stool is missing its coloration, i.e., it becomes pale ("acholic").

Clinical aspects: The clinical course of the disease is closely **dependent on the patient's age** and the presence of other diseases. The older the patient, the more severe is the course of the disease. In toddlers and preschool children, hepatitis A is often asymptomatic. Clinically apparent hepatitis A starts after an incubation time of 15 to 50 days with **unspecific influenza-like and gastrointestinal symptoms** such as fever, joint pain, tiredness, loss of appetite, nausea, diarrhea, loss of weight, and upper abdominal pain (caused by hepatosplenomegaly). After a few days the patient becomes **icteric** with generalized pruritus. Acholic stools and dark urine can be observed. A fulminant course with coagulation disorders, encephalopathy, and hepatic coma are very rare (0.1% of cases).

Diagnostics: Serum values for GOT, GPT, γ-GT, and with icterus, direct and indirect bilirubin are elevated.

The diagnosis is confirmed by positive verification of **Anti-HAV-IgM antibodies**. They can be detected at the start of the disease. The patient is left with immunity that lasts for years or a lifetime.

Treatment: Causal treatment of the disease is not possible. Treatment is limited to symptomatic measures such as bed rest and particular care. By maintaining recommended hygienic measures (e.g., good personal hygiene, hand washing), spread can be significantly reduced. Patients can be treated at home.

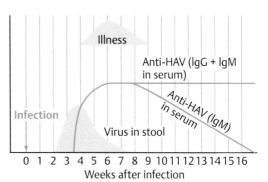

Clinical-serological course of hepatitis A

Prophylaxis: Both passive and active immunizations are available for the prevention of an infection. Active hepatitis A immunization is recommended as an indication vaccination for all at-risk persons (especially hospital staff, childcare facilities; see answer to question 34.5) and before travel abroad. The inactivated vaccine provides immunity for at least 10 years after two applications (on a schedule of 0–6 months). Vaccines against hepatitis A and B are also available; they are administered three times (0–4 weeks–6 months) and provide immunity for at least 10 years (possibly for life). After exposure, the spread of the disease can be prevented by post-exposure prophylaxis vaccination. The immunization is performed with active vaccine and the body's immune response "overtakes" the infection. Passive immunization with immunoglobulin is also possible, e.g., as post-exposure prophylaxis after close contact with the sick person.

Prognosis: The prognosis is good. Individual lengthy courses of the disease can be found, with elevated transaminases for up to 1 year. The lethality of fulminant hepatitis A is 40%.

👥 ADDITIONAL TOPICS FOR STUDY GROUPS
- Hepatitis B

→ Cases 34 Page 35

35.1   What are your first steps?

- **Check suitability to receive immunization:** Medical history (prior intolerance reactions, e.g., to medications, acute/chronic/diseases undergone, allergies) and physical examination (take temperature, examine ear drum/throat/tonsils, palpation of all lymph node stations, auscultation of heart/lungs, search for rashes, → to rule out a severe infection, e.g., pneumonia, otitis media, angina tonsillaris)
- **Informing parents:** about the disease to be avoided, the possibilities of treating it, utility of immunization, type of vaccine (active, passive, components such as chicken albumen), performance of vaccination, duration of immunity, procedure after vaccination, contraindications, possible side effects and complications of vaccination, necessity of booster vaccinations

35.2   Are the parents right? Name the general contraindications for vaccination.

- **No,** the parents are not right. Commonplace infections—even with temperatures up to 38.5°C—are not a contraindication (a frequent error). For other incorrect contraindications, see Comments/Contraindications.
- **General contraindications for active vaccination:** Up to 14 days after severe illness or surgery, adverse drug effects in chronological association with a previous vaccination, allergy to a component of the vaccine (e.g., to neomycin, streptomycin, chicken albumen), immunization with live vaccine in congenital or acquired immune deficiency syndrome and in pregnancy.
- **Contraindications for passive vaccination:** Hypersensitivity reactions to homologous immunoglobulins or components of the product.

35.3   What is meant by the adverse effects of vaccination? What is your reaction to the parents' assertion? What reactions to vaccination can the parents expect?

- **Damage caused by vaccine injury:** Post-vaccination reaction that exceeds the normal severity; requires immediate notification to the Board of Health. These reactions are very rare (< 1% depending on vaccine).
- The parents' statement is correct; the possible vaccine injuries include, among others, encephalopathy (especially in children < 3 years), screaming attacks (cri encéphalique; often as symptom of encephalopathy), chronically weak resistance (e.g., relapsing

middle ear inflammation), Guillain–Barré syndrome, seizures, epilepsy, hypersomnia, character change, delayed speech development, abnormal behavior. In recent years there have been many discussions on whether immunization can be correlated to the onset of diabetes mellitus, multiple sclerosis, or autism. No studies have been able to establish scientific proof of the correlations.

- **Vaccination reactions:** Reactions that are considered "normal" responses to the vaccine, including local reactions (redness, swelling, and pain at the vaccination point) and general reactions (fever, overall feeling of illness, nausea, vomiting, self-pity, sleepiness). They appear within the first 72 hours after vaccination and are very frequent (30%–70%). After live vaccine, so-called **vaccination disease** can occur 1 to 3 weeks after inoculation; this is a normal vaccine reaction. The symptoms are the same as for wild virus infection in weakened form, e.g., mild parotid swelling, measles- or varicella-like rash or joint pain after measles–mumps–rubella and varicella vaccination.

35.4   Must the parents' permission be recorded in writing? How do you proceed in vaccinating the child?

- No, permission for a routine vaccination does not need to be given in writing. On the other hand, refusal of permission must be recorded in writing. The parents must sign a statement that they take responsibility for all possible consequences—including the child's death—since they have refused the treatment recommended by the physician. However, it is always advantageous to have another person, e.g., a nurse, present when the parents give their permission.
- **Vaccinating the child:** Disinfect the skin over the vastus lateralis muscle (anterolateral thigh), i.m. injection of the tetanus vaccine (active immunization), and i.m. administration of tetanus immunoglobulin (a different vaccination site on the other side). Simultaneous vaccination is necessary in this case because the child has not received an immunization but immediate protection is needed because of the injury, i.e., immunoglobulin is administered to achieve immediate protection and tetanus toxoid is given to provide long-term protection. For this purpose, two injection sites are needed, since the effect would be reversed by antagonism if both vaccines were injected at the same site.

Vaccination schedule for infants, children, adolescents, and adults (according to CDC 2017) Recommended vaccination age and minimum interval between vaccinations

Vaccine	Birth	1 mo	2 mo	4 mo	6 mo	9 mo	12 mo	15 mo	18 mo	19–23 mo	2–3 yr	4–6 yr	7–10 yr	11–12 yr	13–15 yr	16 yr	17–18 yr
Hepatitis B (HepB)	1st	← 2nd→			← → 3rd												
Rotavirus			1st	2nd	see *1												
Diphtheria, tetanus, and acellular pertussis (DTaP: < 7 yrs)			1st.	2nd	3rd			← 4th →				5th					
Haemophilus influenza type B (Hib)			1st.	2nd			3rd or 4th										
Pneumococcal conjugate (PCV13)			1st.	2nd	3rd			← 4th →									
Inactivated polio (IPV)			1st.	2nd	←		3rd	→				4th					
Influenza (IIV)					Annual vaccination (IIV) 1 or 2 doses									Annual vaccination (IIV) 1 dose only			
Measles, mumps, rubella (MMR)							← 1st →					2nd					
Varicella (VAR)							← 1st →					2nd					
Hepatitis A (HepA)							← 2-dose series → see *2										
Meningococcal														1st		2nd	
Tetanus, diphtheria. & acellular pertussis (Tdap ≥ 7 yrs)																	
Human papilloma virus (HPV)														2-dose series see*3			

*1: Rotavirus (RV) vaccines (Minimum age: 6 weeks for both V1 [Rotarix] and RV5 [RotaTeq]). Administer a series of RV vaccine to all infants as follows: (1) If Rotarix is used, administer a two-dose series at ages 2 and 4 months; (2) if RotaTeq is used, administer a three-dose series at ages 2, 4, and 6 months. The maximum age for the first dose in the series is 14 weeks 6 days, and the maximum age for the final dose in the series is 8 months 0 days.

*2: Routine vaccination: Initiate the two-dose-HepA vaccine series at ages 12 through 23 months; separate the two doses by 6 to 18 months. Catch-up-vaccination: The minimal interval between the two doses is 6 months.

*3: Routine and catch-up vaccination: Administer a two-dose-series of HPV vaccine on a schedule of 0, 6 to 12 months to all adolescents aged 11 or 12 years. The vaccination series can start at age 9 years. Administer HPV vaccine to all adolescents through 18 years who were not previously adequately vaccinated. The number of recommended doses is based on age at administration of the first dose. For persons initiating vaccination before age 15, the recommended immunization schedule is two doses of HPV vaccine at 0, 6 to 12 months. For persons initiating vaccination at age 15 years or older, the recommended immunization schedule is three doses of HPV vaccine at intervals of 1, 2, and 6 months.

Case
35

→ Cases 35 Page 36

- **Documentation of vaccination**: Record lot number, name of vaccine, date, stamp, and signature of the physician on the vaccination card (obligatory)

35.5 **According to the recommendations of the United States Centers for Disease Control and Prevention (CDC), a 15-month-old child has normally already received various immunizations. What are they? List the ages at which these immunizations are normally given.**

Complete basic immunization (see vaccination schedule) is usually done

- with 5-fold vaccine (against diphtheria, pertussis, tetanus, poliomyelitis, and *Haemophilus influenzae* type B) at 2, 4, 6, and 15–18 months
- Postpartal, 1 to 2 months, and between 6 and 18 months vaccine against hepatitis B, in addition to passive simultaneous vaccination of a newborn of a mother with hepatitis B
- Measles–mumps–rubella (MMR), vaccination ages: 12–14 months
- Varicella (VAR), vaccination ages: 12 to 15 months, booster shot at 4 to 6 years
- Influenza (IIV), annual vaccination one or two doses

Comments

Possibilities for infection prophylaxis: Infections can be prevented by exposure and disposition prophylaxis.

Exposure prophylaxis prevents transmission of pathogens to the individual. This includes measures such as isolation of the sick individual (quarantine), disinfection, or sterilization.

Disposition prophylaxis aims at reducing susceptibility to the disease. This can be achieved by general, unspecific measures (e.g., adequate intake of sufficient calories and vitamins, good environmental conditions) and specific measures such as passive and active immunization. With high vaccination coverage, regional elimination of certain pathogens (e.g., poliomyelitis, diphtheria in industrialized nations) and finally worldwide elimination (e.g., smallpox) is possible. Patients with contraindications for vaccination are protected from disease indirectly by high vaccination coverage rates. Other diseases, such as tetanus, will not be eradicated by vaccination, since the pathogen, *Clostridium tetani*, occurs everywhere in the soil and will remain a permanent source of infection. This makes lifelong, regular vaccination necessary.

Passive immunization: In this process, specific antibodies that a donor has already generated (animals: heterologous antibodies; humans: homologous antibodies) are transmitted to a non-immune person, which creates **immediate** immunity against the corresponding infectious disease. However, the effect only persists for a few weeks or months; no immunological memory is formed. This can only be generated by the body if the immune system itself was able to confront the pathogen and thus to create its own antibodies. Immunoglobulins are foreign bodies for the body and are broken down by the body after a certain time. Therefore, they are only present and efficacious against the pathogen for a limited time.

Passive immunization is indicated for persons with a disrupted immune reaction (e.g., congenital and acquired immune deficiency [e.g., AIDS], immunosuppressive treatment, malignant tumor) and acute endangerment by infection or in the context of simultaneous immunizations (simultaneous active and passive immunization), e.g., against tetanus (see case).

Active immunization: Administration of antigens (toxoids, killed pathogens [dead vaccines], weakened living pathogens [so-called attenuated pathogens], genetically engineered antigens) causes an intact immune system to generate specific protective substances (antibodies) that lead to adequate immunity, often lasting over a long period of time (months to decades). The vaccines can be single (monovalent) or combined (polyvalent) vaccines without a loss of antigen efficacy. Live vaccines can be administered simultaneously. If they are not administered simultaneously, there should be a minimum interval of 4 weeks between the vaccinations in order to give the immune system sufficient time to react, thus creating long-lasting protection. There is no minimum interval for vaccination with killed vaccine.

Primary vaccination and booster shots: A primary vaccination (basic immunization) is the number of vaccine doses required for immediate protection and the formation of an immunological memory. Basic immunization should be started early. This means immediately postpartum (hepB) and then at the beginning of the ninth week of the infant's life, to ensure immunity is built up. In the second year of the child's life, protection through immunization should be complete, since from this age on, the child begins to "learn about the world" and is thus open to increased risk of infection. And vaccinations are repeatedly delayed because of numerous infections, so it is important to have sufficient lead time.

After completion of basic immunization, the necessary immunity must be maintained by regular booster shots that reactivate the immunological memory. The CDC (Center for Disease Control and Prevention; information at **www.cdc.gov**, including a detailed page on vaccines and immunizations) publishes a regularly updated vaccination schedule for infants, children, and youths with recommendations for vaccination age and minimum intervals between individual vaccinations.

Contraindications: See answer to question 35.2. Frequently indicated vaccinations are omitted because certain situations are erroneously understood to be contraindication. The "false contraindications" include commonplace infections with temperatures < 38.5°C, seizures in the family, fever seizures in the medical history of the patient to be vaccinated, chronic diseases, and non-progressive CNS diseases as well as being born prematurely.

Practical procedure: Before a vaccination, the person to be vaccinated must be checked for suitability to be vaccinated (medical history and physical examination), i.e., the above-mentioned contraindications (see answer to question 35.2) must be ruled out. In addition, **careful information** (see answer to question 35.1) is important.

Before administration, check the expiration date of the vaccine and see that the ampoule is correctly closed and dry. The vaccine is injected after an adequate period of disinfection (approximately 10–20 s) of the injection site in the deltoid muscle or, if this muscle is not yet sufficiently developed (in newborns and children under the age of 3 years, for example), in the vastus lateralis. There should be no vaccine adhering to the tip of the needle, since this makes the injection painful. It also spreads the vaccine in the injection channel, which guarantees an inflammatory reaction.

It is important for the child to be held securely during the injection, preferably by a physician's assistant or nurse. At the first vaccination, children are still fairly relaxed, because they do not know what is ahead of them. Depending on how this vaccination goes, they have an idea at their next visit to the doctor or the next vaccination what to expect and that there is going to be another one of "those" shots. It is also useful to position the child on its stomach for a vaccination in the vastus lateralis, so that the needle is out of sight. Usually the shot hurts less that way. But in spite of all the efforts at distraction, the injection should be carried out as quickly as possible. Afterwards, one can make peace with the child with a reward, maybe a certificate of bravery, a colorful band aid, or a treat.

After the vaccination, the parents should see to it that the child doesn't put too much of a load on the injected arm or leg.

Vaccination reactions appear within the first 72 hours after vaccination. One to 4 weeks after the measles–mumps–rubella vaccination, there can be a slight "vaccination illness" with measles- or mumps-like symptoms.

Adverse drug reactions (e.g., allergic reactions over and above normal vaccination reactions) are extremely rare. Diseases that occur at the same time as the vaccination can seem to be side effects and must therefore be carefully explored by differential diagnosis. This is precisely a point where it is important to provide the parents with information. If there are still adverse drug reactions or if some vaccination injury occurs, these can be reported to the Food and Drug Administration. Reporting is voluntary in the United States.

Generally recommended vaccinations: See vaccination schedule. In the United States, there is great variability in coverage for immunizations.

Indicated vaccinations: These are vaccinations that are only recommended for certain indications. This includes, for instance, danger of rabies, FSME, pneumococcus, and meningococcus B.

Unwillingness to vaccinate and counseling: The unwillingness to vaccinate is associated with social determinants and is increasing overall because more and more people are of the opinion that the diseases covered by the vaccinations no longer exist. Thus diseases like diphtheria or poliomyelitis have lost their ability to terrify because at the moment there are few if any new cases. But they do not consider the fact that due to a lack of vaccination coverage, these diseases can flare up again or be re-imported from countries with a high prevalence of the disease and very low vaccination coverage rates. Many parents are of the opinion that struggling with the pathogen strengthens the immune system, but they forget that severe bouts of illness can leave the child with lasting damage. A good example for this is measles infection: If a child falls ill with measles, in 1 out of 1,000 to 2,000 cases there will be a severe case of measles encephalitis. Twenty percent to 30% of these cases have a fatal outcome or involve permanent damage in a large proportion of the cases. Measles encephalitis can also occur as a complication of vaccination, but the risk is only 1:40,000.

Thus: There is a vital need for exploration of the problem. It is important to have a discussion, depending on the situation and the argument put forward by the parents. It must be made clear to

→ Cases 35 Page 36

the parents that, on the one hand, this is a matter of **individual protection** (protection of the child against infectious disease by vaccination) and on the other, of **collective protection** (the vaccinated protect not only themselves, but also indirectly those who are not vaccinated, since they can no longer transmit an infectious disease that is spread from person to person). For this protection to take place, a **vaccination coverage** of at least **90%** is required.

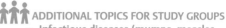 ADDITIONAL TOPICS FOR STUDY GROUPS
- Infectious diseases (mumps, measles, rubella, etc.)
- *Pneumococcus* vaccination before/after splenectomy or in asplenia
- Tetanus

36 Alcohol intoxication and alcohol abuse

36.1 What is your suspected diagnosis?

Moderate alcohol intoxication; rationale: third-party medical history (going-away party the evening before), vomiting, unconsciousness, smell of alcohol, hypoglycemia, hypothermia

36.2 What acute measures do you initiate?

- Hospital admission: Monitoring vital parameters (pulse rate, blood pressure, respiration)
- Undress (because clothes are damp) and warm patient (at temperatures > 32°C, passive warming is sufficient): Rub until warm and dry with warmed towels in a well-heated room, heating blanket, warmed blanket
- Continue looking for possible injuries with clinical indications, e.g., in suspicion of aspiration, thoracic X-ray
- Infusion therapy with glucose–electrolyte solution to balance hypoglycemia
- Laboratory: Alcohol level, acid-base balance (BGA), electrolyte, blood sugar check

36.3 What do you do next?

- If possible, obtain third-party medical history, e.g., speak with a classmate/parents: Alcohol (how much, what, over what period of time), patient's condition, duration of loss of consciousness; "experimenting" or chronic abuse, psychosocial problems (school, friends)
- After sobering up: **Conversation with patient** about psychosocial situation and alcohol abuse (history of addiction: Addictive substance, first contact, first full intoxication, regular/one-time consumption, context of use, attitude of friends to addictive substances, drug use among friends, subjectively experienced effect of alcohol, previously negative experience with consequences of alcohol consumption in school, family, psychosocial context, etc.), informal counseling conversation (teaching about alcohol, e.g., effect, abuse: avoid reproaches)
- Cooperation with parents, avoid reproaches, demonstrate dangers of alcohol use

Comments

General: Use and abuse of alcohol and drugs is frequent in youths and can have serious consequences. In the age group of 15 to 24, alcohol and drug consumption plays a role in 50% of mortalities (through accidents, murders, suicide). The disinhibiting effect of psychotropic substances promotes increased aggressive behavior (e.g., assault, rape).
Steps of youth experience with alcohol and other drugs:
1. Abstinence (no consumption)
2. Trial and experimentation
3. Agreeable feelings
4. Captivation by agreeable feelings, regular/repeated use for relaxation and compensation of problems
5. Feeling normal only on drugs, abuse, and dependence

Trial and experimentation do not necessarily lead to alcohol or other drug dependence. There is an increased risk if there are alcohol-dependent family members.

Reasons for alcohol consumption: Alcohol consumption and intoxication by children and youths are usually caused by curiosity and underestimation of the effect of alcohol. The use of alcohol has cultural, social (e.g., belonging to a group), familial (e.g., consumption habits), and personal (e.g., congenital personality factors) aspects. Especially the combination of curiosity in the young and social pressure makes it difficult to say No. However, it is rare in this age group that alcohol is used in solving psychic problems (e.g., anxiety, depression) or to make up for the lack of positive social capabilities.

Sources: Alcohol (Syn.: Ethyl alcohol) occurs chiefly in alcoholic drinks but also in cosmetics, cleaning, and solvent products (e.g., methylated spirits) as well as medications. Especially for little children, there is a danger that liqueurs that taste good, alcohol-containing medications, and alcoholic mixed drinks could be consumed in large quantities. Individual cases are known in which intoxication occurs after external use of ethanol as a rubbing compound to lower fever.

Kinetics and metabolism: Alcohol is quickly and completely absorbed orally, by inhalation, and dermally. The maximal plasma concentration (blood alcohol concentration) is attained after 30 to 120 minutes. Therefore, in relevant intoxication, symptoms only set in after 30 to 45 minutes, at the latest after 2 hours.

Calculation of the estimated blood alcohol concentration (BAC):

$$\frac{\text{"Alcohol in g (or alcohol in mL} \cdot 0.8)\text{"}}{\text{"Body weight in kg} \cdot 0.7\text{"}} \times 10 = \text{expected BAC (in \%)}$$

The elimination rate is approximately twice as high as in adults and equals 0.024%–0.039%/h.

Alcohol directly inhibits gluconeogenesis and glycogenolysis in the liver so that hypoglycemia can develop. As the alcohol is broken down, lactate and pyruvate utilization break down, which leads to formation of metabolic acidosis (lactate acidosis).

Toxicity: Symptoms of intoxication can arise with blood alcohol concentration under 0.05%, from concentrations of 0.15% to 0.2%, children and youths are already unconscious, in contrast to adults. The lethal dose of pure absorbed alcohol in children as opposed to adults is approximately 1.3 to 1.8 g/kg body weight (adults 5–8 g/kg body weight). The lethal alcohol dose related to body weight can be found in the table (see Tab.).

A bottle of wine (0.7 L) with 12 vol% alcohol contains approximately 67 g alcohol; a bottle of beer (0.5 L) with 5 vol% contains about 20 g alcohol.

Body weight in kg	Lethal alcohol dose in g
20 kg	26 g
30 kg	39 g
40 kg	52 g
50 kg	65 g
60 kg	78 g

Clinical aspects: **Mild intoxication** (< 0.07%) leads to euphoria, disinhibition, and ataxia (*caution:* risk of injury by falling) as well as mild hypoglycemia in individual cases. At low alcohol concentration, breathing becomes more rapid.

In **moderate-to-severe poisoning** (0.07%–0.3%) there is vomiting, double vision, nystagmus, limited vigilance as far as coma. Reflexes are weakened or suppressed. There is an increased tendency to seizures. Hypoglycemia and metabolic acidosis regularly occur. Higher alcohol levels depress respiration and increase acidosis (combined respiratory and metabolic acidosis).

In **severe to potentially life-threatening intoxication** (> 0.3%) there are also disorders of central regulation with hypothermia, hypoxia, respiratory depression, circulatory failure, and cerebral edema.

Moreover, alcohol causes peripheral vasodilation. If they stay for a moderately long time in a cool environment, patients are at risk for hypothermia.

Diagnostics: Blood should be taken to determine blood sugar, blood gases (BGA), electrolytes (Na, K), liver and kidney parameters (GOT, GPT, γ-GT, creatinine, urea), and, if possible, the alcohol level. Imaging (e.g., ultrasound, X-rays) should be performed if there is suspicion of concomitant injuries by falling. In case of collapse or seizure episodes, ECG and EEG should be performed.

Treatment: For acute treatment, see answer to question 36.2. **Mild intoxications** usually need no extra treatment. In **moderately severe and severe intoxications**, patients must be observed as inpatients (vial parameters/blood gases/blood sugar) and, if necessary, treated. Hospital admission is sometimes difficult because patients are not cooperative. If necessary, the patient must be sedated (strict establishment of indication), e.g., with haloperidol. The symptoms of acute alcohol intoxication usually last a short time; patients generally recover within 12 hours. Infusion therapy (glucose 5% + electrolytes, e.g., Jonosteril Ped II solution) is administered as a supplement. Glucose infusions (5%) lower the lactate concentration and thus have a positive alkalizing effect on the acid-base balance. Vomiting is reduced, and hypoglycemia prevented or eliminated.

If more than 1 g/kg body weight pure alcohol was consumed, not more than 1 to 2 hours previously, primary elimination of poison can be considered. In patients who are awake the alcohol can be removed with a gastric tube or through induced vomiting (syrup of ipecac, dose: < 2 years 10–15 mL, 2–3 years 20 mL, > 3 years 20–30 mL); in case of unconsciousness, it can be removed through gastric lavage after prior intubation. High, life-threatening blood alcohol concentrations (> 0.4%) are an indication for peritoneal dialysis or hemodialysis.

After treatment of the acute symptoms, further procedure is chiefly limited to waiting and monitoring

→ Cases 36 Page 37

vital parameters. Naturally it is also important to look for the causes of alcohol excess (see answer to question 36.3). The question should chiefly be the patient's current situation and not the alcohol consumption itself. It is sensible not to have this conversation until the patient has sobered up, and it should be with the patient alone. Questions about the patient's circle of friends, success and weakness in school or at work, and about the specific circumstances of intoxication are all of interest. Particular attention must be given to patients who seem to be unimpressed by the event. In such a case, competent help should be offered to the parents as well, e.g., conversations with psychologists and social workers experienced with this problem. Parents are often helpless in this situation. One should always be intent on cooperation with the parents, avoiding reproaches.

👪 ADDITIONAL TOPICS FOR STUDY GROUPS
  ■ Drug addiction (e.g., amphetamines, ecstasy, cannabis)

37　Intoxications

154

Case
37

37.1　The father asks you what he should do now. What additional information do you ask for on the telephone and what advice do you give the father?
■ **Additional information to request:**
  – How is the child? Have any symptoms developed (e.g., vomiting)?
  – Father's name, telephone number, and time of the call (to be documented)
  – Child's weight
  – Time of admission
  – Have any measures been taken yet?
■ **Advising the father about first aid:**
  1. Stay calm; do not give in to panic.
  2. Do not induce vomiting! No salt water (or other home remedies, since it is not known what the child drank!) No mechanically induced vomiting (risk of injuring the throat cavity and risk of aspiration → additional life threat).
  3. Immediately go to a pediatric practice/children's clinic, bring the original bottle.

❗ 37.2　Approximately how much of the active agent has the little girl consumed? How do you estimate the toxicity of the active agent consumed?
■ Estimate the amount of active agent consumed:
■ An unopened bottle contains 100 mL. Approximately two-third of the content is missing. There is medication on the child's face, hands, and T-shirt. Therefore, estimated amount consumed will be a maximum of 50 mL.
■ 5 mL paracetamol syrup contains 200 mg paracetamol; 50 mL contains 2 g paracetamol.
■ The child weighs 11 kg, amount consumed per kg body weight: 2 g; 11 kg = 180 mg/kg body weight.
■ Paracetamol has a toxic effect when an amount in the range of 100–140 mg/kg body weight/d is consumed.
■ *Caution:* The cumulative daily dose counts. Even at a normal dose, but with frequent consumption (> every 6 hours) poisoning is possible.

37.3　What symptoms must you expect with paracetamol poisoning?
■ After 6 to 14 hours: Sweating, lethargy, gastrointestinal symptoms (e.g., nausea, vomiting, diarrhea, abdominal pain)
■ Transient improvement of symptoms for 24 to 48 hours with increasing transaminases (GOT, GPT) and incipient coagulation disorder
■ After 36 to 48 hours: Liver damage (clinical: upper abdominal symptoms, icterus, tendency to bleeding, hepatic encephalopathy, kidney damage with renal failure, acute pancreatitis)

37.4　What measures do you initiate?
■ **Hospital admission:** ALWAYS!
■ Paracetamol is rapidly absorbed from the gastrointestinal tract; therefore, rapid primary poison removal is advisable. Medication of choice: Activated charcoal 0.5 to 1 g/kg body weight if the medication was not consumed longer than 4 hours ago.
■ **Laboratory:** determination of the paracetamol level (closest special laboratory) earliest 4 but at most 8 hours after ingestion; liver/renal retention/coagulation parameters
■ For paracetamol serum level > 150 µg/mL, 4 hours after ingestion, or in case the determination of the paracetamol serum level cannot be carried out so rapidly, even prophylactically (if possible within the first 8 hours after ingestion—efficacy decreases after this time): Antidote therapy with N-acetylcysteine (e.g., ACC 150 mg/kg body weight in 5% glucose as short infusion over 15 minutes; then 50 mg/kg body weight in 5% glucose over 3 hours; then 100 mg/kg body weight over 16 hours, total dose 300 mg/kg body weight/20 h. If the patient is conscious and cooperative ACC p.o. [at the earliest 2 hours after administration of charcoal, or dose increase by 40%] 140 mg/kg body weight as effervescent tablet, then 70 mg/kg body weight every 4 hours (a total of 17×), that is a total of 1,330 mg/kg in 72 hours). N-acetylcysteine promotes regeneration of glutathione, which is used for detoxification (conjugation with

glutathione) of the toxic degradation product of paracetamol (N-acetyl-benzoquinoline); in addition, general anti-inflammatory effect on the liver cells and prophylactic effect against cerebral edema in hepatic encephalopathy; N-acetylcysteine itself is not poisonous, but particularly when administered i.v., it can trigger allergic reactions (especially flush, pruritus after 15–75 minutes). Therapy: cortisone.

37.5 Give your reasons for the preferred use of activated charcoal for primary elimination of the poison. However, for what kinds of poisoning is activated charcoal without effect or contraindicated?
Activated charcoal has a high binding capacity for a variety of substances, primarily lipophilic. Repeated administration is possible and sometimes useful, e.g., to interrupt enterohepatic circulation. Activated charcoal is non-toxic and has few side effects. It is not efficacious in intoxication with inorganic substances, alcohols, glycols, and heavy metals. It is contraindicated for ingestion of acids, alkali, or other caustic substances. A drawback is the fact that children rarely take activated charcoal willingly (black color, sandy taste). Therefore, taking the charcoal must be made as pleasant as possible for the patient by stirring it into yogurt or fruit juice. Usually these supportive measures are useless, so that the activated charcoal must be administered through a gastric tube. *Caution:* If there is vomiting, the position of the gastric tube must be checked; if it is aspirated, activated charcoal can cause bronchiolitis obliterans.

Comments

General: Ingestion by children is frequent and usually harmless. Poisoning through ingestion of toxic substances, on the other hand, is rare.

Children often eat or drink medications for cardiovascular problems that belong to their parents or grandparents, tasty cough syrups, antihistamines, paracetamol or dimenhydrinate (Vomed) syrup, cleansers (chiefly toilet bowl cleaner), cigarettes, cigarette butts, batteries, (dyed) lamp oil, parts of plants or berries.

Clinical aspects: The poisoning symptoms depend on the substance consumed but are often uncharacteristic (e.g., vomiting, diarrhea, coma, seizures, coughing, dyspnea, circulatory and organ failure). The degree of severity of the poisoning is generally classified as follows (see Tab.).

Classification of severity of poisoning

Degree of severity		Symptoms
0		No symptoms or clinical signs
1	Mild	Mild, transient, and self-limiting symptoms
2	Moderate	Marked or persistent symptoms requiring treatment
3	Severe	Severe or life-threatening symptoms
4	Death	Death as causal consequence of the poisoning

Diagnostics: It is particularly important to find out as much as possible about the substance ingested. If possible, when the child comes to the doctor, the packaging of the ingested substance, the substance itself, or a plant part should be brought along. If it is not clear whether the ingested substance is dangerous or what measures should be taken, a poison control center should be called. The American Association of Poison Control Centers supports the nation's 55 poison centers and offers free medical advice through the Poison Help line at 1-800-222-1222.

To help in estimating the extent of the danger, a careful medical history must be recorded. All the important information is obtained with the "W questions."
- **Who** took the poisonous substance (age and weight)?
- **What** was consumed?

- **What quantity** was consumed?
- **When** did it happen?
- What was the **route of consumption** (oral, rectal, dermal, etc.) of the substance?
- **Why** did this happen?
- **Which symptoms** have already set in?
- What has already been **done**?
- **Which risk factors** or comorbidities are present?

When recording the medical history, it is important to keep in mind that because they are upset, parents will often give imprecise answers. Therefore, the exact time the substance was taken or the amount consumed can only be estimated, since the child was unobserved while consuming it. Information can also be downplayed out of fear of consequences (from partner or from the law) or because the parents are tormenting themselves with reproaches. But the information can also be dramatized out of concern for the child.

→ Cases 37 Page 38

In the physical examination, attention must be given to particular symptoms, depending on the substance ingested. State of consciousness (e.g., awake, oriented, agitated, tired, comatose), bad breath, pupil size (e.g., mydriasis, miosis), skin (e.g., pale, red, sweaty, turgor, temperature), mucosa (e.g., erosions, discoloration), heart (e.g., frequency, rhythm), blood pressure (hypotonic, hypertonic), respiration (e.g., cough, dyspnea, bronchospasm), gastrointestinal tract (e.g., pain, peristalsis), urogenital tract (e.g., urinary retention), neurological deficit manifestations (e.g., reflexes, speech, movement), etc.

On admission, routine laboratory work should be performed (blood panel, hepatic and renal retention parameters, coagulation status, blood sugar, Astrup) and—if possible—the amount of the ingested substance should be estimated.

Treatment: For first aid to be taken by parents, see answer to question 37.1. In addition, a poison information center or a pediatrician should be called up, and the advice given should be followed. In the meantime, immediate administration of 5 to 10 g activated charcoal is advised. After this, a pediatrician (practice, clinic) should be consulted (if still possible). In 9 of 10 cases, no other medical measures are necessary.

First medical measures at the accident site:
- ABC (verification of vital functions)
- Medical history
- Activated charcoal
- Provoke vomiting
- Exception: gastric lavage
- Analytics
- Antidote therapy

If available information is unclear, consulting a poison center is helpful. Primary poison elimination is contraindicated for ingestion of acids, alkali, or caustic chemicals. The mucosa is already damaged by the act of swallowing the substances, and therefore, vomiting would lead to repeated and further damage to the mucosa. It is important to dilute the ingested substance immediately by drinking a large amount of fluid (alcohol- and carbonation-free beverages like water, tea; *caution:* no milk, since it can induce vomiting).

The means of choice for **primary elimination of poison** is administration of activated charcoal p.o. (0.5–1 g/kg body weight, but at least 1 g/100 mg of ingested substance). In the past, induced vomiting or gastric lavage was considered the standard measures. However, clinical studies did not demonstrate any advantage of these very invasive measures, compared to simple administration of charcoal. They should only be applied after a strict indication has been established, within the first 60 minutes

after ingestion and after consulting a poison information center. For this procedure, the patient must be awake, with intact protective reflexes; otherwise, prior intubation is indicated. Vomiting may only be induced under a physician's supervision with ipecac syrup (dosage depends on the child's age: 1–2 years 10–15 mL, 2–3 years 20 mL, > 3 years 20–30 mL; then have the patient drink copiously. If there is no vomiting, after 20 minutes at the latest, a half of the previously administered dose may be repeated). If activated charcoal was previously administered, ipecac syrup is not efficacious, since it binds strongly to activated charcoal. In exceptional cases, apomorphine (0.07–0.1 mg/kg body weight s.c.; faster action. *Caution:* Depressed respiration, hypotension) can be given. Laxatives are no longer routinely recommended because they can increase absorption of the poison by stimulating peristalsis.

Clearly impaired children must be promptly transferred to a hospital, accompanied by a physician. Original containers, plant sprigs, etc. should definitely be brought along.

First aid measures in the hospital also include stabilizing vital functions. After obtaining information (third-party history, poison information center), the primary poison elimination is performed with activated charcoal (see above) or gastric lavage or induced vomiting. The patient must be monitored and, as appropriate, be treated according to symptoms and with antidotes, if necessary.

If primary poison elimination (activated charcoal, induced vomiting, gastric lavage) is no longer possible but poison elimination is still necessary, secondary poison elimination must be performed. This involves forced diuresis or an attempt, by administration of cholestyramine, to interrupt the enterohepatic circulation. Hemodialysis or perfusion may be necessary.

Prevention: In this emergency situation, parents are extremely worried and self-reproachful, so that it is not appropriate to subject them to additional reproaches and reprimands. After the danger has been averted and the child is discharged from the hospital and returns home, there should be a conversation, if the parents have not asked about it already, about the need to store medications, cleaning agents, etc. out of reach of children in cupboards that can be locked. Children should know that medicine is only taken by someone who is sick, even though it tastes delicious. Unfortunately, there is a great danger because of the delicious taste of children's medicines. Medications should never be left in the kitchen as a matter of convenience, or standing next to the lemonade.

Many pediatricians advise parents, at health screening visits, about general sources of danger and how poisoning and accidents can be avoided. For instance, it is useful to install special door locks for cupboards so that dangerous substances can be stored safely.

Moreover, parents should know the number of the nearest poison center, so that in an emergency they can immediately call and start giving first aid if necessary.

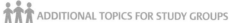 ADDITIONAL TOPICS FOR STUDY GROUPS
- Effective antidotes to poisons (e.g., deferoxamine for iron poisoning)
- Emergency measures (ABC rule, emergency medications)

---

38 Neonatal icterus (Hyperbilirubinemia)

38.1 What is your suspected diagnosis?
Neonatal icterus and breastfeeding and **polyglobulia** caused by dehydration as well as hypoglycemia with insufficient liquid intake: icteric skin color, scleral icterus, tiredness, fatigue, total bilirubin ↑ ↑; polyglobulia (hematocrit ↑ ↑) caused by dehydration (weak suckling) and hypoglycemia (blood sugar ↑ ↑)

38.2 Explain the causes of the clinical picture to the worried parents.
- There is increased breakdown of fetal hemoglobin in the first days of the newborn's life.
- Hepatic immaturity (glucuranyl transferase not completely mature) causing delayed transformation (glucuronidation) of the indirect (unconjugated) to the direct (conjugated) and thus excretable bilirubin
- Indirect bilirubin collects, leading to neonatal icterus
- Probable additional inhibition of glucuronyl transferase by mother's milk

38.3 What do you do next? What are the possible complications if the clinical course is unfavorable?
- **Procedure:** Hospital admission for
  - **Phototherapy** (Indications: bilirubin in fully developed newborns from 20 mg/dL) to decrease bilirubin level to under 20 mg/dL, see Comments
  - **Infusion therapy:** Improve breastfeeding management, i.e., complement with formula milk. In the case of continued insufficient intake, infusion therapy (5% glucose solution) accompanying phototherapy and to compensate for dehydration
- **Complications:** Kernicterus with severe cerebral damage (e.g., choreoathetosis, intelligence deficit, deafness) and possible death; damage irreversible (see Comments); dehydration due to suckling weakness, only in disorder of blood–brain barrier (see below)

Comments

Definitions: Physiological neonatal icterus begins on the third day of the newborn's life, peaks by the fifth day, and then decreases slowly. Bilirubin values may rise to a maximum of 18 to 20 mg/dL. A rise in serum bilirubin over 20 mg/dL is classified as icterus gravis. If a total bilirubin value of > 12 mg/dL is measured in the first 36 hours of the newborn's life, the classification is icterus praecox. Persistence of neonatal jaundice beyond the second week of the newborn's life is labeled icterus prolongatus.

Etiopathogenesis: See answer to question 38.2. Factors more likely to cause icterus in the newborn are premature birth, dyspnea, bleeding and hematomas, polyglobulia, drug interaction (sulfonamide, salicylate, ceftriaxone, digoxin, furosemide, and diazepam), hunger, blood group incompatibility (hemolytic disease of the newborn), neonatal infection, breastfeeding, metabolic changes (e.g., hypothyroidism), etc.

In the example case, the physiological hyperbilirubinemia is most likely reinforced by breastfeeding.

This phenomenon is often observed. The cause is not yet completely understood. It is suspected that mother's milk inhibits the activity of glucuronyl transferase. Dehydration resulting from ineffective suckling leads to polyglobulia. This also intensifies the icterus.

Clinical aspects: Icteric skin color occurs in hyperbilirubinemia of from approximately 5 (3–12) mg/dL, scleral icterus from approximately 2 mg/dL. Children are tired and listless and do not drink enough.

Kernicterus as a complication: Lipophilic bilirubin invades all body structures, including the brain; at high concentrations (> 25–30 mg/dL) it can cause irreversible nerve cell damage by inhibiting neuronal metabolism, especially in the basal ganglia, globus pallidus, and caudate nucleus. When the blood–brain barrier is damaged, e.g., as a result of asphyxia, hypoxia, infection, neonatal meningitis or if the albumin binding capacity is exceeded because the bilirubin concentrations are too high (indirect bilirubin is bound to albumin and cannot cross the blood–brain barrier), as well as in hypalbuminemia, there is a danger of kernicterus. Certain drugs, such as ceftriaxone, digoxin, furosemide, and diazepam, can displace bilirubin from its bond to albumin, thus increasing the risk of kernicterus. Bilirubin encephalopathy develops, with apathy, hypotension, ineffective suckling, and vomiting, weakened newborn reflexes, and shrill crying, opisthotonus, and seizures. A late consequence is often bilateral deafness, motor disorders, and mental retardation.

Diagnostics: In addition to a blood panel, total bilirubin, and direct bilirubin (to rule out cholestasis, e.g., due to bile duct atresia. In cholestasis, the proportion of conjugated bilirubin is at least 10% of total bilirubin), the diagnostic procedure for a newborn with icterus should include determination of mother's and child's blood groups, as well as a direct Coombs test and total protein in the child. If there has not yet been a TSH screening, thyroid values must also be determined.

Treatment: Special safety limits and bilirubin curves for healthy and sick newborns and premature babies have been set in the guidelines established by the GNPI (German Society for Neonatology and Pediatric Intensive Medicine). In uncomplicated full-term newborns, the phototherapy limit is 20 mg/dL after the age of 72 hours. If gestational age is less than 38 weeks, phototherapy limits are calculated according to the following formula: Phototherapy limit = gestational age (in weeks) −20.

When the safety limits are exceeded, treatment is with phototherapy, either continuous or at intervals. The blue light region of the light spectrum (wavelengths from 420 to 480 nm) transforms the bilirubin deposited in the skin into water-soluble bilirubin isomers that can be excreted in the bile and urine without glucuronosylation. The largest possible skin areas should be irradiated (do not use diapers). The child must be turned regularly, every 4 hours, since the bilirubin diffuses into the non-irradiated areas. The bilirubin value is checked for the first time 6 hours after the start of phototherapy. If it has continued to rise, the treatment must be intensified. This is done by continuous irradiation with two photo lamps. The child is placed on a bilirubin mat (emits blue light) and the incubator is lined with aluminum foil. The irradiation can be stopped when bilirubin level is about 10 to 15 mg/dL (depending on the child's age; the younger, the lower).

Possible **side effects of the phototherapy** are diarrhea and increased loss of fluid with dehydration. For this reason, the treatment is accompanied by infusion therapy. This will also promote renal excretion of bilirubin isomers. Newborns must wear protective goggles to prevent radiation damage to the retina.

If the bilirubin concentration is > 10 mg/dL in the cord blood of healthy newborns or > 29 mg/dL in the serum (> 24 mg/dL in premature babies) or if it continues to rise in spite of phototherapy, a blood exchange transfusion with compatible donor whole blood is performed, preferably through an umbilical vein catheter.

An interruption of nursing is not recommended until values reach > 30 mg/dL.

Prognosis: With thorough diagnostics and early initiation of the appropriate treatment, the prognosis is good. If the bilirubin values are under 30 mg/dL, there are normally no further complications. If the bilirubin values are higher, the baby's hearing must be tested with a BERA examination (Brainstem Evoked Response Audiometry).

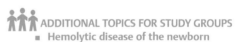 ADDITIONAL TOPICS FOR STUDY GROUPS
- Hemolytic disease of the newborn
- Rhesus incompatibility
- ABO incompatibility

39 Gingivostomatitis herpetica (ulcerative)

39.1 What is your suspected diagnosis?
Ulcerative herpetic gingivostomatitis; rationale: high fever, refusal of nourishment, multiple whitish blisters and ulcers on the oral mucosa and tongue, gingiva swollen and bleeding, fetid mouth odor, painful cervical lymphadenopathy

39.2 Explain the etiology of the disease.
Usually primary infection is with type 1 *Herpes simplex* virus (HSV-1).

39.3 What further measures do you initiate?
- Hospital admission for **Infusion therapy** (see case 4) caused by dehydration in food refusal
- Local **anesthetizing** solutions (e.g., dynexan gel), if needed rinse the mouth with chamomile or sage tea, panthenol solution, or cream
- Antipyretics/analgesics (e.g., paracetamol)
- Systemic acyclovir administration (3 × daily 10 mg/ kg body weight i.v. for 10 days): in suspicion of generalized infection or severe disease course

39.4 The little girl's brother is 3 weeks old. The worried mother would like to know whether there is any danger for the little boy.

- Newborns are **not in danger** if the mother has had herpes simplex before the pregnancy (medical history) and thus has developed antibodies against HSV-1 that could be transferred to the child diaplacentally; in this case, hygienic measures (mask over mouth, hand disinfection) are sufficient but in the example case, this would be difficult to do.

Therefore, the 3-year-old girl should be isolated from the 3-week-old brother as much as possible.

- Newborns are **particularly in danger** of contracting a *Herpes simplex* infection (herpes neonatorum; clinical aspects: various disease courses: localized infection of skin, mucosa, or eyes; herpes encephalitis or disseminated systemic infection) if the mother has **not** had a herpes simplex infection. In that case, observe child. Treatment: with corresponding clinical symptoms, systemic acyclovir (3 × *daily* 10 mg/kg body weight i.v. for 10 days).

Comments

Etiopathogenesis: Herpes simplex viruses (HSV) belong to the group of human pathogenic herpes viruses. There are two types: HSV-1 usually causes diseases and inflammations of the skin and mucosa above the navel, HSV-2 below the navel (especially in the genital area). After the infection, the viruses persist in the cells of the regional sensory ganglia and can be reactivated by a variety of stimuli (e.g., febrile infections, UV sunlight irradiation, menstruation, and immunosuppression).

The **first herpes simplex virus infection** is usually not apparent. In small children, the primary infection often manifests as (ulcerative) herpetic gingivostomatitis. The incubation time is 2 to 12 days. Transmission is by close skin and body contact.

Epidemiology: The rate of endemic infection with herpes simplex virus is very high (90%) because of its pronounced contagiousness.

Clinical aspects: Numerous little blisters and painful ulcers on the lips and oral mucosa are characteristic for herpetic gingivostomatitis. High fever, refusal of food, difficulty swallowing, and regional swollen lymph glands can intensify the clinical picture.

The course of **neonatal herpes infection** is almost always symptomatic. There are either localized skin, eye, and mucosal infections, a CNS infection (herpes encephalitis), or very rarely, disseminated, systemic infection (sepsis-like clinical picture) with and without CNS involvement. At first, the symptoms of neonatal herpes infection can be quite unspecific and resemble sepsis (lethargy, hyperexcitability, vomiting, apnea, etc.). Approximately 60% of newborns exhibit herpetiform, possibly zoster-like, exanthema. In one-third of cases, there are lesions on the oral and pharyngeal mucosa. With CNS involvement, there are seizures and coma.

A *Herpes simplex* superinfection of an existing exanthema is called eczema herpeticum. Children with atopic dermatitis are affected particularly often. Herpetiform blisters are formed on the atopic or eczematous skin. The general condition of the child is severely impaired.

Diagnostics: The diagnosis is established clinically.

Treatment: Treatment is only symptomatic (see answer to question 39.3). Systemic treatment with acyclovir is only indicated in neonatal infection, a severe disease course (e.g., immunodeficiency, eczema herpeticum) or complications (e.g., herpes encephalitis).

Prophylaxis: Pregnant women with a genital herpes infection should be treated with acyclovir; with infection after the 34th week of pregnancy, the child should be delivered by cesarean section. Breastfeeding is permitted if the nipples are not affected by the infection and if hygiene is properly observed (hand disinfection, mask).

Because of the poor prognosis of herpes neonatorum, it is advisable to treat at-risk and premature children prophylactically with acyclovir if they have contact with fresh herpes efflorescences and lack maternal passive immunity, even in the absence of manifest herpes infection.

Children with herpetic gingivostomatitis should not be together with other children, i.e., they should not be allowed to go to kindergarten or school.

Prognosis: Later recurrence of herpetic gingivostomatitis takes the form of **orofacial herpes**. In this condition, there is localized oral reddening with itching, burning, and a feeling of tightness, which develops into papules, blisters, and crusts. These lesions heal within a few days, without scars.

The prognosis for the infection in newborns depends on the time when treatment is begun and the form in which the infection manifests. Nevertheless, it is very poor in spite of treatment in the disseminated, systemic form (lethality of more than 60%).

ADDITIONAL TOPICS FOR STUDY GROUPS
- Herpes zoster
- Perinatal infections

159

Case

39

→ Cases 39 Page 40

40.1   What is your suspected diagnosis? What other typical symptoms or findings do you look for?
- **Suspected diagnosis: Down syndrome**; rationale: slanted eyes, epicanthus, increased skin at back of neck, short, plump hands and feet, bilateral transverse palmar crease, space between first and second toes
- **Other possible morphological abnormalities:** Short stature, enlarged tongue, usually with gaping mouth, brachycephalic skull, anomalies of the external ear (folded helix), broad, flat nasal bridge, high palate, Brushfield spots (whitish stromal thickening in the iris), cataract, strabismus, excessively flexible joints, low muscle tone, prominent iliac wings, coxa valga, brittle nails, rough, dry, often mottled skin
- **Malformations and functional disorders of internal organs:** Cardiac (e.g., atrial and ventricular septal defects), gastrointestinal (e.g., duodenal stenosis, Hirschsprung disease, anular pancreas), immune deficiency, hypothyroidism, cryptorchism, male infertility

40.2   What is at the basis of the clinical picture?
Numerical chromosomal aberration of autosomes: The following forms exist:

- **Free Trisomy 21** (> 90%): There are three copies of chromosome 21, so the number of chromosomes is 47.
- **Translocation trisomy** (5%): Presence of two free copies of chromosome 21; the third Chromosome 21 is fused in the form of a central fusion with another acrocentric chromosome; the number of chromosomes is 46.
- **Mosaic trisomy 21** (in 2%): In addition to a cell line with trisomy 21, there is another cell line with a normal chromosome configuration.

40.3   What do you know about the prognosis for this disease?
The average life expectancy is decreased; only 10% of patients live to be older than 60. The life expectancy depends primarily on the severity of internal malformations and immune deficiency. These factors influence primarily heart failure, elevated susceptibility to infection, and an elevated risk of leukemia. However, the patients' life expectancy is rising appreciably since it has become possible to treat even severe heart disease and metabolic disorders. Furthermore, intelligence is decreased, and the incidence of Alzheimer disease is increased.

Comments

Epidemiology: Trisomy 21 is the most frequent chromosomal abnormality. It occurs with a frequency of 1:600–800 live births. The risk of trisomy 21 rises with the age of the mother (see Tab.).

The risk of repetition depends on the type of trisomy: In free trisomy, the risk of repetition is 2%; in translocation trisomy the risk is between 10% and 100%, depending on the type of translocation. In mosaic trisomy, the risk of repetition is exactly as frequent as in the first birth, since spontaneous mutations are involved.

For forms, see answer to question 40.2. Usually it is a free trisomy 21, but translocation or mosaic trisomy also occurs. In mosaic trisomy, the clinical symptoms can be less pronounced.

Clinical aspects: The children are remarkable for their **typical phenotype** (see case and answer to question 40.1). Malformations of internal organs occur frequently. Every second child with Down syndrome exhibits cardiac abnormalities (principally septal defects, atrioventricular canal defect). Low muscle tone usually results in marked nursing weakness in infancy. Intelligence is decreased (IQ usually < 50), development retarded. Mostly, reading and writing can be learned and simple tasks can be accomplished.

Diagnostics: The diagnosis is confirmed by **chromosome analysis**. It can usually already be established prepartally. Ultrasonography in the 12th to 14th week of pregnancy can establish neck edema from the neck transparency measurement. If the finding arouses suspicion, the diagnosis can be confirmed by **amniocentesis or** with a first-semester screening. This entails a coupling of the neck transparency measurement with a blood test, whereby the concentration of PAPP-A (pregnancy-associated plasma protein A) and β-HCG in the mother's serum is determined. The probability of a chromosomal aberration can be established from the results of this testing.

Mother's age in years	Incidence
20	1:1,925
25	1:1,205
30	1:885
35	1:365
40	1:110
45	1:32
49	1:12

Chorionic villus sampling and **chromosome analysis**, if the parents wish for termination of pregnancy in case of a positive result.

Treatment: Organ malformations such as heart defects or gastrointestinal atresia must be treated in accordance with severity. Adequate treatment is best ensured in special centers with interdisciplinary care.

For long-term care, the support of parents and family is of primary importance. There are numerous parents' associations and self-help groups. The child should receive physiotherapeutic (because of low muscle tone) and early ergotherapeutic and speech therapy to promote psychological-intellectual, linguistic, and psychomotor development. The strength of the patients lies especially in the concrete, cognitive area and in social behavior. They can be well encouraged here. It is desirable to place them in integration facilities. These institutions provide age-appropriate integrative kindergartens (contact with "healthy" children is important for encouragement), special integrative schools or, later, workshops or simple tasks in businesses.

Information and counseling for parents: See also Ullrich–Turner syndrome (case 35).

Always explain truthfully but gently. Explanation to the parents should always be provided by an experienced colleague. It is important for the parents to learn everything about the disease. This will often require several detailed conversations. It is important to check repeatedly whether the parents have understood everything and whether they need more help to process the information. In this way, the parents are given the opportunity to come to grips with the situation. It can be helpful to introduce the parents to self-help groups or to other families afflicted by the same tragedy.

Prognosis: See answer to question 40.3.

ADDITIONAL TOPICS FOR STUDY GROUPS
- Other clinical pictures resulting from gonosomal or autosomal chromosomal abnormalities (e.g., Edwards syndrome, Patau syndrome, Turner syndrome)

---

41 Pediculosis capitis (Head lice)

41.1 What is your suspected diagnosis?
Pediculosis capitis; rationale: patients' age; traces of scratching; eczema-like changes in scalp and neck (medical history and Fig. b [example case]); intense itching; little whitish eggs firmly attached to the hair near the scalp (Fig. a [Example case]).

41.2 How can you confirm the diagnosis?
Diagnosis on examination: Evidence of nits and lice, with the nits easier to recognize because of their white color. They resemble dandruff, usually stuck to the hair, and cannot be scraped off with the fingernails. Furthermore, a louse and nit comb can be used. This makes it possible to comb out the lice and especially nits, which are then stuck to the comb.

41.3 What treatment do you initiate?
- One-time treatment of scalp and hair with **antiparasitic drugs** (e.g., permethrin, pyrethrum, or dimeticon). Repeat after 7–9 days, depending on the preparation, to interrupt the development cycle of the lice (lice hatch after 8 days and are sexually mature after 2–3 weeks).
- **Nits:** Wash hair with warm vinegar water (one part food-grade vinegar 6% to two parts warm water, leave on 10 minutes), comb with fine comb.
- **Treatment of eczema caused by itching:** The approach is to wait; usually the eczema heals spontaneously since the itching decreases with the antiparasitic shampoo treatment, and scratching stops; if the eczema does not heal after about 5 days → local therapy with antiseptics (e.g., octenisept) and/or corticosteroid solutions.
- **Treatment of itching:** In case of intense itching, treatment with antihistamine preparations, e.g., loratadine (5–10 mg/d in one individual dose); the itching stops with time, since the lice die after treatment with antiparasitic drugs, and thus produce no more excreta and no longer suck blood (see Comments);

→ Cases 41 Page 42

recurrence of the itching after 5 to 8 days (due to hatching of lice from the nits) is prevented by repeating treatment with antiparasitic drugs (see above).

41.4 What additional recommendations do you give the family?
- Examination and, if necessary, treatment of all family members.
- Body hygiene, change bed clothes and wash in hot water (> 60°C), in winter wash head covering as well, place combs/brushes in hot water (temperatures over 60°C kill lice), pack non-washable articles in airtight bags for 2 to 4 weeks (lice starve under these conditions) or freeze for 2 days at –10°C.
- If infestation is repeated, inform kindergarten or school (examine and, if necessary, treat school-/ playmates).
- One day after correctly performed antiparasite treatment (the first shampoo and nit removal) children can return to public facilities.

Comments

Etiopathogenesis: A head louse (pediculus capitis) is a 2- to 4-mm long wingless, blood-sucking insect. Human beings are the only natural reservoir, i.e., transmission is from person to person. Poor hygiene promotes the spread but is not a condition of infestation. There are frequent "small epidemics" in kindergartens and schools.

Sexually mature females attach approximately 150 to 300 eggs (called nits) to hair with water-insoluble adhesive in the course of a lifetime (14–28 days). The lice hatch about 8 days later. They feed on blood which they suck every 2 to 3 hours. After 2 to 3 weeks, these lice are sexually mature and lay eggs in their turn. The itch is triggered when the lice suck blood and excrete a substance that causes an allergic reaction.

Clinical aspects: Intense itching is the cardinal symptom of infestation with head lice (Pediculosis capitis). Head lice invade head hair. In adolescents and adults, they can also infest beard and pubic hair; in children, eyelashes and eyebrows. Their bites produce raised red papules, especially behind the ears and on the neck. Scratching leaves scratch marks. Secondary infections are frequent, usually with *Streptococci* or *Staphylococci*, with purulent skin changes and swollen lymph nodes.

Diagnosis: See answer to question 41.2. The diagnosis is established by detection of nits and lice. Nits look like dandruff scales but are not as easy to brush off. Lice prefer to crawl around the hair shaft on the scalp, behind the ears and on the neck. They are easy to remove with tweezers and can then be examined with a magnifying glass or under a microscope (see Fig.).

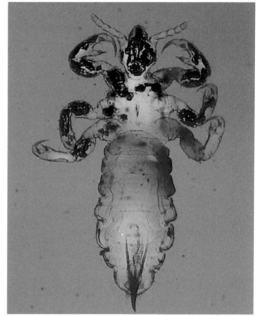

Head louse

Treatment: In addition to hygienic measures, treatment includes the use of antiparasitic preparations (see answer to question 41.3). Pemethrin seems to be the most efficacious, but other preparations, such as pyrethrum extract and remedies made from plant extracts such as coconut or neem are suitable treatments. Dimeticon is also a very effective treatment; it blocks the breathing apparatus of the louse, causing it to suffocate. Nowadays, the recommendation is not to use lindane-containing products because they are toxic. Use and treatment instructions should be

162

Case

41

→ Cases 41 Page 42

followed exactly. Treatment must be repeated after 7 to 9 days in order to catch any newly hatched lice. Nits must also be removed. This is best done with a fine-tooth comb (nit or louse comb), after the hair is washed with vinegar water. The vinegar diluted with water dissolves the adhesive.

Other family and household members are checked for lice and treated if necessary (see answer to question 41.4). This can prevent reinfection. To limit dissemination of the lice, patients should be isolated until the antiparasitic treatment has been completed.

Shaving the head, which used to be the usual and necessary treatment for louse infestation, is no longer indicated today because the current remedies work better and faster than the former ones.

Prognosis: It is very good, at the latest after the second treatment, the lice and nits are gone.

ADDITIONAL TOPICS FOR STUDY GROUPS
- Scabies
- Pediculosis vestimentorum and pubis

---

42   Sudden infant death

42.1   What is meant by "sudden infant death?" What does the acronym "SIDS" stand for?
- Sudden and unpredictable death of a healthy infant in its sleep (often in the early hours of the morning)
- On autopsy, no adequate cause of death can be recognized/demonstrated
- SIDS = Sudden infant death syndrome

42.2   How is the risk for this newborn of sudden infant death assessed? What do you explain to the parents?
The risk for siblings of a child that died of sudden infant death is increased by a factor of 1.6 to 5.
It is especially important to have a calming effect on the parents, and to make it clear to them that the risk is extremely low if risk factors that can be controlled are avoided (see answer to question 42.4 and Comments). In addition, careful training of parents in reanimation methods is very important (see case 65). For psychological reasons, the indication to watch the child with a home monitor should be broad. However, this does not decrease the risk; again and again, children die in spite of monitor supervision.

42.3   What diagnostic or treatment consequences result for the newborn?
- **Clinical examination of the child:** Rule out organ malformations/regulatory disorders; no abnormalities are found in SIDS children in comparison with "healthy" infants; particular attention should be given to breathing (rate, rhythm) so as to detect breathing disorders such as increased periodic breathing or extended breathing pauses. These can be signs of central disorders of respiratory regulation.
- **EKG:** An extended QT interval is a risk factor for SIDS.
- **Laboratory:** Differential blood count, calcium (↑ or ↓), blood sugar (↓)
- If necessary, **EEG:** cerebral attacks
- If necessary, **polysomnography** (electrophysiological examination in the sleep laboratory: EKG + EEG +

respiratory excursion + oxygen saturation + respiratory flow through nose and mouth): Recording of obstructive and central apnea, bradycardia, hypoxemia; indications: in siblings of SIDS children, ALTE (see Comments), unexplained attacks of cyanosis, suspicion of obstructive apnea
- **Further tests if necessary:**
  - If there is a family history of congenital metabolic disorders associated with breathing disorders (see Comments/Differential diagnosis)
  - Skull sonography: structural abnormalities (e.g., Dandy–Walker malformation), space-occupying lesions, signs of cerebral pressure (expanded ventricular spaces)
- If necessary, home monitoring: if there is a family history of ALTE or other risk factors for possible SIDS (see Comments) to monitor respiratory/cardiac frequency and oxygen saturation (optional)
- **Parents must be familiar with resuscitation techniques!**

42.4   What do you recommend to the parents in order to decrease the risk of sudden infant death?
- In the first year, infants should sleep on their backs on a firm mattress that does not give under their weight. There should be no pillow or cushioned bumper "nest" (see Fig.).
- Infants should be placed in bed in such a way that their heads cannot be covered with the bedding; to prevent entanglement/strangulation in the bedding, a baby sleeping bag is recommended.
- Infants should sleep in their parents' bedroom, but in their own beds.
- Infants should grow up in a smoke-free environment.
- Room temperature should be at 18–20°C; blanket and night clothes should be neither too warm nor too cold for the child.
- Breastfeeding and pacifiers can also have calming effect on the child.

→ Cases 42 Page 43

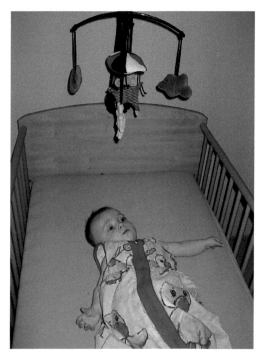

Optimal sleeping position for an infant

| **Comments**

Definition: See answer to question 42.1.

Epidemiology: Sudden infant death is the most frequent cause of death and accounts for approximately 40% of deaths in the first year of a child's life in the industrialized world. The peak frequency lies between the second and fourth months; 95% of infants die from SID following the neonatal period (first 4 weeks) and before the tenth month. Boys are somewhat more frequently affected than girls (♂ : ♀ = 60%: 40%). Two-thirds of SID cases occur in the cold, high-infection time of year. Since 1994, a broad-based campaign has brought about a 50% decrease in SIDS in the United States.

Etiology: The cause of sudden infant death is still unexplained. At present, it is assumed that the genesis is multifactorial, i.e., both endogenous (e.g., instability of autonomic central regulatory mechanisms such as respiratory and circulatory) and exogenous factors (e.g., prone position, overwarming, low oxygen while the infant is sleeping) play a role.

Risk factors: Epidemiological studies have found a number of factors that appears significantly more often in children who died of SIDS. The two most important risk factors are:

- **Child sleeping in prone position** (risk increased tenfold) and
- **Mother younger than 21 years** (risk also increased almost ten-fold). The mother's age does not play a medical or biological role but is significant only because of insufficient knowledge about the background and risk factors of sudden infant death.

Additional risk factors are:
- Child sleeping on its side, because this makes it easier to roll into prone position.
- Soft sleeping surface.
- Excessive warmth while the child is sleeping.
- Sleeping in the parents' bed.
- Sleeping alone in a room.
- Smoking during pregnancy, because this leads to poor circulation in the placenta and thus to undersupply to the child. It is thought that this influences the respiratory center of the brain and reduces the frequency of arousal reactions.
- Forgoing breastfeeding (breastfeeding is also associated with a decrease in the risk of infection).

Children have a higher risk:
- If they have already suffered a seeming or obvious apparent **li**fe-**t**hreatening **e**vent (**ALTE**, near miss event) of unclear etiology. The associated symptoms include apnea, paleness and/or cyanosis, and listlessness.

→ Cases 42 Page 43

- If they come after a sibling who has died of sudden infant death (see answer to question 42.2.).
- If they are born prematurely with bronchopulmonary dysplasia, symptomatic apnea, or bradycardia.
- If they have smoking or drug-dependent parents.
- If they grow up among smokers.

Diagnosis: See answer to question 42.3.

Differential diagnoses of sudden infant death (explainable causes): Disorders of respiratory regulation; central, obstructive, or mixed apnea; cerebral space-occupying lesions associated with breathing disorders (e.g., lack of carnitine, lack of pyruvate dehydrogenase); foreign body aspiration; disturbed cardiac rhythm; infanticide.

Prophylaxis: See answer to question 42.4. It is important to reduce risk factors since at present this is the only way to decrease the danger of sudden infant death. By preventing infants from sleeping on their stomachs, the number of SIDS has decreased approximately 50%. Sleeping on the side, which is an unstable position, should also be avoided for the child. Most importantly, the child's head should not (be able to) be covered by the bed clothes, since this results in increased rebreathing of CO_2, displacement of the upper airways, and over-warming of the child. Heat can no longer be dissipated from head and face. Arousal reactions become less frequent.

The place where the child sleeps also influences the SIDS risk. If the child sleeps in its own bed in the parents' bedroom, the risk of SIDS is minimized. There is no plausible explanation for this fact. Nevertheless, it is possible that parents can more easily pick up subtle symptoms because they are so close to the child. *Caution:* Sleeping in the parents' bed increases the risk of SIDS.

Measures to be taken in suspicion of respiratory arrest: The first step is a careful attempt to wake up the child and if this fails, resuscitation (see case 65).

Conduct if SIDS occurs: If one is called as a physician to an infant who has died suddenly and there are sure signs of death, no further attempts at resuscitation should be undertaken. The parents must be told that their child has died and that the suspected cause of death is SIDS. Since the cause of death is unclear, it must be listed on the death certificate as "unclear." It must be explained to the parents that this does indicate any sort of suspicion. It must be made clear to the parents that the police will be involved and that the public prosecutor's office can order an autopsy to be performed on the child in order to clarify the cause of the child's death. The parents should then be given the opportunity to say goodbye to their child. In caring for the parents, it can be helpful to connect them with other parents who have suffered such a loss, for instance, through support groups like the CJ Foundation for SIDS or SIDS America.

43 Lobar pneumonia

43.1 What possible diseases are you considering? What studies do you order to arrive at a diagnosis?
- **Differential diagnoses:**
  - Gastroenteritis; rationale: abdominal pain, vomiting, fever
  - Acute appendicitis; rationale: high fever, vomiting, tense abdomen, diffuse pain on pressure
  - Pneumonia; rationale: fever, cough, tachypnea, flaring nostril breathing, moderate-to-fine crackles over the right lung, abdominal pain, inflammatory parameters ↑
  - Sepsis; rationale: high fever, poor general condition, inflammatory parameters ↑
  - Urinary tract infection/urosepsis; rationale: high fever, abdominal pain, inflammatory parameters ↑
- **Diagnostics:**
  - Laboratory: triple blood cultures (pathogen detection), possibly sputum test, or throat swab (pathogen detection), urine status (exclusion of urinary tract infection)
  - Thoracic X-ray: infiltrates as sign of pneumonia

  - Abdominal ultrasound: exclusion of appendicitis, free fluid, blocked renal pelvis

43.2 Describe what you see on the survey radiograph of the thorax. What is your diagnosis on the basis of the medical history, clinical picture, and diagnostic findings?
- **Thoracic X-ray:** Homogeneous, sharply outlined shadow on the upper right field of the lung (see Fig. case), otherwise, unremarkable thoracic X-ray
- **Diagnosis:** Lobar pneumonia right upper field

43.3 What pathogens do you suspect in the child? Which pathogens are quite commonly typical for the disease at this age? Which pathogens do you expect in newborns or school children?
- Principally typical for the disease at the patient's age are viruses (see below), but **lobar pneumonia** is chiefly caused by **pneumococci** (*Streptococcus pneumoniae*)

→ Cases 43 Page 44

- **1 month to 5 years:** Principally viruses (RSV, influenza, parainfluenza, adeno-, ECHO-, coxsackie-, rhinoviruses), bacteria (*Streptococcus pneumoniae, Haemophilus influenzae, Moraxella catarrhalis, Staphylococcus aureus* [especially in infants])
- **Newborns:** B-Streptococci, Staphylococci, Gram-negative enterobacteria (e.g., *E. coli, Klebsiella*), *Chlamydia*
- **School children:** Principally viruses (see above), *Mycoplasma pneumoniae, Chlamydia pneumoniae, Streptococcus pneumoniae, Haemophilus influenzae*

43.4 Name additional forms of this disease. Which pathogens do you expect in these forms?
- **Bronchopneumonia:** Principally viruses
- **Interstitial pneumonia:** Principally viruses, mycoplasms

43.5 What treatment do you initiate?
- **Hospital admission:** i.v. fluid replacement required (the boy is hardly eating or drinking), i.v. antibiotic treatment necessary (inflammatory parameters ↑)
- i.v. **antibiotic treatment** with cefuroxime (75–100 mg/kg body weight/d in 2–3 individual doses)
- **Symptomatic measures:** Bed rest, sufficient fluids (infusion therapy), humidified air, oxygen administration in case of hypoxia, inhalation therapy with 0.9% NaCl solution, and breathing exercises for secretolysis

Comments

Definition and forms: Pneumonias are inflammatory diseases of the pulmonary parenchyma. They are among the frequent airway diseases in children.

Pneumonias are classified as bronchial, lobar, or interstitial pneumonias, depending on the morphology. **Bronchial pneumonia** is the most frequent form of pneumonia in children. The inflammatory changes affect the respiratory pathways and the neighboring portions of the pulmonary parenchyma. The boundaries between bronchitis and bronchial pneumonia are fluid. In lobar pneumonia, the inflammatory changes are limited to the pulmonary parenchyma of a lung segment or lobe. In interstitial pneumonias, it is primarily the perivascular or interalveolar connective tissue that is inflamed.

Etiology: The pathogen spectrum of community acquired pneumonia varies as a function of age (see answer to question 43.3). Transmission of the pathogens is primarily through droplet infection. Pneumonias contracted by hospitalized patients are usually caused by more or less resistant hospital germs (Gram-negative bacilli, *Staphylococci*, fungi, etc.). Secondary pneumonias develop as a result of immunosuppression (e.g., immune deficiency syndromes, chemotherapy), underlying diseases (e.g., cystic fibrosis, tuberculosis, AIDS), or foreign body aspiration.

Clinical aspects: Clinical symptoms of pneumonia are coughing (first dry, then productive), fever, abnormal breathing (dyspnea, tachypnea, flared nostrils, labored breathing [air is audibly expressed from the lungs], with accompanying obstruction, thoracic retractions), and possible cyanosis (oxygen saturation < 90%) and chest pains (with associated pleuritis). The feeling of illness can be more or less intense. Often there are associated symptoms such as tiredness, vomiting, loss of appetite, and often abdominal pain ("pneumonia stomach" is an accompanying inflammatory reaction of the peritoneum in pleuritis). *Note:* In every case of acute abdomen in children, the possibility of pneumonia should be considered.

Bacterial pneumonia is usually more severe and is associated with high fever and more intense signs of inflammation.

Diagnostics: The diagnosis is usually established clinically and radiologically. On auscultation, fine crackles, on percussion, circumscribed dullness. In the thoracic X-ray, in lobar pneumonia the affected lobe is shadowed, with sharp borders; in interstitial pneumonia, there is an increased network or stripe pattern in the lung tissue. In bronchial pneumonia, the typical X-ray shows multiple, confluent consolidation; the perihilar stripe pattern is often also intensified. Laboratory tests of the blood picture, inflammatory parameters (CRP, sedimentation rate), blood gas analysis (BGA) are obligatory; if the course is severe, the pathogen should be confirmed in blood culture, by a throat swab, or sputum.

In pneumococcal or staphylococcal pneumonia, sonographically demonstrable pleural effusions or pleural empyema can form.

The "pneumonia abdomen" can be seen in the thoracic X-ray as a distended transverse colon with a small number of haustra, covering the stomach.

Differential diagnoses: See answer to question 43.1.

Treatment: In treatment, the age (typical pathogen spectrum, see answer to question 43.3) and particularly the clinical picture must be kept in mind.

Differentiation between bacterial and viral origin is often difficult. Usually, treatment is with antibiotics, also to avoid bacterial superinfection in viral pneumonia. Where the course of the disease is severe or in the case of young infants, antibiotic treatment should be administered intravenously; in less severe courses, treatment can be oral. Depending on the clinical picture and the probable pathogens, macrolides are used (e.g., erythromycin 40–60 mg/kg body weight/d), and cephalosporins efficacious against *Staphylococci* (e.g., cefuroxime 75–100 mg/kg body weight/d) or penicillins (50,000–100,000 IU/kg body weight/d) may be used over 7 to 14 days.

In addition, **supportive measures** are employed, such as oxygen administration in hypoxia, inhalation treatment with salbutamol and ipratropium bromide in bronchial obstruction, analgesics (e.g., ibuprofen) in case of associated pleuritis (suppression of painful cough can otherwise lead to retention of secretions) as well as sufficient fluids (if necessary infusion therapy) and physical measures such as nebulizer inhalation with table salt solution and physiotherapy for secretolysis. High fever is reduced, for instance, with paracetamol.

Pleural effusions or empyema must be drained.

Prognosis: Pneumonia in the newborn used to be a severe clinical picture with a poor prognosis and a high mortality rate. Because of good monitoring and treatment options, the prognosis today is usually good if treatment begins early. After the newborn period, the prognosis is very good with early and adequate treatment.

ADDITIONAL TOPICS FOR STUDY GROUPS
- Foreign body aspiration
- Tuberculosis
- Cystic fibrosis
- Bronchitis/mild airway infections
- Bronchiolitis

44 Urinary tract infection and vesicoureterorenal reflux

44.1 What do you do next?
- **Hospital admission:** For further diagnostics and i.v. antibiotic treatment if necessary
- **Laboratory:**
  - Verify urinary tract infection: For methods of obtaining urine, see case 24; urine status (leukocytes, erythrocytes, nitrite, albumin), urine microscopy (erythrocyte morphology, casts), urine bacteriology (urine culture)
  - Blood: Blood panel, inflammation parameters (CRP, sedimentation rate), creatinine, urea
- **Sonography of kidneys and urinary bladder:** Blockage at renal pelvis, malformations, urine transport disorders
- **In confirmed urinary tract infection:**
  - i.v. antibiotic treatment for 7 to 14 days: initial calculated antibiotic treatment with cephalosporins (e.g., cefuroxime); after receipt of antibiogram, possible change, e.g., to ampicillin (80–300 mg/kg body weight/d) in combination with aminoglycoside antibiotic (e.g., gentamicin 3–5 mg/kg body weight/d)
  - Infusion therapy: to "rinse" the kidneys and efferent urinary tract
  - Antipyretics and analgesics: paracetamol or ibuprofen

44.2 Explain the course of the examination.
- **Principle:**
  - Retrograde filling of the urinary bladder through bladder catheters (insert under sterile conditions) or suprapubic catheter (chiefly in suspicion of urethral valve) with contrast medium
  - Urination under fluoroscopy with evaluation of bladder volume, bladder wall, urethra, reflux
- **Indications:** Suspicion of subvesicular obstacle (urethral stenosis, diverticulum), vesicoureterorenal reflux
- *Caution:* **Voiding cystourethrography (VCUG)** should only be performed 4 to 6 weeks after a urinary tract infection has healed, since infection-dependent functional bladder disorders can lead to false-positive examination results. If possible, the examination should be conducted with antibiotic prophylaxis to avoid iatrogenic urinary tract infections.

44.3 Interpret the finding from the MCU (see Fig.). Explain the stage classification of the disease.
- **MCU:** Grade III vesicoureterorenal reflux right, i.e., backflow of urine from the urinary bladder into the urethra, slight dilation of the ureter, slight dilation of the renal pelvis
- Stage classification of the vesicoureterorenal reflux (see Tab. and Fig.)

44.4 What additional treatment do you recommend for this patient?
Grade I to III vesicoureterorenal reflux:
- Antibiotic prophylaxis of urinary tract infection for 6 months (e.g., with cefaclor 10 mg/kg body weight or trimethoprim 1–2 mg/kg body weight in one single dose evening)

→ Cases 44 Page 45

- Then repeat MCU:
  - Result unchanged or worse: Collagen injection of the affected ureter or anti-reflux plasty with ureteral reimplantation
  - Result improved: Continuation of urinary tract prophylaxis for another 6 months, then check-up
  - Urinary tract infection during long-term prophylaxis: Immediate check-up

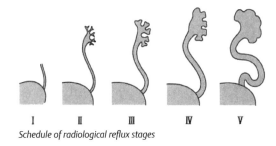

Schedule of radiological reflux stages

Stage classification of the vesicoureterorenal reflux (according to International Reflux Study Group)	
Grade I	Reflux only into ureter
Grade II	Reflux into the ureter and the renal pelvis calyx system without dilation
Grade III	Beginning dilation; slight or moderate dilation of the renal pelvis and slight or moderate blunting of the calyces
Grade IV	Increasing dilation and tortuosity of the ureter; moderate dilation of the renal pelvis and calyces; complete blunting of the fornices
Grade V	Marked dilation and meandering tortuosity of the ureter; marked dilation and plumping of the entire renal duct system

Case
44

Comments

Definition: A urinary tract infection is characterized by colonization or invasion of the urinary tract and kidneys by bacteria and subsequent significant bacteriuria. This results in local or generalized signs of inflammation (for instance, leukocyturia, fever).

Etiopathogenesis: The most frequent pathogens of urinary tract infections are Gram-negative germs from the intestinal tract. *Escherichia coli* can be found in more than **80%** of cases, *Proteus* varieties, *Enterococci, Klebsiella,* etc. in 10%. In anatomical or functional urine transport disorders, *E. coli* are less frequently found. Here the most frequent form is *Pseudomonas aeruginosa.*

Usually it is a matter of ascending infections via the urethra and urinary bladder. In newborns and infants, the colonization of the urinary tract is usually hematogenous in the context of bacteremia or newborn sepsis.

A confirmed, febrile urinary tract infection should always trigger further diagnostics in order to rule out malformations of the urinary tract, e.g., obstructions or obstacles to outflow (e.g., urethral valves, cystoceles) as well as vesicoureterorenal reflux as a cause.

In **vesicoureterorenal reflux** (VUR) urine flows out of the urinary bladder back into the ureters as far as the kidneys. **Primary VUR** occurs in 0.5% to 1% of all children. Girls are more often affected than boys. Usually the closure mechanism of the ureteral

ostium is defective as a result of a deformed junction (e.g., ectopic junction) of the ureter with the bladder. According to an international classification, VUR has 5 degrees of severity (see answer to question 44.3). The reflux itself does not cause any difficulties. It only becomes symptomatic as a result of recurring urinary tract infections. Complications arise through the spread of germs from the bladder into the renal duct system. At higher degrees of reflux severity, there is a risk of pressure damage to the renal parenchyma. **Secondary VUR** results from increased internal bladder pressure due to outflow obstacles or in acute or chronic cystitis caused by edematous swelling of the ureteral ostium.

Clinical aspects: The clinical signs of a urinary tract infection depend on the patient's age and the location of the infection. Infants usually exhibit unspecific clinical symptoms such as a high fever, vomiting, weakness in drinking, and swollen abdomen (see case 24). In older children, fever and abdominal pain as well as renal beds that are painful on percussion suggest pyelonephritis. Alguria, dysuria, pollakisuria, and secondary enuresis (bed wetting) indicate infection of the lower urinary tract.

Diagnostics: Diagnosis of a urinary tract infection can only be established if there is **significant bacteriuria.** A **urine culture** with clean urine must be

→ Cases 44 Page 45

performed. For older children, this can usually be obtained spontaneously with mid-stream urine; with toddlers and infants the urine is best obtained by bladder puncture or catheterization. A urinary tract infection is considered confirmed if a culture of mid-stream urine contains more than 10^4 germs. In urine obtained by bladder puncture, any germ growth indicates an infection. In a urinary tract infection, the urinary status exhibits bacteriuria, leukocyturia, and at least a microhematuria. Nitrite (e.g., in *E. coli*) is often positive and indicates a urinary tract infection. There are also bacteria (e.g., *Pseudomonas*) that produce no nitrite.

In every case of confirmed urinary tract infection, **sonography** of the kidneys and efferent urinary ducts must be performed. This can provide indications of urine transport disorders such as dilated ureters. In addition, to rule out other malformations of the urinary tract (obstructions/outflow blockage, vesicoureterorenal reflux, etc.), a **micturating cysto-urethrography** (MCU) should be performed.

Treatment: See answer to question 44.1. For treatment of grades I to III vesicoureterorenal reflux, see answer to question 44.4. Grades IV and V are usually corrected with Cohen anti-reflux plasty. In this process, the ureter is replanted in the roof of the bladder after tunneling under the submucosa.

Prognosis: In VUR grades I to III, there is a high rate of spontaneous healing. In grades IV and V, operative treatment is usually necessary in order to prevent development of a shrunken kidney with associated renal function limitation.

ADDITIONAL TOPICS FOR STUDY GROUPS
- Malformations of the urinary tract (e.g., urethral valves)
- Urosepsis
- Pyelonephritis
- Acute abdomen

45 Acute lymphatic leukemia

45.1 How do you interpret the findings?

Acute lymphatic leukemia; rationale: paleness, fatigue, coarse, hard lymph node swelling, anorexia, shoulder girdle pain (sign of skeletal infiltration), hepatosplenomegaly, possible weakened resistance to infection (which could result in bronchopneumonia); laboratory: normochromic anemia, leukocytes ↑, LDH ↑, thrombocytes ↓, uric acid ↑; blood smear: lymphoblasts

45.2 What further diagnostic measures do you initiate?

- **Bone marrow puncture with smear:** Cytological diagnosis by detection of blasts in the bone marrow smear (proportion of blasts to nucleated cells > 25%)
- **Laboratory (additional):** Potassium ↑, phosphate ↑, calcium ↓ (+ LDH ↑ + uric acid ↑ (see above); caused by increased cell death = tumor lysis syndrome), virus serology (e.g., CMV, EBV → reactivation possible in case of decreased resistance)
- **Abdominal ultrasound:** Hepatosplenomegaly, intra-abdominal lymphomas, kidney infiltration
- **Lumbar puncture:** Rule out/detect CNS involvement (tumor cells)
- **Thoracic X-ray:** Mediastinal enlargement, pleural effusion
- **Skeletal scintigraphy:** Location of bone foci
- **MRI/CT:** In addition to location of involved organs (e.g., lymphoma in thoracic/abdominal space, CNS/bone marrow involvement)

45.3 How will this disease be treated, if your diagnosis is confirmed?

- **Treatment objective:** Cure by destruction of the entire leukemia cell population.
- Chemotherapy in studies with defined protocols; several therapy phases:
  - **Induction therapy (5 weeks), followed up by induction consolidation (4 weeks):** combination of prednisone and several cytostatics such as vincristin, daunorubicin, L-asparaginase, and methotrexate. If necessary, additional cyclophosphamide, cytarabine, 6-mercaptopurin, etoposide, tioguanine; objective: reduction of leukemia cells, regeneration of normal hematopoiesis, < 5% blasts in bone marrow.
  - Extra compartmental therapy (over 8 weeks) in case of remission through induction therapy. It has the objective of destroying further leukemia cells and maintaining remission. Other drug combinations are selected for this purpose, usually with 6-mercaptopurine and methotrexate. During this phase, cytostatics are preventively administered intrathecally (usually methotrexate), and if appropriate, the skull is irradiated. The CNS treatment is repeated in additional treatment cycles.
  - **Reinduction therapy** (over 7 weeks): the course is similar to that of induction therapy with high doses of cytostatic combinations (vincristin, doxorubicin, L-asparaginase, thioguanine, cytarabine, cyclophosphamide, and dexamethasone). The

→ Cases 45 Page 46

objective is to minimize the risk of a relapse by complete destruction of all cancer cells.
- **Maintenance therapy** (up to a total treatment duration of 2 years): last phase of chemotherapy (usually with 6-mercaptopurine or thioguanine and methotrexate). It can usually be administered on an outpatient basis, i.e., attendance at kindergarten and school are most often allowed. The objective is to allow for the longest treatment period possible, to destroy the last surviving leukemia cells in order to prevent relapses.
- **Supportive measures**: For example, treatment of hemorrhages with thrombocyte concentrates or fresh plasma, infection prophylaxis (e.g., antibiotics, antimycotics, vaccinations), mouth rinses to avoid damage to mucosa, pain therapy, psychological and social-pedagogic care.

- **Stem cell transplantation**: Replacement of diseased with healthy bone marrow; in ALL only, if there is a high risk of recurrence (depending on ALL subtype), in poor response to chemotherapy, as well as in high-risk patients (see below); after intensive radiation and chemotherapy (conditioning = all leukemia cells present in the body should have been destroyed) bone marrow stem cells are infused; stem cells can come from the patient (autologous) or from a donor (allogeneic).

45.4 **Name additional risk factors that promote this disease.**
- Genetic factors, e.g., trisomy 21, Fanconi anemia
- Exposure to radiation
- Chemical substances, e.g., benzol, cytostatics

Comments

Definition and forms: Leukemias are malignant diseases of the hematopoietic system. Proliferation of immature hematopoietic cells (blasts) causes suppression of normal hematopoiesis in the bone marrow and infiltration of extramedullary organs.

A distinction is made between acute and chronic forms. Depending on which cell line is neoplastic, a distinction is made between lymphatic and myeloid leukemias.

Acute lymphatic leukemia is a malignant disease of the lymphatic system that manifests in the bone marrow, the peripheral lymphatic tissue, and in all other organs. In **acute myeloid leukemia**, the malignant cells develop from the various precursor stages of granulo-, mono-, erythro-, and thrombocytopoiesis. Disorders of bone marrow function that persist over a long period and develop into acute myeloid leukemia are called myelodysplastic syndrome.

Epidemiology: Thirty percent to 35% of children's cancers are leukemias. Twenty percent of cases are acute lymphatic leukemia (ALL), and 20% are acute myeloid leukemia (AML). The remainder consists of myelodysplastic syndrome and chronic forms. In the United States, there are 3,000 new cases of ALL every year among children and adolescents (0–19). Boys are affected somewhat more frequently than girls. About 500 children and 230 adolescents in the United States are diagnosed with AML each year.

Etiopathogenesis: Predisposing factors are diseases with chromosomal abnormalities, immune deficiency diseases (e.g., trisomy 21, ataxia telangiectasia, neurofibromatosis), and exposure to carcinogens (see answer to question 45.4). Normal hematopoiesis in the bone marrow is suppressed by uncontrolled growth of immature hematopoietic cells.

The consequences are anemia, thrombocytopenia, and granulocytopenia; extramedullary organs are infiltrated.

Classification: Acute leukemias are classified according to cytomorphological, cytochemical, and immunocytological criteria. In addition, immunophenotyping, cytogenetic, and molecular genetic examinations should follow. This permits a distinction between good and poor prognoses, determination of risk groups, and selection of the therapy.

The FAB (French–American–British) cytomorphological classification is based on cell size, cell shape, nuclear chromatin, nucleoli, the fraction of cytoplasm, the basophilia in the cytoplasm, and the vacuoles and granules in the cytoplasm. ALL is subdivided cytomorphologically into FAB types L1–L3, and AML into M0–M7.

The most important subdivision is the one depending on the antigen pattern of the lymphoblasts in ALL into a B (85%)- and a T (15%)-cell line. Various subtypes (Pro-BALL, common ALL, Pre-B ALL, B-ALL, Pro- and Pre-T ALL, intermediate and mature T-ALL) can be identified.

Cytogenetic and molecular genetic examinations almost always provide proof of numerical or structural aberrations in the leukemia genome and this is relevant to the prognosis.

Clinical aspects: The course of acute leukemia varies. Symptoms usually develop within a few days to weeks (usually < 4 weeks). Children complain frequently of fatigue; they are listless and have no appetite. Weight loss, subfebrile temperatures, and elevated tendency to sweat (B symptoms) can occur. Children often complain of bone or joint pain. Smaller

170

Case

45

children, in particular, do not want to walk any more. Neutropenia facilitates infection, and thrombocytopenia may cause petechiae and mucosal bleeding. The illness can also have very few symptoms.

In AML 1–5, lymphadenopathies are more frequent than in ALL. In AML the first manifestation can be accompanied by disseminated intravascular clotting. Gingival hyperplasia and parotid swelling can also point to the presence of AML. Infiltration of tear and salivary glands leads to decreased secretion of saliva and tears (Mikulicz syndrome).

Diagnostics: A suspected diagnosis can often be established by means of the medical history and symptoms. In addition to a blood panel, differential blood panel, and bone marrow study, further blood studies are necessary for establishment of a diagnosis (see answer to question 45.2). The blood picture shows anemia and thrombocytopenia; the leukocyte count can be elevated or lowered. In addition to normal, mature cells, the characteristic blasts, immature leukocyte precursors, can be seen.

Diffuse infiltration of blasts, which suppress normal hematopoiesis, can be seen in the bone marrow smear. The cell picture is monomorphic. In acute leukemia, the proportion of blasts to nucleated cells in the bone marrow > 25%; intermediate steps in myelopoiesis are lacking (leukemia gap).

The single morphological characteristic for leukemia, the Auer rods, is found in AML (see Fig.). For further diagnostics, see answer to question 45.2.

Possible symptoms of ALL and frequency of their occurrence

ALL symptoms	Frequency
Tiredness, fatigue, feeling of illness	Very frequent
Paleness, low capacity, dyspnea due to anemia	Approximately 80% of patients
Fever	Approximately 60% of patients
Increased tendency to infection due to granulocytopenia	Frequent
Swollen lymph nodes (cervical, axillary, inguinal)	Approximately 60% of patients
Abdominal pain, loss of appetite due to enlargement of liver and spleen	Approximately 60% of patients
Tendency to hemorrhage due to thrombocytopenia	Approximately 50% of patients
Bone and joint pain due to skeletal infiltration	Approximately 20% of patients
Neurological symptoms such as headache, vision disorders, cranial nerve paralysis, vomiting due to cerebral attack	Approximately 5% of patients
Dyspnea, inspiratory stridor due to enlargement of thymus, mediastinal lymph nodes	Approximately 5% of patients
Testicular enlargement due to leukemic infiltration	Very rare
Exophthalmos due to retrobulbar infiltration	Very rare

Treatment: Treatment of acute leukemia is administered in the context of studies with defined therapeutic protocols, in centers for pediatric oncology. The objective of treatment is complete destruction of all leukemia cells in the body, thus giving the bone marrow the opportunity to resume its function as a blood-forming organ. The most important component of therapy is intensive polychemotherapy. In some patients, supplementary skull irradiation is necessary. The selection of therapeutic form is determined according to the risk group into which the patient falls, from which sub-form of ALL the patient is suffering, how aggressively the cancer cells have spread throughout the body, and how well the disease is responding to the treatment. In high-risk patients (infants, children > 10 years, high leukemia cell count at the time of diagnosis, initial CNS involvement, translocations [9;22] and t[4;11], non- or late-responder to chemotherapy) a supplementary **bone marrow transplant** may be indicated. It usually takes place within 3 months after a remission is achieved. Even for patients who have already experienced a relapse and for whom there is a high risk of relapse after a second remission, stem cell transplantation presents the only chance for a cure.

Chemotherapy is administered in several cycles so that leukemia cells that were in the resting phase

→ Cases 45 Page 46

during the first cycle can be destroyed in one of the next cycles. In the resting phase between therapy cycles, the body can regenerate healthy tissue that was also destroyed. Resistance to the chemical therapeutic agents is combatted by rotation of drug combinations. Since cytostatics cannot cross the blood–brain barrier, they must also be administered **intrathecally.**

If a CNS involvement is already detected at the time of diagnosis, the intrathecal administration of cyto-statics is supplemented with skull irradiation.

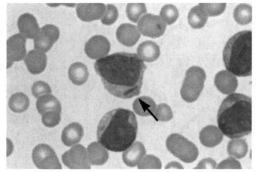

Bone marrow smear: Acute myeloid leukemia. Four blasts that are larger than lymphocytes, whose nuclear structure seems loose and some of which contains nucleoli. In the cytoplasm of one cell there is a reddish rod (arrow), an Auer rod.

In addition to the antileukemic therapy, treatment must also be provided for complications of leukemia and adverse effects of the therapy (e.g., nausea, vom-iting, hair loss). Thus, for instance, where there is a tendency to hemorrhage or anemia, it can become necessary to administer whole blood or thrombo-cyte concentrates, to isolate the patient temporar-ily for infection prophylaxis (at leukocyte counts

< 2,000/µL), or antibiotic or antimycotic therapy (protection against the patient's own microflora).

The diagnosis of "Leukemia" produces the most contradictory emotions in parents and child. Many people equate this diagnosis with a death sentence. But childhood leukemia has a very good chance of a cure. This should be emphasized in conversation. It goes without saying that the explanation of clinical picture, situation, and prognosis must be open and honest. The diagnosis must also be communicated to the child, in an age-appropriate way so that they can understand and cooperate in the need for the invasive therapeutic measures. The long hospital stay presents a particular psychological burden due to the loss of the child's accustomed environment (friends, family, school). Interdisciplinary teamwork with clergy, psychologists, social workers, and sup-port groups is very important for the wellbeing of parents and patient. The disease is often a heavy burden for the family. For this reason, both parents should be equally included in the treatment process.

Prognosis: Without treatment, the prognosis of acute leukemia is unfavorable. With adequate treat-ment the overall prognosis for relapse-free survival of ALL is approximately 80% to 85% and of AML approximately 40%. Infants, children > 10 years, and patients with high leukemia cell mass at the time of diagnosis or initial CNS involvement have a poorer prognosis.

ADDITIONAL TOPICS FOR STUDY GROUPS
- Chronic leukemias
- Myelodysplastic syndrome
- Malignant lymphomas
- (Non-Hodgkin lymphoma, Hodgkin disease)

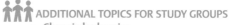

46   Kawasaki syndrome

46.1   What is your suspected diagnosis? What treatment do you initiate?
- **Measles**; rationale: morbilliform exanthema, fever, conjunctivitis, cervical lymph node swelling, child's age
- **Treatment:** Symptomatic (measles is a viral disease) with bed rest, antipyretic measures (e.g., parac-etamol, leg wraps)

46.2   What diagnosis must now be considered?
- Measles infection complicated by superinfection; rationale: persistent high fever, deterioration of the general condition, conjunctivitis, exanthema

- Toxic shock syndrome: high fever, poor general condition, exanthema
- Kawasaki syndrome; rationale: therapy-resistant fever > 4 days, conjunctivitis bilaterally, reddened oral mucosa, swollen cervical lymph nodes, morbill-iform exanthema over whole body, inner surfaces of hands and feet reddened/swollen
- Systemic juvenile chronic arthritis; rationale: very sick child with joint pain and fever > 39°C, polymor-phous exanthema, hepatosplenomegaly
- Other forms of collagenosis, e.g., juvenile derma-tomyositis; rationale: joint involvement, fever, exanthema

- Toxic allergic exanthema (due to drugs); rationale: exanthema, paracetamol ingestion

46.3 What is the most likely diagnosis? What is the underlying cause? How do you confirm this diagnosis?

- Kawasaki syndrome (def.: acute or subacute systemic vasculitis of the small and medium arteries)
- Five of the six cardinal symptoms are sufficient to establish a diagnosis; in the patients described, all six cardinal symptoms are present
- **The six cardinal symptoms are:**
  1. antibiotic-resistant fever > 5 days (remitting with peaks over 40°C, which indicates antipyretics)
  2. Conjunctivitis bilaterally
  3. Changes in oral mucosa and lips (exanthema, "chapped lips," "strawberry tongue," marked reddening of the oropharyngeal mucosa)
  4. Palmar and plantar erythema and edema with large flaking of finger and toe tips in the second to third week of illness
  5. Polymorphous exanthema, particularly on the trunk
  6. Swollen cervical lymph nodes
- The following pathological **laboratory** values are found: Sedimentation rate ↑, CRP ↑, leukocytosis

with left shift, anemia, thrombocytosis (often > 1 M/µL) in the third week of illness

46.4 What complications should you expect if your suspected diagnosis is correct?

- Heart: Pan-, myo-, or pericarditis (19%), formation of coronary aneurysms (6%–65% depending on the time the treatment was started) with a risk of thrombosing, myocardial infarction, rupture, and sudden cardiac death
- Kidneys: Proteinuria, hematuria (38%)
- Liver: Moderate hepatitis and icterus (45%), gallbladder hydrops (15%)
- CNS: Aseptic meningitis (17%), encephalopathy
- Joints: arthritis, oligo-/polyarthritis

46.5 What treatment do you initiate if your suspected diagnosis is correct?

- Hospital admission: For immunoglobulin therapy and diagnostics (see Comments)
- Immunoglobulin administration (once 2 g/kg body weight i.v.)
- Acetylsalicylic acid (ASA; 30–100 mg/kg body weight/d in four doses) until fever is gone, then 3 to 5 mg/kg/d for 6 to 8 weeks for inhibition of thrombocyte agglomeration
- Bed rest is not required!

Comments

Definition: Kawasaki syndrome (Syn.: mucocutaneous lymph node syndrome) is an acute or subacute systemic vasculitis of the small and medium arteries. There is also a systemic inflammation of many organs.

Epidemiology: The peak frequency occurs 1 and 2 years of age; after 10 years of age, the Kawasaki syndrome occurs only very rarely. The incidence in the United States is 4,200 children a year.

Etiology: The cause of the disease is not known. An infectious origin is under consideration, but no germ has so far been identified. Probably various pathogens interacting with a genetic basis lead to the disease picture.

Clinical aspects: The full disease is present when five of the six cardinal symptoms (see answer to question 46.3) or four of the six cardinal symptoms are present with coronary aneurysms. Other typical features are gastrointestinal complaints (e.g., diarrhea, vomiting, abdominal pain) as well as liver (e.g., hepatitis with icterus) and joint involvement (e.g., arthritis).

The disease progresses in three stages: The typical cardinal symptoms occur in the **acute phase** (7–14 days). In the second or third week of illness (**subacute phase**), fever, lymphadenopathy, and exanthema diminish. Coarse flaking of finger and toe tips as well as thrombocytosis of > 1 million/µL sets in. This is also the critical time for formation of arterial aneurisms, especially of the coronary artery.

Extracardiac arteries (e.g., proximal arm and leg arteries, mesenchymal, renal, and intracranial arteries) can also be affected, but this is much rarer.

This is followed by the **convalescence phase** (sixth to tenth week of illness, can last up to several months) with disappearance of all clinical signs, often even the aneurysms, and normalization of the blood sedimentation rate.

Caution: There are also atypical or incomplete courses of the disease.

For complications: See answer to question 46.4.

For diagnostics: See answer to question 46.3. For atypical or incomplete courses, the diagnosis is hard to establish; therefore, mistaken diagnoses are frequent (see case). Abdominal sonography can provide an important indication: A gallbladder hydrops develops in 15% of affected patients. Echocardiograms should be regularly done for early recognition

→ Cases 46 Page 47

of coronary aneurysm formation. Further diagnostics are determined by the clinical symptoms, e.g., lumbar puncture in suspicion of meningitis, EKG in suspicion of carditis. Blood cultures, throat smears, ANA screening, and serological examinations can be helpful for demarcation of the differential diagnoses.

Differential diagnoses: See answer to question 46.2. Scarlet fever, leptospirosis, EBV infection, measles, vasculitis syndromes, Still's disease.

Treatment: See answer to question 46.5. With failure to react to immunoglobulin, the dose can be repeated. If the second dose does not succeed, treatment with methylprednisolone is recommended. After the fever

is gone, a low dose of ASA (3–5 mg/kg body weight/d) is administered for at least 6 weeks for inhibition of platelet aggregation. If there are signs of coronary aneurysms, long-term therapy with a low dose of ASA for at least 8 weeks is necessary.

Prognosis: The prognosis is decisively influenced by cardiac involvement and the formation of coronary aneurysms. The risk can be decreased by adequate early treatment, preferably in the acute phase.

 ADDITIONAL TOPICS FOR STUDY GROUPS
- Exanthematic infectious diseases (e.g., measles, scarlet fever)
- Systemic juvenile chronic arthritis

47 Nephrotic syndrome

47.1 Make a suspected diagnosis. Name other findings and symptoms typical of your suspected diagnosis.
- **Suspected diagnosis: Nephrotic syndrome**; rationale: swollen face, particularly eyelid edema
- **Other findings and symptoms:** Generalized edema (particularly eyelid edema, calf edema), possibly ascites/pleural effusion (then also dyspnea), oliguria, possibly lack of appetite, fatigue, nausea, vomiting, diarrhea (due to edema in the gastrointestinal tract), vulnerability to infection, tendency to clotting

47.2 How do you confirm the diagnosis?
- **Laboratory:**
  - Urine: "major" proteinuria (> 1 g/m² body surface/d [for determination of body surface, see Comments], evidence in the 24-hour urine collection), hyaline casts, transitory microhematuria, leukocyturia, oliguria
  - Blood: Hct ↑, total protein < 50 g/L, immunoglobulins (α_2/β ↑), albumin ↓ (see Fig. Protein electrophoresis), blood sedimentation rate ↑, creatinine normal or ↑, cholesterol ↑(↑), C_3-fragment normal, double strand DNA antibodies negative
- **Sonography:** Abdomen (ascites), kidneys (size, morphological abnormalities), pleural effusions
- **X-ray:** Thorax (pleural effusion)

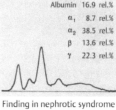

Albumin	55-70 rel.%
α_1	2-5 rel.%
α_2	5-10 rel.%
β	10-15 rel.%
γ	12-20 rel.%

Albumin	16.9 rel.%
α_1	8.7 rel.%
α_2	38.5 rel.%
β	13.6 rel.%
γ	22.3 rel.%

Normal finding   Finding in nephrotic syndrome

Protein electrophoresis

47.3 List the most frequent causes of this disease.
Minimal-change glomerulonephritis

47.4 How do you treat the disease in this child?
- **Hospital admission:** diagnostics, treatment (duration of hospital stay usually until remission, i.e., approximately 2–3 weeks)
- **Glucocorticoids** (initially i.v., later oral) according to the following schedule: prednisolone 60 mg/m² body surface/d for 6 weeks, additional 6 weeks 40 mg/m² body surface/d every 2 days
- Symptomatic measures (intake and output monitoring: moderate fluid intake [urine volume + 400 mL/m² body surface], albumin and diuretic only for marked edema, in infections, early antibiotic treatment, if necessary, thrombosis prophylaxis [seldom required])
- If therapy fails, see Comments

Comments

Definition and epidemiology: Nephrotic syndrome is characterized by the symptom triad of **edema**, **"serious" proteinuria** (> 1 g/m² body surface/d), and **hyperlipidemia**.

The age maximum for nephrotic syndrome lies between the ages of 1 and 10 years. Boys are approximately twice as frequently affected as girls.

Forms, etiopathogenesis, and clinical aspects: A distinction is made between primary (idiopathic) and secondary (symptomatic) nephrotic syndrome.

In 90% of cases it is a matter of a **primary nephrotic syndrome**. The cause are glomerular lesions, most frequently minimal change glomerulonephritis. Sometimes the disease is preceded by a viral infection. The loss of protein in the urine is due to increased permeability of the glomerular membrane to low-molecular-weight protein (albumin, transferrin, AT III, IgG). As a result, the serum protein concentration (particularly albumin) falls, and with it, the oncotic pressure. As a result, intravascular fluid is displaced into the interstitium. Edema, ascites, and pleural effusions form with simultaneous hypovolemia and oliguria. Children become increasingly thirsty. The danger of thrombosis is increased by hypercoagulability (caused by loss of AT III) and lack of intravascular volume. Vulnerability to infection is caused by the loss of immunoglobulins. Children are particularly endangered by sepsis and, in case of ascites, by peritonitis.

The less frequent **secondary nephrotic syndrome** (10% of cases) occurs as the result of systemic diseases (e.g., Lupus erythematosus, Schoenlein–Henoch purpura), chronic infections (e.g., hepatitis B HIV, EBV, post-streptococcal glomerulonephritis), metabolic diseases (e.g., diabetes mellitus), or drug-induced diseases (gold, D-penicillamine).

Diagnostics: Typical clinical aspects and examination results (see answer to question 47.1) can point the way. **Laboratory tests** confirm the diagnosis (see answer to question 47.2).

Blood lipids, especially cholesterol, can be massively elevated due to the high synthetic activity of the liver (to make up for the albumin deficiency). Determination of C_3 complement and double-strand DNA antibodies makes the differentiation of other, rarer forms of glomerulopathies (secondary nephrotic syndrome) possible.

A **kidney biopsy** is not indicated primarily but can be necessary for explaining the cause if therapy fails. Often, in steroid-resistant cases, a focal sclerosis is diagnosed, a serious glomerulopathy of unclear genesis.

Differential diagnoses: Other causes of generalized edema, e.g., angioneurotic edema, heart failure, protein malnutrition edema caused by insufficient nutrition or enteral loss.

Treatment and prognosis: An attempt at treatment is started with prednisolone according to a set schedule (see answer to question 47.4) Prednisolone is dosed according to body surface area. This surface area is calculated according to a normogram (see appendix/Nomogram). The body height is entered on the left axis and body weight is entered on the right. The two points are connected with a line. The intersection with the central axis gives the body surface.

In addition, in severe edema, fluid and salt intake must be reduced in order to prevent the occurrence of any further edema. Fluid levels must be carefully balanced. In severe cases, water excretion is induced by administration of human albumin followed by furosemide.

In 90% of cases the nephrotic syndrome is **steroid sensitive**, i.e., the symptoms decrease on this treatment.

Protein excretion in the urine continues to be monitored daily, for instance, with urine strips. A third of steroid-sensitive patients are healthy after the first episode. In another third of cases, there is a relapse or repeated relapses after the prednisolone is discontinued. The last third are steroid dependent, i.e., the children only remain symptom free if they receive steroid therapy. The first relapse is again treated with glucocorticoids. Further recurrences and steroid dependence are an indication for therapy with cytostatics (cyclophosphamide, cyclosporine A).

Forms that do not respond to cortisone are called steroid-resistant (10% of cases). No efficacious therapy for these is known. In consultation with a pediatric nephrology center, it is possible to consider therapy attempts with ACE inhibitors, cytostatics, or cyclophosphamide. The success of treatment is controversial. A serious course leads to kidney failure in a few years, with the need for dialysis and kidney transplantation.

👪 ADDITIONAL TOPICS FOR STUDY GROUPS
- Nephritic syndrome
- Glomerulonephritides

→ Cases 47   Page 48

48.1 Interpret the laboratory values. What causes associated with the medical history and clinical examination are you considering?

- **Laboratory:** Microcytic normochrome anemia (MCV ↓, MCH, and MCHC normal), reticulocytosis (evidence of hypergenerative erythropoiesis; possible causes: hemolytic anemia, hemorrhagic anemia)
- **Suspected diagnosis: Spherocytosis**; rationale: paleness, splenomegaly, scleral icterus, laboratory (see above), positive family history
- **Differential diagnoses:** Other hemolytic anemias (e.g., elliptocytosis, enzymatic defects [e.g., glucose-6-phosphate dehydrogenase deficiency])

48.2 How do you confirm the diagnosis?

Spherocytosis: Blood smear (evidence of spherocytes [spherical cells] and reticulocytes), decreased osmotic resistance of erythrocytes, if necessary electrophoretic and immunological examination of the erythrocyte membrane, additional laboratory tests (LDH ↑, haptoglobin ↑, indirect bilirubin ↑, direct bilirubin/GOT/GPT normal), abdominal sonography (liver/spleen size, gallstones)

48.3 What is your diagnosis?

Spherocytosis (hereditary spherical cell anemia); rationale: see answer to question 48.1; in blood smear,

evidence of spherocytes and reticulocytes (see Fig. example case)

48.4 Explain the pathogenesis of the disease.

- Membrane defect of the erythrocytes leads to altered ion permeability with resulting increased water flow into the cell → spherical shape of the erythrocytes.
- Pathologically deformed cells cannot pass through the splenic sinus quickly enough and are therefore broken down prematurely.

48.5 How can the disease be treated? What should be kept in mind here?

- Splenectomy with relapsing hemolytic crises
- If possible only after the age of 6 years because of the increased danger of infection resulting from asplenia; triple immunization preoperatively (*Pneumococci, Hemophilus influenzae B, Meningococci*); in children < 10 years, additional postoperative antibiotic prophylaxis with penicillin V for 2 years because of the danger of fulminant septicemia (OPSI = overwhelming post-splenectomy infection), particularly by encapsulated pathogens such as *Pneumococci, Meningococci,* and *Hemophilus influenzae*
- In a mild course: No additional treatment necessary
- With severe anemia: If appropriate, blood transfusion

Comments

Definition: Spherocytosis is caused by a **defect in the erythrocyte membrane**. Because of this defect, the erythrocytes assume a spherical shape, which makes them less susceptible to deformation. For this reason, they are prematurely broken down in the reticuloendothelial system (RES), especially in the spleen.

Epidemiology: At 1:5,000, spherocytosis is the most frequent hereditary hemolytic anemia in central Europe.

Etiopathogenesis: Inheritance is normally **autosomal-dominant** (75%); spontaneous mutations (25%) occur. The cause is a **defect in the erythrocyte membrane protein.** The chief component is usually spectrin; more rarely, ankyrin is quantitatively decreased. This leads to a change in ion permeability with an inflow of sodium and water into the erythrocytes, which then become spherical and less easily deformed. The spherical erythrocytes are phagocytized in the splenic sinus. Erythrocyte survival time is decreased.

Clinical aspects: In half of the cases, the disease already manifests in **newborns as severe**

hyperbilirubinemia (icterus gravis, prolongatus, praecox). Later the icterus is pronounced to varying degrees. Often (bilirubin) gallstones are detected in childhood. The children are pale and almost always exhibit splenomegaly. Infections (e.g., parvovirus B19 [fifth disease]) can trigger hemolytic and aplastic crises that are associated with severe icterus, nausea, fever, and upper abdominal pain.

Diagnostics: See answer to question 48.2. Microcytic normochrome anemia (Hb concentration usually between 6 and 10 g/dL), numerous spherocytes and reticulocytes in the blood smear, splenomegaly, and positive family history make the diagnosis of spherocytosis seem likely. Decreased osmotic resistance of the erythrocytes confirms the diagnosis. Additional characteristic laboratory changes such as reticulocytosis (6%–20%), (indirect) hyperbilirubinemia, elevated LDH, and decreased haptoglobin are an expression of hemolysis. The latter is also a cause of (bilirubin) gallstones that can sometimes already be sonographically verified in 4- and 5-year-old children. An enlarged spleen (splenomegaly) is regularly seen in sonography.

Treatment: The indication for transfusion is strictly set. It should only take place in aplastic or life-threatening crises.

In the case of gallstones, removal of the gallbladder may be necessary.

The folic acid requirement is elevated because of increased erythropoiesis. The disease can only be "cured" by **splenectomy**. This is indicated in relapsing hemolytic crises and repeated need for transfusion but should not be performed before 6 years of age because of the danger of **postsplenectomy sepsis**, and only after immunization (see answer to question 48.5). Preoperatively, spleen scintigraphy should be performed to rule out the presence of possible accessory spleens. These must also be removed in the operation. Splenectomy removes the "filter" that eliminates the deformed erythrocytes from the blood prematurely. After removal of the spleen, the erythrocyte survival time is normalized, although the corpuscular defect and the formation of spherical cells persist. After extirpation of the spleen, a transient thrombocytosis develops that usually requires no treatment.

Prognosis: After the splenectomy, the prognosis is usually good. Especially in girls, aplastic crises often develop in puberty because of hormonal changes and menstruation; these are hard to treat.

👥 ADDITIONAL TOPICS FOR STUDY GROUPS
- Neonatal icterus
- Other hemolytic anemias
- Inoculations
- Forms and causes of anemias/anemia diagnostics

49   Medulloblastoma

49.1 You examine the child once more, in great detail. What do you look for in particular?
- **Signs of dehydration:** Check skin turgor (skin tenting), moistness of oral mucosa
- **Abdomen:**
  - Palpation: Resistances, pain on pressure, protective reaction, peritonism
  - Auscultation: Lacking or intensified intestinal sounds as a sign of ileus
- **Neurological examination:** Signs of meningism, pupil width and reaction, check intrinsic muscle reflexes, polysynaptic reflexes (Babinski reflex, abdominal skin reflex), strength, coordination (Unterberger test, Romberg test, finger–nose test, tightrope walker test, 1-leg stand) and sensory test

49.2 What differential diagnosis are you considering now that you have this new information? What diagnostic measures do you take to distinguish between the differential diagnoses?
- **Differential diagnoses:**
  - Brain tumor: Headache, vomiting, personality changes, clumsiness
  - Meningitis/encephalitis: Vomiting, headache, elevated temperature
  - Metabolic disorders in diabetes mellitus Type I: vomiting, personality changes
  - Defective vision: difficulties in school, clumsiness

- **Laboratory:** Signs of inflammation (differential blood picture, CRP, sedimentation rate), electrolytes (electrolyte shift because of vomiting), blood gas analysis (metabolic acidosis), blood sugar (hyperglycemia)
- **Abdominal ultrasound:** Exclusion of invagination and ileus
- **EEG:** Imaging of focal changes as evidence of inflammatory or space-occupying processes
- **Inspection of ocular fundus:** Papilledema as evidence of cerebral pressure
- **Cranial imaging, e.g., MRI, CT:** To rule out a cerebral space-occupying lesion
- **Lumbar puncture:** After exclusion of cerebral pressure to rule out meningitis, encephalitis

49.3 An MRI of the skull with contrast medium is performed. (see Fig. MRI in Cases). Describe the result.
Large, inhomogeneous tumor that concentrates contrast medium, in the posterior cranial fossa, distended inner subarachnoid spaces

49.4 What will the further treatment be?
- Operative resection of the tumor, histological examination
- Depending on the histology, further treatment such as postoperative radiation therapy, chemotherapy if appropriate

Comments

Definition: Medulloblastomas (or primitive neuroectodermal tumors [PNET]) are undifferentiated, rapidly growing embryonic cerebellar tumors. The histological picture is characterized by a rosette arrangement of the tumor cells.

→ Cases 49 Page 50

Epidemiology: Medulloblastoma is the most frequent malignant cerebellar tumor in children. The peak manifestation time lies between the ages of 4 and 8 years. Boys are affected somewhat more frequently than girls. Every fifth medulloblastoma appears beyond the age of 15, with a peak age of 30 years.

Pathogenesis: The medulloblastoma starts at the cerebellar vermis, grows rapidly, and infiltrates both halves of the cerebellum, the brainstem, the fourth ventricle, and the meninges. So-called drop metastases develop in the subarachnoid space. Extraneural metastases are observed, but rarely, in the bones/bone marrow.

Clinical aspects: The most important clinical symptoms are signs of **cerebral pressure** such as headache, nausea, and vomiting on an empty stomach, changes of behavior and impaired consciousness. The symptoms described in this case are suggestive of a brain tumor until this is proven wrong. Signs of a cerebellar tumor are ataxia (Romberg test), Unterberger step test (tightrope walker gait), and intentional tremor (finger–nose test). Seizures, motor deficits, and apraxia can occur.

Diagnostics: The first step toward finding a diagnosis is the taking of a detailed history. This is followed by a careful clinical and neurological examination (see answer to question 49.1). This is followed by **skull imaging**, possibly with contrast medium. The most informative method is MRI, which provides the best visualization of soft tissue. If there is suspicion of metastasis (MRI), cytological examination of the CSF should also be performed. But it may only be done if cerebral pressure (papilledema?) has first been ruled out.

Differential diagnoses: Other intracranial space-occupying lesions (e.g., hematomas, brain abscesses), and inflammatory diseases of the brain (e.g., meningitis, encephalitis, cerebellitis).

Treatment: The first step is the most complete possible **resection of the tumor**, since local space occupying lesions and CSF circulation disorders are life threatening for children. Life threatening increase in cerebral pressure is treated by extreme drainage of the cerebrospinal fluid. Continuing treatment of the tumor depends on the age of the child and the stage of the tumor: locally limited, **non-metastasized tumors in children under the age of 4 years** are only treated with chemotherapy. The agents used are cyclophosphamide, vincristin, methotrexate, carboplatin, VP16. The treatment is best carried out in the context of a study.

Non-metastasized medulloblastomas in patients **older than 4 years of age** are chiefly irradiated. This is followed by chemotherapy with cisplatin, CCNU, and vincristin, over several cycles.

If there is already metastasis at the time of diagnosis, a poor prognosis must be expected. Experimental treatment approaches are needed.

Prognosis: The prognosis for medulloblastoma depends very much on the operability of the tumor and the child's age, i.e., the older the child, the better the prognosis. The 10-year survival rate is at approximately 60% but one must also count on late relapses even after 10 years. Long-term sequelae may be caused by treatment (most of all radiation therapy) and by the destructive growth of the tumor. They manifest in the form of paresis, coordination disorders, neuroendocrinological disorders (e.g., lack of growth hormone with short stature), and neuropsychological disorders such as disorders of concentration, short-term memory, learning, etc.

👪 ADDITIONAL TOPICS FOR STUDY GROUPS
- Other pediatric brain tumors (e.g., astrocytomas, craniopharyngioma, brainstem tumors)
- Other malignant pediatric tumors
- Hydrocephalus
- Meningitis

50 Acute appendicitis

50.1 **By questioning the parents and the child, try to narrow down the possible causes. What causes are you thinking of and what do you ask about?**
- **Acute gastroenteritis:** Stool frequency, consistency, abnormal stool odor, abnormal pain with defecation, consumption of spoiled food (similar symptoms in persons who ate the same thing?) or salmonella-contaminated food (e.g., eggs, milk, ice cream, mayonnaise)
- **Acute pancreatitis:** Belt-shaped pain radiation from the upper abdomen into the back
- **Constipation:** Stool frequency, food habits, fluid intake
- **Urinary tract infection:** Frequent need to urinate, pain on urination, known deformities of the urinary tract, prior urinary infections
- **Referred pain from the respiratory tract:** Catarrhal symptoms (coughing, congestion, sore throat)

→ Cases 50 Page 51

- **Acute appendicitis:** Wandering pain (often begins in epigastric or periumbilical region, later pain moves to right lower abdomen; *caution:* in children the symptoms are often very unspecific)
- **Insufficient pain localization** in angina, otitis media, coxitis, etc.; because the body schema is not yet developed in children, the pain is often projected into the abdomen
- **Invagination:** Sudden start of pain, repetitive vomiting, pain-free interval, recurrent screaming, bloody stools
- **Mesenteric lymphadenitis:** Status post gastroenteritis
- **Meckel diverticulitis:** Bloody stools, colic-like pain

50.2 What diagnostic measures should you use next in order to establish a diagnosis?

- **Clinical examination:**
  - Head/Neck: Throat examination, otoscopy, palpation of the lymph nodes to rule out ENT diseases
  - Heart/Lung: Auscultation to rule out pneumonia, bronchitis
  - Abdomen: Palpation to rule out acute appendicitis (see Comments)
  - Extremities: Mobility, exanthema
  - In addition: Temperature measurement → axillorectal temperature difference > 1°C suggests acute appendicitis
- **Laboratory diagnostics:** Blood picture, inflammatory parameters (sedimentation rate, CRP), lipase, amylase, GOT, GPT, electrolytes, blood sugar, blood gas analysis, urine status
- **Abdominal sonography:**
  - Double cockade: Indication of invagination
  - Evaluation of intestinal mobility, wall thickness, and filling: Indication of acute gastroenteritis
  - Markedly filled intestinal loops: Indication of constipation
  - Edematous wall thickening (cockade)/congested lumen/fecalith in the vermiform appendix: Indication of acute appendicitis
  - Free fluid: Indication of ascites, inflammatory process, or perforation
  - Evaluation of abdominal lymph nodes: To rule out mesenteric lymphadenitis
  - Evaluation of the pancreas: Swelling, necroses, calcification
  - Evaluation of the kidneys: Indication of pyelonephritis, concrements, renal obstruction

50.3 What do you do next?

- Admit the child to hospital for observation
- Examine child repeatedly for early detection of changes/deterioration of the general condition and local symptoms
- Enema to mobilize possible "stationary" painful fecaliths
- Request collaboration of a surgical colleague
- Appendectomy if signs of acute appendicitis increase (Laboratory: inflammatory parameters [sedimentation rate, CRP, leukocytes] ↑, sonographic indications [see answer to question 50.2 and Comments], typical examination findings [see Comments])

50.4 What complications should you expect if this is acute appendicitis?

- Perforation/migratory peritonitis (in children, preoperative perforation is frequent because of atypical/rapid course, but the prognosis is good)
- Abscess formation (so-called perityphlitic abscess)
- Paralytic ileus

50.5 What additional differential diagnoses would you have to consider if the patient were a 15-year-old girl?

Gynecological causes such as ovarian cysts, ovarian torsion, adnexitis, extrauterine pregnancy, menarche, hematometra/hematosalpinx with hymenal atresia, ovulation

- **Clinical aspects:** Lower abdominal pain, nausea, vomiting, possible shock
- **Diagnostics:** Laboratory (β-HCG, inflammatory parameters), sonography, gynecological/surgical consultation

Comments

Definition and etiopathogenesis: Acute appendicitis is an inflammation of the vermiform appendix.

The cause is displacement of the vermiform appendix lumen, e.g., by hyperplasia of the lymphatic tissue in the appendix, emptying disorder (e.g., by fecaliths), worms (e.g., *Oxyuris vermicularis*), or intestinal kinking and local bacterial infection.

Epidemiology: The peak onset age is between the 4 and 12 years of age.

Clinical aspects: Acute appendicitis typically has a **short history** (12–24 hours).

Pain accompanied by nausea begins principally in the epigastrium. In the course of the disease, the pain wanders into the right lower abdomen; in addition, vomiting can occur. At first, the pains are only intermittent and then a steady pain develops. Shortly before perforation, pain stops again. There is usually no diarrhea, but its presence does not rule out acute appendicitis. *Caution:* The course is often atypical in children and very rapid.

Diagnostics: Diagnosis can be difficult, especially in toddlers. Often there are only non-specific clinical and laboratory findings. Leukocytosis and axillo-rectal temperature difference (see below) may not be present.

For this reason, in case of unspecific abdominal pain—independently of localization—the possibility of appendicitis must always be considered, especially if there are additional signs of inflammation (leukocytosis, sedimentation rate, and CRP ↑). It is always important to ask about the course of appendicitis in the family, especially among siblings, because the course of an illness is often similar within a family.

Classical examination results when the appendix is in typical position (see Fig.):
- **McBurney point:** Pressure pain halfway between navel and superior anterior iliac spine, right, position of caecum with outflow of appendix
- **Lanz point:** Pressure pain at transition between middle and right third of a line connecting the two superior anterior iliac spines

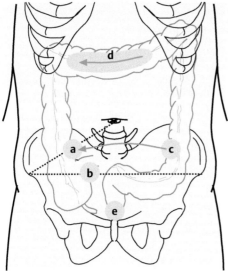

a McBurney Point **d** Rovsing Sign
b Lanz Point **e** Douglas Pain
c Blumberg Sign

Pressure and pain points in acute appendix

- **Blumberg sign:** Contralateral rebound pain in already existing peritonitic irritation
- **Rovsing sign:** Retrograde stretching of the colon leads to pain in the right lower abdomen
- **Psoas sign:** Painful irritation of the psoas fascia leads to pain relief posture by bending the right leg in the hip joint; extension produces stretching pain
- **Concussion pain:** Hopping can cause protective limping
- **Douglas pain:** Pain on rectal palpation as evidence of peritoneal irritation; right intestinal is more painful during examination as other locations

Caution: In a child with abdominal pain, rectal examination should never be omitted. However, rectal examination is particularly unpleasant for children. Therefore, the examination should always be explained to children in advance. It may be that it is useful to compare it to rectal temperature measurement or application of suppositories. The child should be distracted during the examination (e.g., talking about kindergarten or a favorite sport. If possible, the examination is performed with the fifth digit and only with Vaseline).

Additional findings associated with the classical picture of acute appendicitis are **axillorectal temperature** difference of more than 1°C in 50% of cases as well as a laboratory finding of **elevated inflammatory parameters** (leukocytes, CRP, sedimentation rate). **Abdominal sonography** can only supplement the clinical diagnosis. The image of ulcerophlegmonous appendicitis is readily recognized. In cross section, the inflamed appendix has the appearance of a cockade with a total diameter of over 6 mm; in longitudinal section, there is a dead end tubular structure, possibly with contents (e.g., concrement). In perforation, the appendix is surrounded by free fluid. *Caution:* A negative sonographic finding does not rule out acute appendicitis.

Treatment: If the findings are unambiguous, appendectomy, either laparoscopic or conventional, must take place immediately. If a perforation or inflammatory involvement of the peritoneum has already taken place, antibiotic treatment (e.g., Amoxicillin 50–100 mg/kg body weight/d) is administered in addition to the operation. The patient can usually be discharged from the hospital after 3 to 5 days, depending on the intensity of the local symptoms.

If the diagnosis cannot be established without question, the patient is admitted to the hospital for observation with regular examination of the abdomen and monitoring of the inflammatory parameters. Surgical colleagues should be included in the case. The child receives infusion therapy and remains in fasting until it is clear whether an operation is necessary. Antipyretics and analgesics, e.g., with paracetamol or an ice pack on the abdomen should be provided as support. An enema is always to be recommended (only if there is no contraindication [ileus, perforation]). If constipation is at the root of the symptoms, relief can be produced with a laxative. Many findings that arouse suspicion of appendicitis improve in 1 to 2 days.

🚶🚶🚶 ADDITIONAL TOPICS FOR STUDY GROUPS
- Meckel diverticulitis
- Invagination
- Oxyuriasis

51.1 Justify your suspected diagnosis on the basis of the medical history and the clinical picture.
Chassaignac's "paralysis" (Syn.: dislocation of the elbow joint, subluxation of the radial head, Chassaignac's disease); rationale: Typical history (sudden pull at the child's arm), clinical picture (affected arm seems to be paralyzed, arm is held in pronation, seems to be painful, and is no longer used even to reach for a candy)

51.2 What other possible injuries should you be considering? How can you distinguish between these and your suspected diagnosis?
- **Differential diagnoses:** Joint luxation, fracture
- **Possibilities for definition:** Not a typical accident, if appropriate, X-ray of the elbow joint in two planes

51.3 Explain the mechanism of injury for your suspected diagnosis.
Usually the child is held by the hand and, for instance, abruptly pulled upward when there is something in the way; the sudden traction on the child's arm, which is extended and pronated at the elbow joint (see Fig. Injury mechanism) causes subluxation of the radial head from the upper part of the anular ligament.

51.4 What do you do next?
In the typical history and clinical picture, as presented here, no additional X-ray studies are necessary. Repositioning by passive supination and bending of the lower arm with simultaneous pressure on the head of the radius can follow immediately (see Fig. Repositioning maneuver). After this, the child is once more free of symptoms, and additional therapy or immobilization is not necessary. *Tip:* An attempt at repositioning is only painful for a short time. Therefore, one should take the child by surprise: For instance, explain to the little patient that you want to start by tickling the sick arm carefully, to find out why it can't move anymore. At the same time, feel for the head of the radius and without much warning, quickly perform the repositioning. The child notices that the arm can move again and so forgives the painful action (at least mostly).
A long announcement or possibly even sedation only draws the matter out unnecessarily and scares the child even more. No damage can be done during the repositioning attempt. Complications only occur when the repositioning does not succeed right away, especially if one pulls too carefully. This is usually the case the first time one has to perform a repositioning alone. Then, unfortunately, one has to try again and bear the child's screams and the parents' skeptical looks.

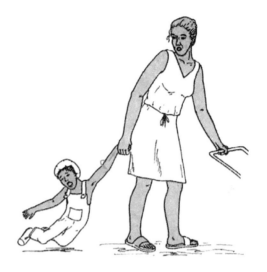
Injury mechanism

181

Case
51

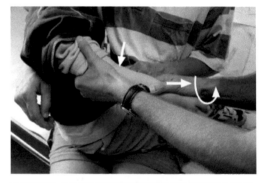

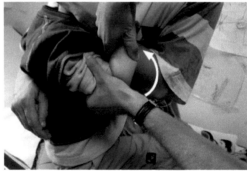
Repositioning maneuver

→ Cases 51 Page 52

Definition: Chassaignac's paralysis is a painful subluxation of the head of the radius within the annular ligament of the radius.

Epidemiology and etiopathogenesis: Between the first and fourth year, Chassaignac's paralysis is an extraordinarily frequent injury. For the typical etiopathogenesis, see answer to question 51.3. But subluxation can also be caused by indirect (e.g., a fall) or direct trauma (e.g., in sports [judo]), especially in older children.

Clinical aspects: The noticeable appearance is a pain-dependent impediment to movement of the lower arm in the elbow joint with fixation in pronation. The arm is protected (see case).

Diagnosis and treatment: With a **typical history** and clinical picture, no further diagnostics are required. An attempt at **repositioning can take place immediately** (see answer to question 51.4.). The success of the treatment is tested by holding the healthy arm tight and extending a toy or something

similar. *Caution:* Before and after treatment, circulation, motor function, and sensory perception (CFS) should always be tested. If no typical event is reported in the history or if there has been a trauma, elbow luxation or fracture must be considered. The indication for an X-ray of the elbow in two planes (a.p. and lateral) should then be broadly defined (see answer to question 51.2).

Prophylaxis: The parents should avoid jerking the child's arm (for instance, when crossing wide streets or if the child suddenly takes off). And the child should not be swung in the air by the arms, since this could cause Chassaignac's paralysis.

Prognosis: A relapse is possible, since the ligamentary apparatus can be loosened. However, the prognosis is good. From preschool age, Chassaignac's paralysis is very rare.

ADDITIONAL TOPICS FOR STUDY GROUPS
- Fractures in childhood (e.g., greenstick fracture)

52 Migraine

52.1 Which differential diagnoses are you considering? What is the most likely diagnosis? What is your rationale?
- **Acute migraine attack** (migraine with aura): Most likely diagnosis; rationale: neurological blackouts as aura, strictly unilateral headache, associated autonomic symptoms
- **Inflammatory diseases** (e.g., meningoencephalitis, neuritis, transmitted ENT diseases): Inflammation of the meninges can lead to headache and nausea; neurological blackouts are untypical
- **Vascular disorders** (e.g., aneurysm): Ischemia or increased blood flow can lead to vision disorders and headaches
- **Subarachnoid hemorrhage:** Very intense headaches accompanied by vomiting, nausea, sweating, and light sensitivity, followed by disturbed vigilance ranging to coma; neurological blackouts before the headaches are not typical
- **Tumors** (e.g., astrocytoma, meningioma: Elevated cerebral pressure can cause headache, nausea, neurological deficits)
- **Tension headache:** Headaches caused by muscle tension can (rarely) be associated with autonomic symptoms such as vision disorders
- **Psychogenic causes:** e.g., with depression, anxiety

52.2 What further tests would you consider useful?
- **Laboratory:** Blood picture, CRP, sedimentation rate, electrolytes, clotting parameters (to rule out inflammation, electrolyte or clotting disorder)
- **EEG:** Very variable disorders, e.g., basic rhythm changes, slowing, focal general changes (to rule out focal changes as evidence of inflammatory or space-occupying processes)
- **Possibly MRI or CT:** Always if there is suspicion of elevated cerebral pressure or visible focal changes in EEG; to rule out space-occupying lesions, cerebral hemorrhage

52.3 What treatment do you initiate?
- **Treatment of acute migraine attack:**
  - Hospital admission, rest, protection against irritation (darkened room, no television or reading, no loud noises)
  - Antiemetic (e.g., metoclopramide 0.1 mg/kg body weight every 4–6 hours)
  - Analgesics (e.g., paracetamol 10–15 mg/kg body weight every 6–8 hours or ibuprofen 8–10 mg /kg body weight every 6–8 hours)
  - In severe attacks: Sumatriptan 10 to 20 mg intranasal

→ Cases 52 Page 53

- **Migraine prophylaxis:**
  - Keeping a headache calendar to gather data on possible triggers
  - Behavioral therapy for reduction of attack frequency and mitigation of associated vegetative symptoms

  - Relaxation techniques (e.g., progressive muscle relaxation according to Jacobson, autogenic training)
  - Prophylactic drug treatment (see Comments)

Comments

Definition and epidemiology: The International Headache Society defines migraine as recurring headaches, with or without aura, that last from 2 to 48 hours. Usually the headaches occur on one side and are pulsing in character; the intensity is moderate to high and is intensified by physical activity. Frequent accompanying symptoms are nausea, vomiting, photo- and phonophobia. Childhood migraines are shorter and often more atypical than adult migraines. Thus in affected children, the pains are bilateral and frontotemporal; often the attacks are accompanied by abdominal pain.

The incidence of migraine is 250 per 100,000 inhabitants. In 10% of cases, the first attack takes place in childhood. At preschool age, boys and after puberty, girls are more frequently affected.

Etiopathogenesis: The pathological mechanism of migraine is not yet completely understood. In 70% to 90% of patients, there is a family history of migraine.

The pain arises in the trigeminovascular system. Secretion of vasoactive substances (calcitonin, substance P, nitrogen monoxide) from the ends of the trigeminal nerve causes vasodilation and development of a sterile inflammation. There are trigeminal stretch and pain receptors in the walls of cranial blood vessels. Stimulation of these receptors leads to the typical headache. The anticipatory aura can be explained as inhibition of cortical activity that gradually spreads from occipital to parietal and temporal. Involvement of additional brain stem centers, such as the area postrema, explains the accompanying autonomic symptoms (nausea and vomiting).

A migraine attack can be triggered by stress, lack of sleep, change of time zone, consumption of alcohol or certain foods (e.g., chocolate, cheese, nuts, bananas), or hormones. Often the migraine attack also occurs in the relaxation phase after stress ("weekend migraine").

Clinical aspects: The most frequent course is **migraine without aura**, which occurs as gradually increasing headaches, usually one-sided but not always constantly affecting one side. It usually persists for 4 to 72 hours (in childhood, 2 to 48 hours) and is associated with nausea, vomiting, light and noise sensitivity, as well as other autonomic symptoms.

Twenty percent of cases, like the case presented here, are **migraine with aura.** The aura precedes the headache attack. This involves reversible, focal neurological symptoms that develop gradually and do not persist for more than 60 minutes. The most frequent associated symptoms are visual, such as flickers, visual field deficits, distorted perceptions, but other focal symptoms, such as paresthesia, (hemi-) paresis, or speech disorders, are possible.

A migraine is called complicated if the neurological deficits persist for more than 7 days after a migraine attack (Status migrainosus).

Diagnostics: In addition to a thorough physical and neurological examination and a laboratory examination for orientation, instrumental examinations (EEG, imaging) may become necessary to define the important differential diagnoses (see answer to question 52.2).

Differential diagnoses: See answer to question 52.1.

Treatment: See answer to question 52.3. In migraine, it is decisive to treat early and with a sufficiently high dose. In an **acute attack**, in addition to protection against irritation, the recommended treatment is administration of an **antiemetic** (e.g., dimenhydrinate, domperidone [from the age of 10 years], metoclopramide [from the age of 12 years]). This reduces the associated autonomic symptoms such as nausea and vomiting, stimulates intestinal peristalsis, and thus leads to better absorption of the analgesic. To treat pain, an analgesic is administered, if possible, 15 to 20 minutes after administration of the antiemetic: paracetamol (10–15 mg/kg body weight) or ibuprofen (8–10 mg/kg body weight). From the age of 12 years, acetyl salicylic acid can be given (contraindicated at an earlier age because of risk of Reye syndrome), preferably as an effervescent tablet (takes effect sooner).

For adults with severe migraine attacks, serotonin receptor agonists (triptans) have proven successful for years. Their efficacy in youths has also been demonstrated in clinical studies; children under the age of 12 years do not seem to benefit from the treatment. Sumatriptan nasal spray at a dose of 10 mg is approved for youths from the age of 12 years.

→ Cases 52 Page 53

To determine whether prophylaxis is necessary, it is necessary to keep an **attack journal**, in order to find possible triggers (see Etiopathogenesis). A record is made over a period of weeks of occurrence, location, quantity, and quality of the headache pains and their treatment.

Then these triggers must be avoided as much as possible. An orderly daily routine with sufficient sleep should be the objective. Acupressure and acupuncture, behavioral therapy and relaxation techniques can bring relief. If foods (e.g., cheese or chocolate) are identified as attack triggers (very rare), an elimination diet can be tried.

Migraine prophylaxis with drugs for 3 to 6 months should be considered if more than two attacks per month occur, the attacks last for more than 48 hours, or the pain intensity and psychological stress are very severe. This is also the case if the associated symptoms are extreme, the aura is severely prolonged, or there are complications.

For this purpose, in childhood, calcium antagonists (e.g., flunarizine) or β-blockers (e.g., metoprolol 2.5–5 mg/kg body weight/d) can be used. Magnesium and *Petasites hybridus* extract seem to have a favorable effect.

Prognosis: Migraine is not curable but it can be well controlled by prompt, adequate treatment. However, there are cases in which it no longer occurs after puberty.

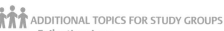 ADDITIONAL TOPICS FOR STUDY GROUPS
- Epileptic seizure
- Headaches

184

53 Undescended testis

Case 53

53.1 **What do you think about the fact that up to now there has never been a diagnosis or a treatment? What advice do you give the parents?**
Testicular dystopia (testicular aberration) in early infancy is physiological. After the first year, 1% to 2% of all boys still have a testicular dystopia. This needs to be clarified and treated. Treatment must be completed **before age 2** since dystopically located testicles are damaged in their exocrine function (fertility) and have a higher risk of degeneration. Diagnosis and treatment should therefore begin immediately for this boy.

53.2 **What did you want to find out when you asked the parents whether the testicle is in the scrotum during bathing?**
This is meant to differentiate between the inguinal testicle and the retractile testis. A retractile testis shifts into the scrotum in warm surroundings, e.g., while bathing.

53.3 **Name and explain the different forms of undescended testis.**
- **Retention of inguinal testis:** The testis is palpable in the inguinal canal.
- **Retention of abdominal testis (cryptorchism):** The testis lies intra-abdominally and can therefore not be palpated.
- **Sliding testis:** The testis lies before the outer inguinal ring in the inguinal canal, can be brought into the scrotum with tension, but when released, it slides back into the starting position.
- **Retractile testis:** Physiological special form of the sliding testis; the testis lies in the scrotum, but is nevertheless sometimes displaced into the inguinal canal by excessive tension on the cremaster muscle.

- **Ectopic testis:** The testis lies outside the physiological descent pathway (e.g., perineum, inner thigh, under the abdominal skin).

53.4 **What could cause an undescended testis?**
The etiology is not yet completely understood. However, anatomical, physiological, and mechanical causes are blamed.
- A lack of gonadotropins in the last weeks of pregnancy
- Defective prenatal androgen secretion
- Testicular agenesis
- Testicular atrophy, e.g., because of intrauterine testicular torsion
- Mechanical obstacles, e.g., in anatomical anomalies
- Within the context of secondary symptom following inguinal hernia surgery

53.5 **What therapeutic possibilities are available for the treatment of undescended testis?**
- Hormone treatment is only indicated if testes do not descend spontaneously by the time the child is 6 months of age.
- **Hormone treatment:**
  - At first with intranasal GnRH application (Kryptokur 3 × 400 µg daily for a period of 4 weeks)
  - If treatment does not succeed hcG injections (Primogonyl 1 × 500–1,500 IU/week i.m. for 3 weeks)
- **Operative treatment:** If conservative treatment fails, the testis is moved into the scrotum with orchidopexy before the age of 1 year; in ectopic testis position, surgery is always the primary treatment indicated.

→ Cases 53 **Page 54**

Definition and epidemiology: Undescended testis (Syn.: Cryptorchism) is an incorrect position of the testis / testes outside the scrotal sack because of incomplete descent (see schematic drawing).

Cryptorchism is found in about 4% of all male newborns. In the course of the first year, there is spontaneous descent in a good half of cases.

Etiology: See answer to question 53.4.

Complications: Unphysiological pressure and temperature conditions outside the scrotal sack cause inhibition of tubulus growth, atrophy of the Leydig cells, and disruption of spermatogonium formation in the testes as early as after the first year of the child's life. In 30% of cases of untreated unilateral failure to descend and 80% of cases of untreated bilateral failure to descend, the outcome is infertility. There is an increased risk of testicular torsion and malignant degeneration, as well as later for psychosexual disorders. The risk of developing a malignant testicular tumor later is a good 5 to 10 times higher in a dystopic testicle than in an orthotopic one.

Clinical aspects: See answer to question 53.3.

Differential diagnoses: Testicular agenesis (anorchia), secondary cryptorchism, e.g., after hernia surgery.

Diagnosis and Treatment: Cryptorchism is a **clinical diagnosis**. The examination should take place in a pleasant and warm environment. First the genital is inspected with the patient standing and/or lying down. Attention should be paid to age-appropriate development and possible deformation, as well as the shape and symmetry of the scrotum.

Then one attempts to feel the testicle with warm hands. For this purpose, older children should sit tailor-fashion (in this position, the cremaster reflex is not triggered and it is easier to distinguish with certainty between a retractile testis and a sliding testis); infants are examined lying down. In the examination, the position of the testis, its size, and consistency are evaluated. It is best to perform the **examination biennially:** If the testis is palpated in the groin, one can try to move it into the scrotum with one hand while the other hand exerts pressure on the outer inguinal ring to prevent the testis from wandering into the inguinal canal. If the testis cannot be moved to the scrotum, it is an **inguinal testis** and must be treated. If the testis can easily be moved into the scrotum and remains there, it is a **retractile testis** and does not require treatment. This must be differentiated from the **sliding testis**, which must be treated. It can only be moved into the scrotal sack with tension on the spermatic cord and when this is released, the testis immediately glides back into the groin. If no testis can be felt, an **ectopic position** of the testis (see Fig.) or an abdominal, **non-descending testis** must be considered.

In the case of an inguinal testis or a non-palpable testis, an attempt is made to visualize the testis **sonographically**. This requires extensive experience and a high-resolution instrument. It is often impossible to visualize the testis, especially if it is located retroperitoneally. Even an MRI does not have an advantage here, because the testes, which are often too small, are not imaged with certainty. In that case, an **exploratory laparoscopy** is indicated. This makes it possible to locate and inspect the testis and if necessary, to mobilize and replace it in the scrotum.

If neither testis can be palpated, an attempt is made to identify functional testicular tissue with an **hCG stimulation test**. The test is positive if the testosterone level rises after i.m. administration of hCG. Evidence of **basal Inhibin B** produced by the Sertoli cells also indicates whether functioning testicular tissue is present. If the clinical laboratory tests are negative, it can be assumed that the patient is suffering from **cryptorchism**. A **laparoscopy** should be performed in any case because atrophied, non-functional testes should also be located and removed because of the risk of malignant degeneration.

185

Case

53

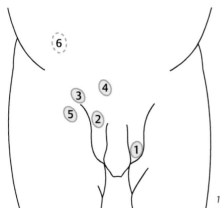

1) Descended testis 2) Gliding testis 3) Canicular testis 4) + 5) Ectopic testis 6) Intra-abdominal testis

For treatment, see answer to question 53.4. The objective of treatment is to return the testis to the scrotum. Because of the negative effects of cryptorchism on spermiogenesis and the increased risk of later testicular cancer developing, treatment should be started as early as possible, preferably in the second half year of the child's life. Treatment must be completed at the latest by the first birthday. The success of hormone therapy is between 20% and 50%. Even after completion of the therapy, the position of the testis must be regularly checked. Often, usually during the first 6 months, there is a relapse that requires a prompt operative correction with orchidopexy.

Prognosis: Drug therapy of the undescended testis is successful in 14% to 50% of cases. Operative treatment is successful in 80% to 90% of cases.

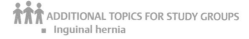 ADDITIONAL TOPICS FOR STUDY GROUPS
- Inguinal hernia

---

54   Diabetes mellitus Type I

54.1 What is your suspected diagnosis on the basis of this medical history? What pathological findings might you gather in the clinical examination if your suspected diagnosis is correct?
- **Suspected diagnosis: Manifestation of Diabetes mellitus Type I**; rationale: patient's age, acutely occurring polyuria and polydipsia, enuresis, weight loss (in spite of sufficient nutritional intake), fatigue, bad mood, abdominal pain, nausea, vomiting
- **Pathological laboratory results**
  - Dry skin and mucosa, sunken eyeballs
  - In ketoacidosis: Pre-coma or coma, acetone odor in exhaled breath (sweetish, like fruit), Kussmaul breathing (deep thoracic breathing), hypovolemic shock (Blood Pressure ↓, HF ↑)

54.2 What examinations do you perform to confirm the diagnosis?
- **Laboratory:**
  - Blood/serum: Blood sugar ↑↑, blood gas analysis (metabolic acidosis: pH ↓, pCO2 ↓, BE ↓), blood count, hematocrit ↑, electrolytes (Na normal, ↑ or ↓; K normal or ↑), creatinine (normal or ↑), urea (normal or ↑), cholesterol, triglycerides (↑), HbA1$_c$ (↑)
  - Urine: glycosuria, ketonuria

54.3 What acute treatment do you initiate? How do you proceed?
- **Treatment:**
  - Hospital admission for monitoring of vital functions (blood pressure, ECG monitoring, breathing, excretion)
  - Rehydration (infusion therapy, initially with NaCl 0.9%, with blood sugar values < 250 mg/dL [13.9 mmol/L] half isotonic NaCl solution with 5% glucose) after onset of diuresis electrolyte replacement (especially potassium) with continuous (every 4 hours) electrolyte monitoring
  - i.v. administration of altinsulin (recommended value: 0.05 IU/kg body weight/h), slow decline

of blood sugar (not more than 100 mg/dL/h [5.5 mmol/L]; *caution:* risk of cerebral edema), for this reason, initial hourly blood sugar control
- **Procedure:** Four pillars of diabetes treatment
  - **Insulin therapy** (conventional, intensified, insulin pump therapy)
  - Balanced **diet**
  - **Activity**
  - **Training** of patient and parents, patient care in the special diabetes outpatient facility, regular medical checkup for late complications (see Comments)

54.4 Explain the etiology of the disease.
- The etiology is unknown but a genetic disposition and an association with certain virus infections (e.g., coxsackie, mumps, CMV, rubella) are assumed.
- Formation of autoantibodies against pancreatic B cells with destruction of the B cells and resulting absolute lack of insulin

54.5 What kind of diet should the child have with this disease? Explain and calculate the energy needs of the 8-year-old boy.
- **Diet:**
  - Balanced and varied, adapted to the child's requirements and habits
  - Foods with high fiber, low fat, high protein content.
  - No rapidly absorbed sugars (e.g., beet sugar)
  - Physical activity lowers the insulin requirement and improves insulin efficacy
- **Calorie requirement:**
  - 1,000 + (age of the child × 100) = total daily calorie requirement
  - Fulfillment of calorie requirement with 50% to 60% carbohydrates, 30% fats, 10% to 20% protein
  - 1 g carbohydrate or protein = 4 kcal, 1 g fat = 9 kcal
  - 12.5 g (= 50 kcal) carbohydrate = 1 bread unit (BU)
  - Calculation of the carbohydrate proportion of the foods used is simplified by using carbohydrate exchange tables

■ **Calorie requirements of the 8-year-old boy:**
  - 1,000 + (8 × 100) = 1,800 kcal
  - 50% to 60% of the calories = 1,000 kcal carbohydrates; 1,000 kcal = 250 g carbohydrates

- In conventional insulin therapy, the daily amount of carbohydrates should be divided among six to seven meals (three main meals, two to three snacks, one late meal)

| Comments |

Definition: Diabetes mellitus is a metabolic disease characterized by an **imbalance in the regulation of the blood sugar level**, with a preponderance of blood sugar elevating factors. In addition to hyperglycemia, there is an increased breakdown of fatty tissue and protein with elevated plasma lipid level that can go as far as ketoacidosis. There are different types, depending on the cause and course (see Tab.).

Epidemiology: Diabetes mellitus Type I is the most frequently occurring metabolic disease in children and youths (prevalence 1:1,000). The peak age of onset is between the ages of 2 and 3 years (20%), the ages of 6 and 7 years (30%), and at the start of puberty (50%).

Etiology: See answer to question 54.4.

Pathogenesis: Insulin lowers the blood sugar level by causing the uptake of glucose, especially in muscle and fat cells; in the liver, it inhibits gluconeogenesis and promotes glycogenolysis. For this reason, an insulin deficiency leads to decreased glucose uptake in the cells and an increased blood sugar level. Gluconeogenesis out of amino acids and glycogenolysis occur to a greater extent. Body protein is broken down to a greater extent. Decreased glucose uptake in the muscle cells and breakdown of muscle proteins lead to muscle weakness. Concentration of glucose in the extracellular space causes hyperosmolarity. The transport maximum for glucose in the kidneys is exceeded; glucose is excreted in the urine. The result is osmotic diuresis (polyuria) with loss of water (dehydration), sodium, and potassium. Fat breakdown is predominant in the fatty tissue. More fats are released into the blood (hyperlipidemia) and transformed in the liver into acetoacetate and β-hydroxybutyric acid. The accumulation of these acids leads to metabolic acidosis. The organism tries to compensate for the acidosis with respiration, by deeper breathing (Kussmaul breathing). In part, the fatty acids are also broken down to ketone bodies that are eliminated in expiratory breaths (acetone odor) and excreted in the urine (ketonuria).

Clinical aspects: The course and degree of severity are very variable. In 80% of cases, the **onset is insidious** with symptoms such as polyuria, severe thirst, increased drinking (polydipsia), and **weight loss**, tiredness, fatigue, poor concentration, irritability, and possibly secondary enuresis (due to polyuria), vomiting, and abdominal pain ("diabetic pseudo-appendicitis"). In 20% of cases the diabetes mellitus presents with **diabetic coma** (see example case). Symptoms are hyperkalemia, clouded consciousness, dehydration, dyspnea, Kussmaul breathing, hypotension, and tachycardia.

Complications: Micro and macroangiopathy (retinopathy, nephropathy, neuropathy, arterial hypertension), skin changes (necrobiosis lipoidica) and joints (cheiroarthropathy = painless limitations of movement, especially in finger joints), poor resistance (especially bacterial [skin] infections), lipid metabolism disorder.

Diagnostics: The classical symptoms and findings of polyuria, intense thirst (with polydipsia), weight loss, and glycosuria, ketonuria, and elevated postprandial blood sugar values (> 200 mg/dL) or fasting blood sugar values (> 140 mg/dL), and a pathological glucose tolerance test (2-hour value > 200 mg/dL) confirm the diagnosis.

The total potassium is decreased by osmotic diuresis. Serum potassium levels can be normal or even elevated (2 mechanisms: 1. Insulin normally stimulates Na–K-ATPase and thus potassium uptake into the cell; 2. in acidosis potassium ions are shifted from the intra- to the extracellular space).

Treatment: See answer to question 54.3. **Acutherapy** has the objective of **eliminating hyperglycemia** and **normalizing energy metabolism** by administration of insulin as well as **balancing the electrolyte and fluid deficit** with constant monitoring of vital parameters.

Prolonged intravenous infusion of normal insulin with constant blood sugar control is used to normalize blood sugar and energy metabolism; a slow decline in blood sugar values is wanted in this process (see answer to question 54.3). If the blood sugar concentration falls too rapidly, thus decreasing the serum osmolality, there is a danger of cerebral edema. The fluid deficit is estimated clinically in percentage of the body weight (see case 4). The deficit must be compensated slowly in order to avoid a volume overload. Excessively rapid rehydration can lead to brain edema through intensified water flow into

→ Cases 54 Page 55

the brain cells. Possible consequences are loss of consciousness and cerebral seizures. Fluid replacement and (especially renal) acidosis correction (only very slight reabsorption of ketone bodies by the kidneys) as well as insulin administration lead to a potassium redistribution from extra- to intracellular. Therefore a sharp drop in serum potassium must be expected in the first hours. After onset of diuresis, potassium must be quickly replaced with constant monitoring.

After equilibration of the acidosis, and if the child shows clinical improvement (awake, adequately reactive, tolerating food again) insulin can be given subcutaneously. Oral antidiabetic agents such as sulfonyl urea are not effective in type 1 diabetes mellitus because they increase the release of insulin from the pancreatic B cells. In type 1 diabetes, the B cells are destroyed, so that an increase in insulin secretion is no longer possible.

The objective of further treatment is to achieve a metabolic situation that is as close to normal as possible, in order to reduce the risk of late complications (see above). The foundation of diabetes therapy is **insulin** replacement, **diet**, **activity**, and detailed **training** of patient and parents. Care by an experienced diabetes team, e.g., in a diabetes outpatient facility, is desirable.

Insulin therapy can be conducted in three different ways:

- **Conventionally**, with two (to three) insulin doses per day, where insulin administration (mixture of delayed release and normal insulin) and meals take place at definite times of day.

Diabetes form	Characteristics
Type 1	Insulin-dependent diabetes mellitus (IDDM), occurring principally in children and youths, **absolute insulin lack**
Type 2	Non-insulin-dependent diabetes mellitus (NIDDM), occurring mainly in older, obese persons, **relative insulin lack**, insulin resistance of target tissues
MODY (maturity onset diabetes in young)	Rare, autosomal-dominantly inherited, not insulin-dependent
Pregnancy diabetes	Manifestation of diabetes mellitus in pregnancy, metabolic disorder usually limited to the period of pregnancy

- **Intensified** according to the basic bolus principle, where delayed release insulin is injected one to two times a day and normal insulin is given at meals that can be taken at flexible times.
- **Insulin pump therapy** with continuous administration of normal insulin, adapted to the body's physiological insulin requirement; at meals, an insulin bolus is demanded.

The choice of therapy selected in the individual case depends on the patient's age, the patient's cooperation, and the blood sugar setting.

The blood sugar must be monitored several times a day. The patient and/or parents are required to keep a blood sugar log in which blood sugar values, doses of insulin administered, if relevant, sugar in urine, or ketone body tests are recorded. About every 3 months, patients should visit their doctor or diabetes outpatient facility for a checkup. The blood sugar target level is determined on the basis of the log; the serum HbA1$_c$ value is determined at the checkup. In this way the insulin regimen can be adjusted and the blood sugar target can be optimized. The physical examination screens especially for diabetes complications, injection sites are evaluated,

physical development (body measurements, stage of puberty) is documented, and blood pressure is measured. More complete blood studies should be carried out once a year (blood lipids, renal values, thyroid values, urine status). Ophthalmological checkups are required once a year at first; if the disease has lasted for more than 10 years, semiannual checkups are required.

Prognosis: The prognosis very much depends on how well blood sugar level targets are maintained. Good target levels with only slight fluctuation of blood sugar values can be achieved by precise metabolism monitoring and patient training. This makes decompensation rare. However, life expectancy is limited by late complications, especially angio-, neuro-, and nephropathy. At present it is at 15 to 20 years below the life expectancy of the normal population.

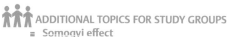 ADDITIONAL TOPICS FOR STUDY GROUPS
- Somogyi effect
- Dawn phenomenon
- Diabetic coma
- Oral glucose tolerance test (OGTT)

55.1 What are the symptoms of respiratory distress syndrome? Explain the etiopathogenesis of respiratory distress syndrome.

- **Symptoms: Respiratory distress** sets in immediately after birth or within the first hours of birth, with thoracic retractions (intercostal, subcostal, jugular, xiphoidal), flaring nostrils, tachypnea (> 60/min), expiratory wheezing, weakened breathing sounds, slight thoracic excursions, rising oxygen need, hypercapnia
- **Etiopathogenesis:**
  - **Surfactant** (phospholipid) is formed by the pneumocytes from the 26th week of pregnancy but only in sufficient amount from the 35th week of pregnancy; it covers the inner surface of the alveoli and decreases the surface tension. This makes development of the alveoli and thus gas exchange possible.
  - A lack of surfactant (primary [usually in immature premature births], secondary [inhibition of surfactant production/increased surfactant usage]) leads to collapse of the alveoli with microatelectases and decreased alveolar ventilation → the residual capacity falls → perfusion disorders in the lungs with formation of intrapulmonary shunts → oxygen uptake decreases → acidosis and hypoxia inhibit surfactant synthesis (a vicious circle); hypoperfusion and increased vascular permeability further lead to a flow of plasma into the alveoli, which leads to formation of protein-containing (earlier: hyaline) membranes with deterioration of oxygen exchange

55.2 How is respiratory distress syndrome treated?

- Slight respiratory distress syndrome (can be diagnosed with a thoracic X-ray): continuous oxygen administration (with continuous monitoring of oxygen saturation) by conducting oxygen into the incubator
- Early (nose or throat) CPAP ventilation can make intubation unnecessary. It should be initiated at the latest with hypercapnia (pCO_2 > 60 mmHg) and oxygen requirement > 40%
- If the CPAP therapy fails: Intubation and controlled ventilation
- Oxygen requirement > 40% or rising ventilation parameters (inspiration pressure > 20 cmH_2O and/or PEEP > 4 cmH_2O) on intubated and ventilated child: endotracheal surfactant application (100 mg/kg body weight) with continuous monitoring (since the ventilation situation improves dramatically after administration of surfactant. But this has the result that when reduction of the ventilation parameters is too slow, there is a danger of barotrauma and cerebral hemorrhage; the effect can fade after 1–12 hours; surfactant administration can be repeated up to three times)

55.3 What disease are the parents thinking of? Describe the clinical picture.

- **Retinopathy of prematurity:** Vasoproliferative disease of the retina in very small premature infants (< 1,500 g)
- **Classification:** Location (3 zones) and degree of severity (5 stages)
- **Etiology:** As a result of a long period of ventilation
- **Pathogenesis:** The immature retina is not yet completely vascularized; high oxygen partial pressure leads to stoppage of retinal vascularization; however, photoreceptors continue to grow and their increased metabolic requirements after termination of oxygen therapy lead to inadequate supply of the not yet vascularized areas. This triggers excessive vascular growth with expansion of vessels in retina and vitreous humor.
- **Clinical aspects:** Depending on the severity of retinal hemorrhage, scar formation, retinal detachment, formation of retrolental fibroplasia with blindness
- **Treatment:** Stage I/II usually heals spontaneously; from stage III, cryotherapy or laser therapy
- **Prognosis:** Stages I to III good; in stages IV and V there is retrolental fibroplasia that leads to blindness
- **Prophylaxis:** Avoidance of oxygen partial pressure that is too high or too low ("as high as necessary, as low as possible"), regular ophthalmological examinations

55.4 What disease is most likely? How can you confirm your suspected diagnosis?

- **Suspected diagnosis: Necrotizing enterocolitis** (NEC); rationale: in premature infants < 1,500 g, NEC is the most frequent cause for an acute abdomen (distended, often shiny abdomen, bilious vomiting, bloody stool, or stool content); previous hypoxia (e.g., because of respiratory distress syndrome) in the child could have led to ischemic damage of the intestinal wall (see Comments)
- **Diagnostics:**
  - **Examination of abdomen:** Visible intestinal loops, lack of peristalsis, pressure pain, protective tension, redness of flanks as a late symptom of peritonitis
  - **Laboratory:** Blood count, blood culture, coagulation, and inflammation parameters (septic disease picture → inflammatory parameters ↑), BGA, electrolytes, stool bacteriology
  - **X-ray:** Abdominal overview in supine and left-side position with horizontal beam path or a.p., hanging (intestinal pneumatosis with string-of-pearls air inclusions, gas in the portal vein system, thickened intestinal walls, dilated intestinal loops, free air in the abdomen as a sign of perforation [see Fig. Necrotizing enterocolitis])

189

Case

55

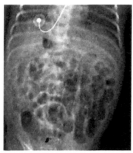

Necrotizing enterocolitis (intramural gas in intestinal loops)

Comments

Premature birth (definition, problems, first care): A birth is called premature when the child is **born before completion of the 37th week of pregnancy**. The immature condition of the child's organs at this stage entails a number of problems. This includes primarily breathing disorders (e.g., respiratory distress syndrome, central breathing disorders), cerebral hemorrhage, persistent ductus arteriosus (PDA), retinopathy of prematurity, and necrotizing enterocolitis (NEC).

The **first care** for (small) premature infants in the delivery room should be given by personnel experienced in neonatology (pediatricians and pediatric nurses). It is particularly important to protect the child from heat loss. The resuscitation unit should be heated in advance, the doors should be closed to avoid draft, and sufficient warmed blankets should be available. The smaller the child, the more carefully the first care must be administered: patting the baby dry instead of rubbing, careful tactile stimulation. At any sign of respiratory distress, a CPAP can become necessary immediately postpartum. The indication for intubation and ventilation must be broadly defined. After stabilization, the child should be transferred as quickly as possible to a neonatal intensive care unit. For this move, the premature baby should be placed in a transport incubator. If there is no neonatal intensive care unit on the spot, transportation to the nearest perinatology center must be organized. Neonatology centers have their own pickup service for such cases.

In **preparing for a premature birth**, the parents should not be forgotten, especially if a very small premature baby (< 1,500 g) is expected. The parents are usually very concerned and anxious and often do not know the characteristics and problems associated with prematurity. When they see the child for the first time, many parents are frightened by how small the child really is and to how many wires and tubes the child is connected. Therefore, when possible, there should be a prepartal visit with the parents. The parents are told what happens during the child's first care, and that later, the child will be placed in an incubator and monitored. Many cables will be used for this purpose. The child may also need ventilation since because of its immaturity, it cannot yet breathe sufficiently on its own. It is very important to speak gently with the parents. Nowadays, the prognosis, even for extremely small and immature infants born prematurely, is relatively good. After the birth, the parents should be encouraged to bond with the child, not to be afraid to touch the baby, and to speak with the premature infant a great deal. Kangarooing in skin-to-skin contact with mother or father should be offered (see Fig. Kangarooing neonate).

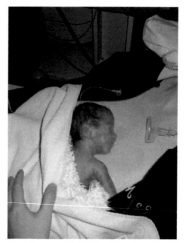

Kangarooing neonate (The child, dressed only in diapers, lies on the mother's unclothed breast. The intensive body contact gives the child a sense of boundary, warmth, and security. The parent–child bond is strengthened, the child's circulatory status is stabilized, and the parents' self-confidence is strengthened.)

→ Cases 55 Page 56

Respiratory distress syndrome: For clinical aspects and etiopathogenesis: see answer to question 55.1 (Syn.: RDS, hyaline membrane syndrome, infant respiratory distress syndrome (IRDS). Surfactant production can be increased with sympathomimetics, thyroxine, stress factors (e.g., premature of the membranes, birth), and cortisone. Inhibition or increased surfactant consumption can be caused, for instance, by maternal diabetes, hypoxia, acidosis, shock, amnion infection syndrome, or meconium aspiration. Therefore, for prevention of respiratory distress syndrome, maternal diabetes mellitus should be optimally managed. If there is a suspicion of amniotic infection, antibiotic prophylaxis is called for, and the birth process should be gentle (avoidance of hypoxic states). If delivery before completion of the 34th week of pregnancy cannot be avoided, an attempt should be made to delay labor for at least 48 hours and to administer dexamethasone to the mother. The steroids reach the fetus through the placenta and stimulate lung maturation. Respiratory distress syndrome is classified into four stages according to radiological criteria (see Tab./Fig. Respiratory distress syndrome).

Retinopathy of immaturity: See answer to question 55.3.

Stage classification of respiratory distress syndrome

Grade	Radiological criteria
I	Fine reticular pattern over the entire lung (microatelectases)
II	In addition, positive air bronchogram
III	In addition, blurred heart shadow and diaphragmatic borders
IV	Radiologically "white lung"

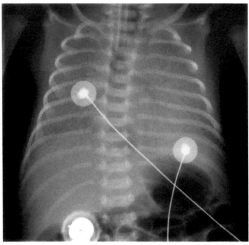

"White lung," respiratory distress syndrome Stage IV

Necrotizing enterocolitis: Clinical aspects and diagnosis: See answer to question 55.4. The cause of this hemorrhagic-necrotizing intestinal inflammation that frequently occurs in preterm infants and often affects the terminal ileum and colon (but involvement of the entire intestine is also possible) is not completely understood. A multifactorial genesis is assumed, e.g., immaturity of the gastrointestinal tract, buildup of diet too rapid, primary or secondary infections, prior damage to the intestinal walls due to insufficient perfusion or hypoxia. Possible risk factors are perinatal stress, hypothermia, shock, hypotension, hypoxemia, organic defects, and persisting ductus arteriosus. As a result of damage to the mucosa, gas-forming bacteria enter the intestinal wall with subsequent submucosal and subserous gas accumulation. This is visible in the abdominal survey radiograph and is labeled intestinal pneumatosis (see answer to question 55.4).

In the beginning stage, **treatment** is conservative with continuous clinical control. This includes parenteral nutrition, removal of gastric secreta with a gastric tube, i.v. antibiotic therapy, and ventilation. Risk factors, for instance, PDA, and the results of sepsis, such as disseminated intravascular coagulation or thrombocytopenia, should be treated. To support the circulation, volume therapy and administration of dopamine can become necessary. As the disease progresses, with perforation and peritonitis, operative resection of the affected intestinal section becomes necessary. Necrosing enterocolitis is associated with a mortality, depending on the degree of severity, from 10% to 50%. In 10% to 30% of patients, stenoses and adhesions arise during the healing process and can lead to relapsing ileus symptoms. In 5% to 10% of cases, short bowel syndrome develops.

Cerebral hemorrhage: An additional fearful and frequent complication of premature birth is cerebral hemorrhage. The germinal matrix with its very vulnerable blood vessels lies in the ventricular region of the preterm baby. It regresses again by the 32nd (−36th week). The risk of cerebral hemorrhage increases with the degree of immaturity. It is increased by fluctuating blood pressure, ischemia, hypoxia, acidosis, and coagulation disorders. Ninety percent of cerebral hemorrhages manifest within the first 4 days after birth. The hemorrhage can take place without symptoms. Sudden deterioration of the overall condition, paleness, hypotension, and cerebral seizures suggest cerebral hemorrhage. The diagnosis is established sonographically. Four degrees of severity are differentiated (see Tab. Cerebral hemorrhage).

The coagulation parameters should be examined and Vitamin K should be administered prophylactically

(0.1–0.2 µg/kg body weight i.v.). The blood pressure should be stabilized and peak blood pressure values should be avoided (*caution:* Bolus administration when hanging catecholamine infusions). Oxygen saturation is maintained within the normal range, which may require intubation. Hypo- and hypercapnia must be avoided since they may have a long-term effect on cerebral perfusion. Administration of sedatives may be medically sensible. The blood sugar level should also be maintained within the normal range. In case of seizures, anticonvulsive treatment must be liberal.

Stage classification of cerebral hemorrhages

Stage	Location
Grade I	Subependymal, at the transition of the head of the caudate nucleus to the thalamus
Grade II	Rupture into the ventricle, bleeding fills < 50% of the ventricle
Grade III	Rupture into the ventricle, bleeding fills > 50% of the ventricle
Grade IV	Additional bleeding into the cerebral parenchyma

Grade I and II hemorrhages require no further therapy. Their prognosis is good. Sometimes small cysts develop in the germ layer without causing neurological symptoms. In a Grade II hemorrhage, there may be a transient imbalance between production and resorption of cerebrospinal fluid with enlargement of the ventricle, but hydrocephalus requiring treatment usually does not develop. From Grade III, cerebral hemorrhages are complicated by formation of posthemorrhagic hydrocephalus that usually

requires a CSF drain. Parenchymal hemorrhages (Grade IV) leave behind cysts (porencephaly) that are the same size as the former hemorrhage and are often associated with neurological defects.

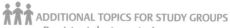 ADDITIONAL TOPICS FOR STUDY GROUPS
- Persistent ductus arteriosus
- CPAP (mechanism of action, indications)
- Causes in mother and child of premature birth

56 Constipation

56.1 How do you explain the alternation between stool retention and diarrhea? What is the cause of the boy's soiled underpants?

This alternation between stool retention and diarrhea is called **paradoxical diarrhea**. The thickened stool is subjected to secondary decomposition by bacteria, creating a foul-smelling, fluid stool that can run out uncontrolled past the hardened stool mass because of the distended rectum. The boy tries to hold the stool back but does not always succeed on time so that some stool can leave the ampulla. This is why his underpants are soiled (**fecal smearing, encopresis**).

56.2 What is your suspected diagnosis? What are the general underlying causes of these symptoms?

- **Chronic constipation and perianal eczema**; rationale: Relapsing episodes of stool retention in the past 2

years, hard stool palpable in the ampulla, paradoxical diarrhea and fecal smearing; perianal erythema, itching with traces of scratching
A distinction is made between:
- **Primary and idiopathic constipation** (95% of cases): In incorrect nutrition (too little to drink, too little fiber), change of diet (particularly in infants), lack of activity
- **Secondary constipation:**
  - Congenital or acquired intestinal diseases, e.g., Hirschsprung's disease, aganglionosis, stenoses in large intestine or rectum (e.g., in Crohn's disease), anorectal malformations, anorectal lesions (e.g., anal fissures), dolichocolon
  - Underlying diseases outside the intestine such as endocrine diseases (e.g., hypothyroidism), chronic fluid loss (e.g., renal tubular acidosis, diabetes insipidus), neurological causes (e.g.,

meningomyelocele, tethered cord), immobilization, medication use (e.g., chronic laxative abuse), metabolic diseases (e.g., cystic fibrosis), hypercalcemia, celiac disease, and infrequently, intra-abdominal tumors
– Situational problems, psychological stress

56.3 **What is your next diagnostic step?**
■ **Detailed medical history:**
  – Onset of symptoms
  – Stool history: Frequency (constipation already in infancy [distinction between congenital and acquired constipation], consistency, caliber of stool (indication of stenosis), amount of stool, blood in stool (indication, e.g., of anal fissure)
  – Eating and drinking habits (alimentary constipation)
  – Enuresis / Urinary tract infection; innervation disorder of bladder and rectum, e.g., in meningomyelocele, spina bifida
  – Chronic diseases: See answer to question 56.2.
  – Psychosocial conflicts, toilet training
■ Taking and recording body measurements in somatogram: Failure to thrive, e.g., as evidence of chronic diseases
■ Abdominal sonography: stenoses, tumors
■ **Laboratory:**
  – Blood (if appropriate to clinical suspicions): blood count, thyroid values, renal values, electrolytes, anti-transglutaminase antibodies

– Urine status: Urinary tract infection (outflow blockage often associated with chronic constipation)
– Anal smear: evidence of, e.g., *Streptococci*, fungi (frequent cause of perianal eczema)

56.4 **What is your next treatment step?**
■ **First measures:** Enema to empty intestine, possibly local anesthetic salve to ease pain of defecation (e.g., xylocaine gel.); if there is evidence of *Streptococci*, systemic antibiotic therapy (Penicillin V 50,000–100,000 IU/kg body weight in 3–4 individual doses) over 10 days; if there is evidence of fungi, local antimycotic treatment (e.g., nystatin salve)
■ **In the days that follow:**
  – One to two times daily intestinal emptying with enemas or glycerin suppositories for 5 to 7 days
  – possibly additional medications to encourage and soften stool (e.g., lactulose, macrogol)
■ **Long-term treatment:**
  – General measures: Diet rich in fiber (e.g., plentiful fruit and vegetables [raw], preferably five times daily), sufficient fluid intake (1–1.5 L/d, especially uncarbonated water, unsweetened tea, juice spritzers; no sweetened lemonades), activity
  – Behavioral training (toilet training) with reward and positive reinforcement
  – Care by a child psychologist

193

Case

56

Comments

Definition and forms: Constipation is stool retention because of incomplete stool emptying and/or defecation problems with hard stool. In **chronic** constipation, the symptoms last for longer than 3 months. A distinction is made between **primary** or idiopathic constipation and **secondary** forms that occur as a result of intestinal diseases or because of neurological or metabolic diseases (see answer to question 56.3).

Etiology: The most frequent cause of constipation is an **incorrect and unvaried diet**. There is frequent acute constipation around Easter and Christmas because of immoderate consumption of chocolate. Other causes are insufficient fluid intake, starvation, changes of life habits when traveling, fluid loss on account of fever, immobilization, stool retention caused by abdominal disease (e.g., remittent gastroenteritis) or painful anal fissure, and drug consumption (e.g., iron preparations). For other causes, see answer to question 56.2.

Clinical aspects: Often constipation is associated with acute, intense abdominal pain and the abdomen can be distended and painful on pressure. The symptoms are reminiscent of an "acute abdomen" (see example case). Often the abdominal pain is accompanied by nausea and vomiting. Patients suffer from meteorism. In chronic constipation, patients complain repeatedly of more or less intense abdominal pain. Fecal smearing, soiling one's pants and alternation between very hard stool and vile-smelling diarrhea are another typical sign of chronic constipation. Blood in the stool is also observed, caused by injury to the mucosa at the anus by hard stool or anal fissure.

Diagnostics: In general, children expel stool daily, but intervals of several days can be physiological. It is therefore impossible to determine "normal" behavior from the stools expelled every day. Rather, the stool quality and quantity as well as changes in stool habits must be taken into account.

As part of the diagnostics, therefore, a detailed history (see answer to question 56.3) is obligatory. A thorough pediatric examination, including rectal examination and recording of body measurements, is also obligatory. In addition, a urine status should be determined, and further laboratory tests may be

→ Cases 56 Page 57

necessary (e.g., blood count, thyroid values, renal values, electrolytes).

If constipation persists in spite of appropriate treatment or in the absence of concrete evidence of a cause, a colon contrast enema, anorectal manometry, or rectal biopsy may be required.

Differential diagnoses: Pseudo-constipation (no stool without symptoms in breastfed infants up to 2 weeks), appendicitis, urinary tract infections.

Treatment: The objective of the treatment is **complete and regular stool emptying**, i.e., a normal stool without encopresis should be expelled daily or at least every second day. To achieve this, stool hardening and rectal stretching must be reversed. The stool must become so soft that expulsion of the stool does not cause pain. Medications such as lactulose or macrogol can be used. In addition to general measures such as change of **diet** (high-fiber diet), **sufficient fluid intake**, and a great deal of **activity**, **behavioral measures** are used, such as toilet training (positive reinforcement such as sending the child to the toilet regularly, giving the child sufficient time, praise for success). In addition, it is particularly important to provide explanations and training for the parents. They should understand the cause and occurrence (e.g., decreased intestinal movement due to insufficient fiber content, insufficient physical activity, thickening of the stool mass because of insufficient fluid, pain during stool expulsion caused by stool hardening leads to stool retention and reinforcement of constipation). They should understand that treatment must sometimes be carried out over a period of months. Psychotherapeutic accompaniment of parents and child can be very helpful in this regard.

If the constipation is secondary, the treatment of the underlying disease must be emphasized, e.g., surgical treatment for Hirschsprung's disease, drug therapy of hypothyroidism, etc.

Prognosis: The prognosis of chronic constipation is very good with consistent treatment, strict management, and information for patients and their parents. If treatment is inconsistent, there is a risk of sequelae in adulthood such as diverticulosis, diverticulitis, and laxative abuse.

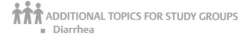 ADDITIONAL TOPICS FOR STUDY GROUPS
- Diarrhea

---

57 Systemic juvenile chronic arthritis (Still syndrome)

57.1 What is your diagnosis? What differential diagnoses are you considering?
- **Suspected diagnosis: Systemic juvenile chronic arthritis** (Still syndrome, Still's disease); rationale: fever, hepatomegaly, generalized lymph node enlargement, laboratory (elevated sedimentation rate, sharply elevated CRP, hypochrome anemia, leukocytosis, thrombocytosis), exanthema, swollen joints
- **Differential diagnoses:**
  - Sepsis: High fever, sharply elevated inflammatory parameters, left shift in the differential count
  - Septic arthritis: High fever, sharply elevated inflammatory parameters, joint inflammation
  - Osteomyelitis: Swollen joints, sharply elevated inflammatory parameters, high fever
  - Leukemia: Generalized lymphadenopathy, hepatosplenomegaly, leukocytosis, thrombocytosis
  - Rheumatic fever: Swollen joints, rash, fever
  - Infectious arthritis: Suspicion of fifth disease
  - Malignant bone disease: Swollen joints, thrombocytosis
  - Kawasaki syndrome: Persistent high fever longer than 5 days, swollen lymph nodes, exanthema, thrombocytosis

57.2 What further tests would you consider useful?
- **Laboratory:** For establishment of diagnosis, monitoring progress; *Caution:* Interpretation only in context of clinical picture, since all laboratory parameters can also turn out to be normal.
  - Blood: Inflammatory parameters (sedimentation rate, CRP): monitoring progress
  - Serology to rule out other forms of arthritis: IgM rheumatoid factor, ANA, HLA-B27, borreliosis titer
  - Blood cultures: Ruling out sepsis
  - Urine: Ruling out urinary tract infection as cause of the fever and the high inflammatory parameters
- **Sonography:**
  - Abdomen: Involvement of visceral organs
  - Joints: effusions, synovial swelling, synovial cysts, tenosynovitis, etc.
- **MRI:** Joints; monitoring progress;
- **ECG/Echocardiography:** Heart involvement (peri-, myocarditis)
- **Ophthalmological examination:** Iridocyclitis, uveitis

How is the disease that you are suspecting generally treated?
■ **Stepwise drug treatment:**
1. Nonsteroidal antiphlogistics (naproxen, indomethacin, ibuprofen, or diclofenac)
2. Disease-modifying drugs:
   – Basic therapeutic drugs (e.g., sulfasalazine)
   – Immunosuppressive agents, cytostatic agents (e.g., methotrexate, etanercept)
3. Glucocorticoids

■ **Supportive measures:**
   – Information and training with regard to the diseases (parents + child)
   – Accompanying physio- and ergotherapy: e.g., cold therapy in case of acute inflammation, heat therapy in the inflammation-free interval
   – Psychosocial care (e.g., psychological family therapy, promoting school lessons, even when the patient is homebound with illness, professional counseling)

Comments

Definition and forms: The Still syndrome is the **systemic form** of juvenile idiopathic arthritis (JIA), a **chronic, destructive joint inflammation**. For other forms of JIA see Tab. in appendix.

Epidemiology: The incidence of JIA is approximately 1 in 1,000 new cases in a given year in the United States. The **onset age** of Still syndrome is usually in toddlers, **between 1 and 4 years of age**.

Etiopathogenesis: The cause of the disease is not known. **Autoimmune disorders** have been considered, with the appropriate genetic predisposition (e.g., HLA-DR4, -5, -6, -8) and a variety of triggering noxae (e.g., parvovirus B 19) or trauma. These lead to chronic synovitis, cartilage destruction, and extra-articular inflammations. The severity of the disease can vary; it occurs in flare-ups in which with time the systemic symptoms become less prominent and the arthritis becomes more prominent.

Clinical aspects: Still syndrome is characterized by **high, intermittent fever for at least 2 weeks, exanthema, lymphadenopathy**, and **usually involvement of internal organs** (e.g., polyserositis, peri-/myocarditis, hepato-/splenomegaly) as well as considerable impairment of the general condition; affected children are very ill. Uveitis that is typical for other forms of JIA does not usually occur in Still syndrome. Often there is also **pain in the cervical spine** that is especially observed at the beginning of the disease and can be misinterpreted as meningism. **Arthritis** can occur at the beginning of the disease or may not follow until months or years later. This often makes diagnosis difficult (see answer to question 57.1). Wrists, elbows, shoulders, hip joints, knees, and ankles are affected particularly often.

Diagnostics: See answer to question 57.2. Indicative factors in the medical history are episodes with **intermittent, septic fever** that occurs especially in the early morning and evening and disappears spontaneously. The patient should be asked about muscle pain,

unwillingness to walk, lack of appetite, weight loss, previous infections, tick bites, and familial diseases of a rheumatic nature. In the physical examination, particularly all joints, including the spine, must be examined in detail. All lymph node stations must be palpated; heart and lungs must be auscultated. Pain on deep inspiration can indicate pleuritis. In palpation of the abdomen, special attention is given to enlarged organs. **Changes in laboratory parameters** are rather unspecific overall. There are high inflammation parameters (CRP, leukocytes, sedimentation rate) and elevated complement factors (C_3 and C_4), thrombocytosis, and hypochromic anemia. Antinuclear factors (ANA, anti-dsDNA, ENA, ANCA) are usually negative; the rheumatic factors are seldom unspecifically elevated. Sonographic evidence of hepato-/splenomegaly and serositis can be found, with possibly evidence in the echocardiogram of pericardial effusion and myocarditis. The extent of joint destruction can be radiologically determined. Uveitis can be excluded (even if rarely in Still syndrome).

Treatment: See answer to question 57.3. A **causal treatment** of the disease is not known. The objective of treatment is complete disappearance of local and systemic inflammation, freedom from pain, and avoidance of deformity and organ complications. Therapy is determined by the extent of the symptoms (stepwise therapy). The medicine of choice is **non-steroidal anti-inflammatories** that inhibit inflammation by influencing prostaglandin synthesis. The pain-relieving effect occurs at once; the inflammatory process is not inhibited after a few weeks. **Glucocorticoids** also have a very efficacious anti-inflammatory effect; they can be administered systemically or locally (intra-articular injection) depending in the degree of severity. The large number and severity of side effects (e.g., Cushing syndrome with central obesity, arterial hypertension, hyperglycemia, tendency to infection, osteopenia, growth retardation, and stunted growth) should always be kept in mind when prescribing.

In addition, so-called **disease-modifying drugs** (DMARD = disease-modifying antirheumatic drugs) such as methotrexate, sulfasalazine, and etanercept are used. These drugs have a positive effect on the course of the disease; this can be measured on the radiologically demonstrable joint changes. The anti-inflammatory or analgesic action of disease-modifying drugs is not primary and immediate, and therefore a combination with non-steroidal anti-inflammatory agents and/or glucocorticoids is usually unavoidable. Such second-line medications as gold, penicillamine, or hydrochloroquin are not used for children because they have little or no efficacy against JIA. In addition to drug therapy, **physio- and ergotherapy** play an important role in the treatment of juvenile idiopathic arthritis, in reducing the secondary joint dysfunctions that arise as a result of pain and protective posture. In intractable monoarthritis a synovectomy can produce improvement, and secondary joint changes caused by a chronic inflammatory process can make reorientation osteotomy necessary. Furthermore, long-term treatment of children suffering from chronic rheumatism requires comprehensive information and training with regard to the disease or mastery of the disease and **psychosocial care** that includes the family.

Prognosis: With early diagnosis and adequate treatment, prognosis for JIA is generally good. In adults, 75% of cases are healed or only demonstrate a small amount of disease activity. Twenty-five percent develop severe joint involvement.

👪 ADDITIONAL TOPICS FOR STUDY GROUPS
- Forms of JIA (oligo-/polyarthritis)
- Effects/side effects of glucocorticoids

58   Inguinal hernia

58.1   Name and justify your suspected diagnosis. What differential diagnoses must you take into account in case of an inguinal swelling?
- **Suspected diagnosis:** (incarcerated) **inguinal hernia right**; rationale: child's age, swelling of right groin, probably very painful (constant screaming)
- **Differential diagnoses:**
  - Hydrocele of the spermatic cord: Bulging elastic swelling in the spermatic cord
  - Hydrocele testis: Bulging elastic swelling in the scrotum
  - Scrotal torsion: Testis painful on pressure and enlarged, possibly livid discoloration of the scrotum
  - Inguinal testis: Small, movable, coarse swelling in the inguinal region
  - Swelling of the inguinal lymph nodes: Coarse, movable inguinal swelling

58.2   There are two forms of this disease. List differences. What form is the infant most likely to have?
- **Indirect inguinal hernia (lateral inguinal hernia):**
  - Usually congenital (through incomplete closure of the peritoneal vaginal process) but also acquired
  - Occurs frequently in premature infants (because of connective tissue weakness)
  - Hernial orifice (= inner inguinal ring) lateral to the epigastric vessels
  - Contents of hernia: mostly intestine, in girls also tube and ovary

- **Direct inguinal hernia (medial inguinal hernia):**
  - Always acquired (herniation takes place due to weak muscle gaps in the abdominal wall)
  - Hernial orifice (= external inguinal ring) medial to the epigastric vessels (inguinal fossa)
  - Rare in children
- The infant in this case is very likely to have indirect inguinal hernia.

58.3   What do you do next?
- The diagnosis is established clinically. Sonography is performed only when the diagnosis is unclear, to rule out testicular torsion or an inguinal testicle
- Thirty minutes after administration of analgesic (e.g., paracetamol suppository), attempt at careful repositioning; practical procedure: place the hands on the hernial sac and attempt to push it further intra-abdominally, if possible when the child is relaxed and not screaming (for instance, when the child is feeding from a bottle or nursing from the breast, during a bath, or while distracted with a favorite toy)
- Operation follows shortly after successful repositioning
- Impossibility of repositioning is an indication for immediate surgery

58.4   List complications of this disease.
Incarceration with ileus/subileus/peritonitis/intestinal gangrene; in girls, herniation of the ovary

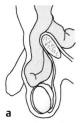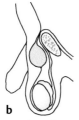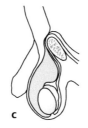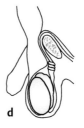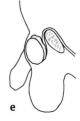

a   b   c   d   e

Causes for swelling around groin and testicles
a) Inguinal hernia b) Hydrocele of spermatic cord with fluid inside the spermatic duct c) Testicular hydrocele with fluid between the layers of the tunica vaginalis d) Testicular torsion e) Inguinal testis

Comments

Definition and epidemiology: Inguinal hernia (Syn.: Inguinal hernias) are protrusions of the peritoneum with contents (e.g., intestine, tube, ovary) in the inguinal canal. The right side is much more frequently affected. But inguinal hernias are often bilateral.

Their incidence is 1% to 2%; in premature infants, the rate rises to 30%. Boys are affected 6% to 8% more frequently than girls. The peak age is within the first year. Inguinal hernias often appear in the first month of an infant's life.

Forms, pathogenesis, and complications: A distinction is made between direct and indirect inguinal hernias (see answer to question 58.2). Indirect inguinal hernia is typical for children.

The testis moves into the scrotum through a peritoneal diverticulum, the peritoneal vaginal process. After the descent is complete, the process is not obliterated, or only incompletely. In girls, the non-obliterated peritoneal vaginal process runs along the round ligament through the inguinal canal. The contents of the hernia passes through the internal inguinal ring along the (in-)completely closed peritoneal vaginal process (the hernial sac). The contents of hernia usually consist of the intestine, and in girls often tube and ovary also.

In case of incarceration of intestinal sections, venous return can be impeded by necrosis of the intestinal wall, subileus, ileus, perforation, and peritonitis.

Clinical aspects: Clinically, there is inguinal swelling that is particularly noticeable when the child is screaming or bearing down. Children who are already presenting with a strangulated hernia exhibit other symptoms in addition to inguinal swelling, such as pain, restlessness, and vomiting.

Diagnostics: The example case shows the importance of a detailed physical examination of the child. For this purpose, it must be completely undressed. If a child is

crying for undetermined reasons, the possibility of an inguinal hernia must always be kept in mind. Other causes of unexplained screaming are often acute otitis media and, in boys, testicular torsion.

Treatment: A careful attempt is made to reposition the contents of the hernia in the abdominal space, but never when this involves the ovary (which can be palpated as a spherical structure in the hernial sac). This may only succeed during a bath or after administration of sedatives (diazepam) and analgesics.

Every diagnosed inguinal hernia must be surgically treated. The operation should be performed early, in order to avoid strangulation. In premature infants, an operation is only performed shortly before discharge to home, when the child weighs enough (> 2,000 g) and the anatomical structures can be more easily seen. Usually the hernial orifice is large enough so that there is no risk of strangulation. But if the hernia is strangulated, surgery is performed regardless of body weight.

If repositioning is impossible, it must be assumed that the inguinal hernia is strangulated or incarcerated. If sections of the intestine are incarcerated, the impeded venous return causes swelling. This makes repositioning of the hernial contents impossible. The incarcerated inguinal hernia is an indication for urgent surgical intervention.

Prognosis: If the diagnosis is established promptly and treatment is adequate, the prognosis is very good. If the diagnosis is established too late, resection of the intestinal sections may become necessary. There is an increased risk of an inguinal hernia on the other side.

 ADDITIONAL TOPICS FOR STUDY GROUPS
- Scrotal torsion
- Umbilical hernia
- Testicular hydrocele

197

Case

58

→ Cases 58 Page 59

59.1 What diagnostic measures do you consider useful to initiate next? What are the grounds for this?

The child has clinical signs of **hemolytic anemia** (sallow, pale, icteric skin color), **blood coagulation disorder** (individual hematomas, skin petechiae), **dehydration** (skin tenting, circles under the eyes), and **gastroenteritis** (diarrhea, vomiting, bloody stools). For this reason, the first measure should be infusion therapy. When the indwelling venous cannula is inserted, blood is taken for **laboratory tests**: blood picture (Hb, hematocrit, leukocytes, thrombocytes), differential, blood smear, serum (urea, creatinine, electrolytes [Na, K, Ca], LDH, bilirubin), coagulation status.

59.2 Interpret the laboratory values. What is your diagnosis?

- **Laboratory:**
  - Blood picture: Anemia, thrombocytopenia, reticulocytosis
  - Blood smear: Distorted, eggshell-shaped erythrocytes (= fragmentocytes)
  - Serum: Renal retention parameters ↑ (urea ↑, creatinine ↑), potassium ↑, LDH ↑
- **Diagnosis: Hemolytic–uremic syndrome** (D⁺-HUS); rationale: child's age; gastrointestinal infection (vomiting, bloody stools for the past week); pale, icteric skin color; petechial bleeding; individual hematomas, neurological symptoms (clouding); anuria; laboratory changes (**thrombocytopenia, hemolytic anemia** [and fragmentocytes], **uremia**)

59.3 Explain the pathogenesis of the disease.

Gastrointestinal infection with **enterohemorrhagic E. coli** (chiefly EHEC Serovar 0157:H7) or other intestinal pathogens (e.g., Salmonella, Shigella) or respiratory tract infection (S. pneumoniae)

↓

Release of bacterial endotoxins (chiefly **verotoxin**)

↓

Damage to the vascular endothelium

↓

Activation of intravascular coagulation (formation of microthrombi and fibrin nets)

↓

Thrombocyte consumption, occlusion, chiefly of glomerular capillaries, mechanical erythrocyte damage

↓

Thrombocytopenia, hemolytic anemia, uremia (acute renal failure)

59.4 How do you treat the girl?

- Only **symptomatic treatment** is possible
- Admission to pediatric intensive care
- Careful **rehydration** (avoid excessive hydration) with infusion therapy with semi-isotonic solution (NaCl 0.9% and glucose 5% 1:1)
- No diuresis after correction of the fluid deficit (renal failure): Administration of furosemide 1 to 2 mg/kg body weight (to a max. of 5 mg/kg body weight i.v.)
- Monitor blood pressure, antihypertensive therapy in case of arterial hypertension (e.g., nifedipin 0.5–2.0 mg/kg body weight or propranolol 1.5–5 mg/kg body weight)
- Continued increasing renal retention values (creatinine, urea): Early renal replacement therapy (peritoneal/hemodialysis)
- With progressing anemia (Hb < 5 mg/dL): Blood transfusion; *caution:* strict establishment of indication; only in case of vital indication because transfusion can reactivate the disease process
- Falling thrombocyte values < 15,000–20,000/μL: Platelet concentrates

---

Comments

Definition and epidemiology: The co-occurrence of **hemolysis, thrombocytopenia**, and **oliguria or anuria** is called hemolytic–uremic syndrome (HUS). This is the most frequent cause of acute renal failure in children. The peak frequency occurs in early childhood (1–4 years of age). An endemic course in summer months (frequent food poisoning) is observed in infection-associated HUS.

Etiopathogenesis: See answer to question 59.3. Frequently, hemolytic–uremic syndrome can be caused by medication (mitomycin, tacrolimus, cyclosporine). It also occurs with tumor diseases, kidney diseases, after bone marrow and organ transplantation, and during radiation treatment.

Clinical aspects: In infection-associated HUS, 1 to 12 days after a case of gastroenteritis or respiratory tract infection, symptoms such as **bloody diarrhea, fever, vomiting, abdominal pain, oligo- or anuria, cerebral symptoms** (e.g., clouded consciousness, seizures) and critical rise in blood pressure are observed. Hemolysis leads to anemia (pale skin color) and hemoglobinuria (beer-brown urine). Platelet destruction causes petechial or **extensive skin and mucosal bleeding**.

Diagnostics: The triad of thrombocytopenia, hemolytic anemia (with fragmentocytes), and increase in serum creatinine, together with the clinical symptoms, leads to the diagnosis.

Differential diagnoses: Acute renal failure caused by other factors, shock, Waterhouse–Friderichsen syndrome.

Treatment: See answer to question 59.4.

Prognosis: Kidney function is impaired in 30% to 60% of cases. Approximately 5% of affected children will require dialysis permanently. There is often a complete cure in infancy.

Worldwide lethality is between 1% and 5%. The prognosis is poor where there is cerebral involvement and severe arterial hypertension.

Prophylaxis: Unpasteurized milk and raw beef should be avoided.

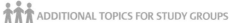 ADDITIONAL TOPICS FOR STUDY GROUPS
- Anemia
- Icterus (forms)
- Gastroenteritis
- Renal replacement therapy

! | 60   Congenital heart defect

60.1   What is your diagnosis on the basis of the clinical and echocardiographic findings?
Patient's echo: Aorta is in anterior position and arises from the right ventricle, pulmonary artery rises from the left ventricle, in the parasternal longitudinal section the **parallel position of the large vessels** (see Fig.) [KR_A060a.tif] is characteristic, resulting in parallel circuit of pulmonary and body circulation. The great **arteries are transposed** (TGA).

60.2   How is this deformity treated?
- Keep the ductus arteriosus of Botalli open or reopen it to ensure perfusion of the body circulation: The systemic circulation does not receive oxygenated blood because of the shunt to the pulmonary circulation; both circulations are connected by the ductus arteriosus. The blood is commingled and the systemic circulation is supplied with mixed blood. To keep the ductus arteriosus open, a continuous prostaglandin-E1 infusion (0.05–0.1 µg/kg body weight/min) is maintained until the time of the operation. *Caution:* Apnea is a possible side effect and intubation and ventilation may become necessary.
- If there is a risk of hypoxemia, emergency Rashkind balloon atrioseptostomy may be necessary (see Comments).
- Arterial switch operation within the first 2 weeks of the infant's life (see Comments).
- Senning or Mustard atrial switch procedure by diversion of the blood flow to the atrium in older patients.

60.3   What do you do next?
- Careful physical examination including palpation of pulses in upper and lower extremities (pulse difference between upper and lower extremities in aortic isthmus stenosis), apex beat ("precordial buzz" by conduction of the heart sound to surrounding tissue), liver size, edema, respiratory frequency, and flaring nostrils (signs of heart failure?).
- Blood pressure measurement at all four extremities: see above.
- EKG: Determination of cardiac axis (in newborns, usually right type because of physiological right hypertrophy, displacement of the cardiac axis as sign of volume or pressure hypertrophy). The most suspicious are axis deviation types; search for bundle branch block, rhythm disorders.
- Echocardiography: Search for heart defects, determination of contractility.

60.4   Diagnose the echocardiogram. What do you determine?
Small ventricular septum defect (VSD); rationale: "Gap" in the perimembranous ventricular septum

60.5   In many congenital heart defects, there is an elevated risk of endocarditis. In this connection, what is meant by endocarditis prophylaxis?
- **Endocarditis** is an inflammatory bacterial (less often fungal) disease of the heart valves, endocardium, or the endothelium of the great arteries close

→ Cases 60 Page 61

to the heart. The turbulent blood flow around a defect, even after its correction, causes lesions in the neighboring endocardium or endothelium, on which thrombotic deposits develop. In particular, Gram-positive bacteria (*Streptococci, Staphylococci*) attach themselves to these deposits. The oropharyngeal space is the main portal for these pathogens.

- **Endocarditis prophylaxis:**
  - Administration of antibiotics (see below) for interventions in the nasopharyngeal, gastrointestinal, urogenital tracts, and skin.
  - In addition, good dental hygiene and regular dental check-ups, determination of cause of fever, in obvious bacterial infections, systematic antibiotic treatment for 8 to 12 days, depending on the pathogen spectrum
  - Instruction of parents and issuing a "heart passport"
- There are various risk groups:

- **Risk group A** (type two atrioseptal defect [ASD II], 6 months after correction of an ASD II or a VSD, status post section of a ductus arteriosus Botalli, mitral valve prolapse without mitral insufficiency): no prophylaxis, low endocarditis risk (flow conditions almost normal, low turbulence in blood flow)
- **Risk group B** (all other heart or vessel malformations [also after surgical correction], mitral valve prolapse with mitral insufficiency, hypertrophic obstructive cardiomyopathy): single dose of antibiotic (penicillin, amoxicillin, or flucloxacillin i.v.) 30 to 60 minutes before procedure
- **Risk group C** (artificial heart valves, other foreign material, aorto-pulmonary shunts, status post endocarditis): antibiotics (penicillin, amoxicillin, or flucloxacillin in combination with gentamycin i.v.) immediately before procedure and once after 8 hours

Comments

Definition and classification: All inborn heart defects are classified as congenital heart deformities. On the basis of hemodynamic characteristics they are classified as:

- Acyanotic heart defects:
  - **Without shunt** with right- or left-sided obstruction of the outflow, e.g., pulmonary stenosis, aortic stenosis, aortic isthmus stenosis
  - **With left–right shunt**, e.g., ventricular septum defect (see below), atrial septum defect, open ductus arteriosus Botalli
- **Cyanotic heart defects** (with right–left shunt): Transposition of the great arteries (see below), tetralogy of Fallot (see below), Ebstein's anomaly, pulmonary atresia, tricuspid atresia, hypoplastic left heart, total anomalous pulmonary vein connection, double outlet right ventricle, common arterial trunk, singular ventricle

Epidemiology: The incidence of congenital heart defects is approximately 6–8:1,000. The most frequent heart defects are ventricular septal defect (30%), atrial septal defect (12%), pulmonary stenosis (10%), persistent ductus arteriosus Botalli (10%), and tetralogy of Fallot (10%).

Etiology: The precise cause is not known; a number of predisposing factors is held responsible, such as chromosomal anomalies (e.g., trisomy 18, trisomy 21, Turner syndrome) as well as viral infections (e.g., rubella, CMV, herpes simplex), medications (e.g., phenytoin, coumadin, lithium) or alcohol abuse during pregnancy.

Transposition of the great arteries (TGA): See answers to questions 60.1 and 60.2. Transposition of the great arteries is one of the cyanotic defects and constitutes 8% of all congenital heart defects. In transposition of the great arteries, the aorta arises from the right and the pulmonary artery from the left ventricle (see Fig. TGA).

As a result, the pulmonary and systemic circulations are not connected in series but in parallel, so that venous blood is pumped back into the systemic circulation and arterial blood back into the pulmonary circulation. Only short-circuit connections (shunts, septal defects, or patent ductus arteriosus Botalli) can ensure oxygen transport from the minor into the major circulation. When there is no shunt, hypoxemia results, and this is not consistent with life. **Shortly after birth**, newborns exhibit **generalized cyanosis** that cannot be reversed with the administration of oxygen. The **hyperoxia test** (patient receives 100% oxygen for 10 to 15 minutes) produces no improvement in oxygen saturation. There is usually no heart murmur. The diagnosis is established by means of echocardiography. The first step after establishment of the diagnosis is first **maintaining the ductus arteriosus Botalli open**, to ensure a sufficient supply of oxygenated blood through the ductus arteriosus. This is done by continual infusion of prostaglandin E1. If there is nevertheless a critical degree of hypoxemia, the cardiac circulation can be stabilized by Rashkind balloon atrioseptostomy (tearing the atrial septum with a balloon catheter). During the first 2 weeks of the infant's life, the heart defect is then surgically corrected in a cardiac center. The preferred method is the **arterial switch operation** in which the great arteries are severed above the sinus and re-anastomosed in the inverted position. In addition, a new implantation of the coronary arteries in the new aorta is necessary. If the switch operation is impossible because of a particular heart defect morphology, an alternative is Senning's or Mustard's atrial switch operation, in which the blood flow is diverted at the atrium.

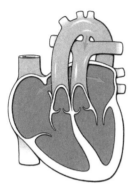

Transposition of the great arteries (TGA). Systemic and pulmonary circulations are connected in parallel. Only additional cross-connections (→), in the form of septal defects or persisting ductus arteriosus, permit partial mixing with oxygenated blood.

Without interventions, the lethality in the first year of a child's life is approximately 90%. However, the **long-range prognosis** after complete correction is good. After the switch operation, stenoses in the anastomosis of aorta, pulmonary artery, and coronary arteries, as well as heart rhythm disorders must be expected. Frequent complications of the atrial switch operation include right ventricular failure, stenoses of the vena cava and life-threatening supraventricular tachyarrhythmia, as well as bradycardia as a result of injuries of the sinus node artery (sick sinus syndrome).

Ventricular septum defect (VSD): The VSD (see Fig. VSD) is the most frequent **congenital heart defect** (25%). It often presents with other defects. Depending on the location, a distinction is made between perimembranous (70%) and muscular defects. After decrease of the postpartally elevated pulmonary resistance, a left–right shunt without cyanosis develops over the septal defect.

The **clinical signs** are largely determined by the size of the defect. Other than a loud systolic murmur in the 3rd/4th left parasternal intercostal space, small (pressure separating) defects generally cause no symptoms ("a lot of noise about nothing"). In larger (pressure-decreasing or pressure-equalizing) defects, it is also possible to hear a diastolic murmur, and at the sternum, a thrill can be felt.

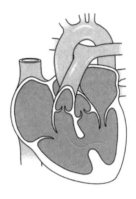

Ventricular septal defect (VSD): Muscular form.

With untreated larger ventricular septal defects, an **increasing (global) heart failure** develops, with symptoms such as tachypnea, tachycardia, hepatomegaly, peripheral edema, difficulty in drinking, sweating, and failure to flourish. In addition, there is a tendency to bronchopulmonary infections. *Note:* In case of relapsing pulmonary infections, a cardiac defect must always be ruled out. In untreated large defects, pulmonary hypertension develops that finally leads to irreversible shunt reversal (**Eisenmenger reaction**). **Small defects** do not require therapy; they usually close spontaneously in most cases. **Large defects** are corrected surgically. In case of pulmonary hypertension and heart failure that is difficult to treat, the operation is already performed in infancy. If no pulmonary hypertension develops and the heart failure can be controlled, the defect is corrected at preschool age. There is an increased risk of endocarditis (Group B). Until the operation is performed, the heart failure is treated with medication, e.g., with diuretics, ACE inhibitors, and digitalis. The defect is then closed with application of a patch ("mending," usually with a Dacron patch) or with a direct suture. The prognosis for the surgically treated ventricular septal defect is good. The most frequent postoperative complication is heart rhythm disorder.

Tetralogy of Fallot: Tetralogy of Fallot is classified in the group of cyanotic cardiac defects with decreased pulmonary perfusion. It occurs at a frequency of 1:1,500 births; the proportion among congenital cardiac defects is 8% to 11%. Boys are most often affected. Classical characteristics are ventricular septal defects, overriding aorta, pulmonary stenosis, and right ventricular hypertrophy (see Fig. Tetralogy of Fallot).

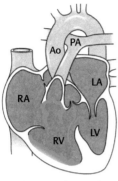

Tetralogy of Fallot (combination of ventricular septal defect with overriding aorta, pulmonary artery stenosis and right ventricular hypertrophy, as well as atrial septal defect)

of the pulmonary artery during the cardiac catheterization.

β-blockers (e.g., propranolol 1–3 mg/kg body weight in 3–4 individual doses/d) are administered until the operation as prophylaxis of hypoxemic attacks. The hypoxemic attack is interrupted by positioning (lateral recumbent, bent legs) and administration of esmolol (0.5 mg/kg body weight, slowly i.v.) and morphine (0.1 mg/kg body weight s.c. or i.v.). Endocarditis prophylaxis is required. Surgical correction should take place as soon as possible after establishment of diagnosis. The VSD is closed with a patch (e.g., Dacron); the right outflow is also widened by piecing. In spite of the best possible correction, there are always residual functional disorders of the pulmonary valve (pulmonary failure or stenosis) that can result in limited capacity and cardiac rhythm disorders. The symptoms increase with age. Pharmacological or surgical therapy (pulmonary valve replacement) may become necessary.

Varying degrees of severity are observed. When the pulmonary stenosis is only slight and the aorta is not significantly overriding, pulmonary perfusion is increased and there is no cyanosis. This is the so-called Pink Fallot. The hemodynamics and **clinical symptoms** are primarily determined by the degree of obstruction of the **right ventricular outflow tract**. In the newborn, the clinical signs are often not distinct; the child may only be noticed because of slight-to-moderate central cyanosis. A loud systolic murmur (pulmonary stenosis) is audible in the second to fourth left paracardiac intercostal space. Typically the cyanosis increases in the course of the first months of an infant's life. From the third to the sixth month of a child's life, so-called hypoxemic attacks can occur. They are triggered by spasms of the hypertrophied infundibular muscles, especially upon awakening or after physical exertion. Children become cyanotic, developing paleness and loss of tone; seizures to the point of unconsciousness are observed. A hypoxemic attack can last from a few minutes to hours. Earlier (but rarely today, because of early surgical intervention) it was often observed that children in a state of exertion squatted, in order to achieve improvement of the hypoxia. Additional symptoms in older children are nail clubbing, drumstick fingers, and polyglobulia because of a chronic oxygen lack.

The **diagnosis** is established by means of **echocardiography**. The ECG shows signs of right cardiac hypertrophy and possible heart rhythm disorder. The thoracic X-ray shows an uplifted cardiac apex, enhanced cardiac waist, and decreased pulmonary vascular markings. In addition, a cardiac catheterization is indicated to determine the morphology of the pulmonary artery and associated deformities. A possible intervention is a balloon valvuloplasty

Persistent ductus arteriosus Botalli: The ductus arteriosus Botalli is a vascular connection between the bifurcation of the pulmonary artery and the descending aorta; it is an important component of the fetal circulatory system. Normally, it closes by contraction of its wall musculature within the first few days of an infant's life and forms the ligamentum arteriosum. If the ductus does not close spontaneously, the condition is called open ductus arteriosus or persistent ductus arteriosus (see Fig. PDA). In premature births, the ductus closes late because of immaturity (immaturity of the ductus tissue and elevated prostaglandin level). A persistent ductus arteriosus in a mature newborn is an anomaly; spontaneous closure is rare. At 8% to 10%, an isolated open ductus arteriosus is a frequent cardiac defect; it also occurs as a complication of more complex defects.

A hemodynamically significant ductus arteriosus leads to a left–right shunt with excess volume loading of the left atrium and left ventricle. Blood flows into the lung even in diastole (lung flooding, danger of pulmonary edema, and [in a premature birth] bronchopulmonary dysplasia). A high blood pressure amplitude with high systolic and low diastolic pressure is the result (high, rapid pulse rate). The systemic circulation is insufficiently supplied (particularly to the abdominal organs and the kidneys). In newborns and premature births, there is also an elevated risk that necrotizing enterocolitis will develop. Cerebral circulation is also decreased; in immature children, there is a risk of periventricular leukomalacia.

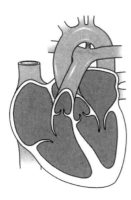

Persistent ductus arteriosus Botalli

The clinical signs depend on the size of the ductus. A **cardinal symptom** is a variation in the loudness of the systolic–diastolic "machine noise" with peak in the second left parasternal intercostal space. Often the heart sound is accompanied by a palpable precordial thrill. The femoral pulses can be felt as heaves because of the high blood pressure amplitude. A large ductus is associated with heart failure with hepatomegaly, edema, and tachypnea. Decreased physical capacity (poor drinking, increased sweating) and failure to thrive are additional characteristic symptoms. When the persistent ductus arteriosus is small and hemodynamically insignificant, the symptoms are restricted to the heart sound. The risk of endocarditis is increased.

The **diagnosis** is established by means of **echocardiography**. Pulmonary flooding can be visualized in the thoracic X-ray. A hemodynamically significant ductus arteriosus is an indication for treatment. In small premature infants (< 1,000 g), treatment is recommended even for subtle symptoms. It includes achieving precise fluid balance, in order to avoid hypovolemia (decreases blood flow to organs) or hyperhydration (increases the volume load of the left ventricle). An attempt to treat with indometacin (over the course of 3 days: Day 1, 0.2 mg/kg body weight; days 2 and 3, depending on age, 0.1–0.25 mg/kg body weight) as a short-term infusion can lead to closure of the ductus by inhibiting prostaglandin synthesis. Excretion must be carefully monitored; transitory renal insufficiency must be expected as a side effect. In addition, there is increased danger of a transient decrease in cerebral and intestinal circulation. If this fails, a second attempt to treat with indometacin can be undertaken. If the second attempt also fails, the ductus must be closed surgically or interventionally. Surgical closure is also undertaken with older infants and children. Two possible therapeutic procedures are available. In an interventional closure, a coil is introduced into the ductus during a cardiac catheterization, thus closing it. If the ductus is large, operative closure is recommended, by ligating or severing it. Ligature and interventional closure have a residual shunt risk of 5% to 20%. The prognosis for the ductus arteriosus after closure is good.

 ADDITIONAL TOPICS FOR STUDY GROUPS
- Additional heart defects (e.g., atrial-septal defect, pulmonary and aortic stenosis)
- ECG

---

61 Tonsillitis, peritonsillar abscess, rheumatic fever

61.1 What is your diagnosis?

Peritonsillar abscess with acute tonsillitis; rationale: Feverish tonsillitis, severe pain on swallowing (refuses food), salivation (saliva is not swallowed because of the pain on swallowing) causing rattling breath sounds, pain radiating to ears, throat examination (swelling of left tonsil with displacement of uvula), swollen glands in neck

61.2 What do you do next?

- High antibiotic doses, e.g., with penicillin V (100,000 IU/kg body weight/d in three individual doses) or cefuroxime (100 mg/kg body weight/d in three individual doses for 10 days), neck ice pack
- **Surgery is indicated** since there is a manifest abscess. Depending on location, patient's condition:

– Abscess tonsillectomy, i.e., abscess incision, emptying, and tonsillectomy in one session; advantage: Patient is only anesthetized once; disadvantage: elevated risk of wound and environmental infection
– or abscess incision; 3 to 4 days later, tonsillectomy

61.3 Name and explain the complications of streptococcal angina.

- **Lymphadenitis colli** (frequent) caused by transmission of the infection into the local lymph nodes (see case 13)
- **Tonsillogenic sepsis** (rare): Severe clinical picture with shivering and septic fever, high-infection parameters (leukocytosis, left displacement, elevated CRP), splenomegaly, septic spread to lungs, skin, and liver

→ Cases 61 Page 62

- **Rheumatic fever:** 2 to 5 weeks after streptococcal angina, there are secondary antigen–antibody reactions ([poly-]arthritis, especially of the large joints, endo-/myocarditis, chorea minor)

61.4 **What is meant by the Jones diagnostic criteria?**
Jones diagnostic criteria: Clinical and paraclinical parameters (see Tab.) are used to establish a diagnosis of rheumatic fever. The presence of two primary criteria or one primary and two secondary criteria make the diagnosis of rheumatic fever very probable.

Jones diagnostic criteria

Primary criteria	Secondary criteria
1. Carditis	1. Fever
2. (Wandering) arthritis	2. Arthralgia
3. Erythema anulare marginatum	3. Extended QT interval in the ECG
4. Subcutaneous nodes	4. BSG and CRP ↑
5. Chorea minor	5. ASL-titer ↑
	6. History of rheumatic fever

Comments

Tonsillitis: Tonsillitis is an acute inflammation of the palatine tonsils caused by **Group A β-hemolyzing Streptococci**, in rare cases also by *Staphylococci*, *Haemophilus influenzae* or *Pneumococci*, or even by viruses. The signs are high fever, difficulty swallowing with severe pain that often radiates to the ears, and swollen neck lymph nodes. Inspection of the throat reveals very red, swollen tonsils, with whitish-yellow coating in case of bacterial infection. The blood inflammation parameters (leukocytes, BSG, CRP) are elevated. A throat smear should be made for microbiological diagnosis of the pathogen. A streptococcal infection can also be diagnosed by the rapid strep test based on detection of an antigen.

If β-hemolyzing *Streptococci* are present, **penicillin** G (50,000 IU/kg body weight in 3–4 individual doses, p.o. or i.v.) **is administered for 7 days.** Alternatively, cephalosporins (for instance, cefuroxime 30–100 mg/kg body weight in three individual doses) can be administered for 5 to 7 days. In case of penicillin allergy, macrolides (e.g., erythromycin 40–60 mg/kg body weight in three individual doses) can be used.

Complications of tonsillitis: **Peritonsillar abscess** is rare but severe complication of tonsillitis that occurs primarily at school age. The inflammation is transmitted from the tonsillar parenchyma to the immediately neighboring tissue. Abscess formation results. The clinical symptoms develop in the course of tonsillitis. Children also complain of severe pain on swallowing that usually radiates to the ears and often leads to refusal of food. Opening the mouth becomes difficult (lockjaw), typically there is a copious flow of saliva and strong, foul bad breath. Speech sounds clumsy. There is associated lymph node swelling of varying degrees. When the throat is examined, which can be difficult because of the lockjaw, the tonsils, palatal arch, and soft palate are red, swollen, and bulge forward; the uvula is forced toward the healthy side. The abscess can be well visualized in the tonsillar region by sonography.

There is a danger that the laryngeal aperture will be shifted, with increasing shortness of breath and danger of suffocation. For this reason, rapid surgical intervention is essential, i.e., the abscess must be lanced. If appropriate, a tonsillectomy is performed at the same time because of the danger of relapse. Treatment with high parenteral doses of antibiotic (where *Streptococci* are found), penicillin V (100,000 IU/kg body weight/d in three individual doses) or cefuroxime (100 mg/kg body weight/d in three individual doses for 10 days).

Another serious complication of streptococcal angina is **rheumatic fever**. In the industrialized world, this disease has become very rare in recent years (incidence 1–5/100,000). This may be attributed to the generous use of antibiotics in infections of the upper respiratory tract as well as the improved socioeconomic level of the population. The peak age for rheumatic fever is around the age of 9 years. It sets in 2 to 5 weeks after an upper respiratory tract infection with β-hemolyzing Group A *Streptococci* as a secondary illness, i.e., not directly caused by infection but as a result of an autoimmune reaction. This means that the rheumatic fever can arise in spite of appropriate antibiotic treatment.

In case of an infection, the specific M protein of certain *Streptococcus* strains (so-called rheumatogenic strains) induces an immune response with formation of antibodies. These exhibit cross-reactivity with the sarcolemmal antigens tropomyosin and myosin. This results in binding of antibodies to myocardium and endocardium (mainly heart valves). At the same time, formation of immune complexes (post-streptococcal glomerulonephritis, see case 18) as well as cross-reactivity of the antibodies with antigens of the caudate and subthalamic nuclei can develop. In addition to general phenomena such as fever, headache, and sweating, this can also cause carditis, arthritis, skin signs, subcutaneous nodules, and chorea minor. The carditis can affect all areas of the heart. Cardinal symptoms are tachycardia and possible heart rhythm disorders. But usually valve involvement (endocarditis) stands out. The principal structures affected are mitral and/or aortic valves. Endocarditis verrucosa is the late form. Combined acquired heart defects with failure and stenosis result. Arthritis is typically acute wandering polyarthritis of the great joints. It is associated with swelling, redness, over-heating, and intense pain. Rare erythema anulare marginatum is the typical skin sign of rheumatic fever. It is characterized by transient, ring, and garland-shaped skin changes, chiefly on the trunk. In addition, subcutaneous nodules can be seen at tendinous sheaths, joint capsules, and periosteum. These are histologically indistinguishable from rheumatoid nodules. Chorea minor sometimes occurs after a long latent period (months

after streptococcal infection) and is characterized by abrupt, jerky, involuntary movements with twisting components that emphasize one side or the other.

The diagnosis of rheumatic fever is established clinically. It is guided by the Jones diagnostic criteria (see answer to question 61.4): The presence of two primary criteria or one primary and two secondary criteria make the diagnosis very probable if at the same time, there is positive evidence of *Streptococci* (culture, rapid test, elevated or rising ASL titer). Treatment includes eradication of *Streptococci* with penicillin V (100,000 IU/kg body weight/d) in three individual doses) or cephalosporins for 10 days, as well as anti-inflammatory treatment and pain therapy with acetylsalicylic acid (60–120 mg/kg body weight/d), ibuprofen (20–40 mg/kg body weight/d in three individual doses) for at least 6 weeks. Severe carditis is treated for 4 to 6 weeks with prednisolone (2 mg/kg body weight/d). Subsequently, relapse prophylaxis with penicillin (penicillin V 40,000 IU/d) must be continued for several years, possibly even for a lifetime.

👪 ADDITIONAL TOPICS FOR STUDY GROUPS
- Differential diagnoses of rheumatic fever
- Additional tonsillitides (scarlet fever tonsillitis, Plaut–Vincent angina, monocytic angina, herpes angina, diphtheria)

205

Case
62

---

62   Cystic fibrosis

‖ **62.1   Describe the abnormalities in the liver ultrasound findings. Which liver disease is probably present here?**
- Abnormalities in ultrasound findings: coarsened echo structure, coarse, lumpy liver contour
- **Suspected diagnosis: Cirrhosis of the liver**

‖ **62.2   In your opinion, what disease does the boy have? What is your rationale?**
Cystic fibrosis; rationale: failure to thrive, relapsing bronchopulmonary infection, liver cirrhosis, abdominal pain

‖ **62.3   What pathophysiological changes underlie this clinical picture? Which organs are particularly affected by the changes?**
- Pathophysiology:
  - Mutation of the CFTR gene (CFTR = cystic fibrosis transmembrane conductance regulator; the gene is located on the long arm of chromosome 7) leads to defective codding of a chloride channel in the epithelium of exocrine glands

  - At present, approximately 1,400 mutations are known; the most frequent CFTR mutation in the Caucasian population worldwide (~ 66%) is ΔF508
  - This causes absence/malfunction of chloride transport with effects on electrolyte and water transport over the cell membrane of the epithelial cell: Chloride secretion is decreased → increased sodium uptake into the cell → increased water inflow into the cell → increased viscosity of mucous secretions → obstruction of glandular excretory ducts→ relapsing inflammation
- Most affected organs: **Sweat glands, lungs, respiratory tract** (especially nasal sinuses), small and large intestines, pancreas, bile ducts
- Less-often affected: Reproductive organs, bones, joints, connective tissue

‖ **62.4   What other studies do you order to confirm this diagnosis?**
- **Sweat test** (see Comments): positive if chloride > 60 mmol/L or sodium 70 mmol/L—a **positive sweat test confirms the diagnosis**; however, a negative test does not rule out the disease.

→ Cases 62 Page 63

- Determination of pancreatic enzymes in the stool (chymotrypsin activity, pancreatic elastase), lipid content of stool: Presence of exocrine pancreatic insufficiency.
- In case of positive findings: Genetic diagnosis (determination of the most frequent diagnoses among Caucasians), measurement of nasal potential difference (see Comments).

Cystic fibrosis is inherited autosomally; the probability that the child will fall ill is 25% in every pregnancy. Prenatal diagnosis (chorionic villus sampling) is possible.

Comments

Definition: Cystic fibrosis (Syn.: Cystic fibrosis, CF) is an **autosomal-recessively** inherited disease of the exocrine glands with increasing respiratory and digestive insufficiency.

Epidemiology: It is the most frequent congenital metabolic disease with early lethality in the white population and is acquired by autosomal-recessive inheritance.

The incidence is 1:1,600–2,500. Both genders are affected at the same frequency. In northern Europe, 5% of the population is healthy (heterozygous) carriers, which means that in 1 of 400 couples, both partners carry a mutated gene. Thus in every pregnancy, there is a 25% probability that the child will fall ill with cystic fibrosis.

Etiology and pathophysiology: See answer to question 62.3.

Clinical aspects: Cardinal symptoms of cystic fibrosis are failure to thrive, **relapsing bronchopulmonary infections,** and voluminous, fatty, shiny stools. Depending on the mutation, the intensity of the symptoms can be variably pronounced. In 10% to 20% of cases, cystic fibrosis can already be seen in the newborn, in the form of **meconium ileus**. Rubbery meconium leads to obstruction of the small intestine, usually around the terminal ileum.

The most severe is the **pulmonary form**. Often there is already bacterial infestation in the infant, particularly by *Staphylococcus aureus*. Later, the disease is complicated by resistant *Pseudomonas* strains and fungi (e.g., *Aspergillus fumigatus* [allergic aspergillosis with asthma-like symptoms]). The result of chronic infection is destruction and modification of the lung tissue with formation of bronchiectasis, fibrosis, and emphysema. Further typical complications are pneumothorax, hemoptysis, and atelectasis. As the disease progresses, it is frequently possible to observe a barrel chest (convexity of the sternum, thoracic kyphosis) and clubbed fingers with hippocratic nails (see Fig.). Increasing respiratory insufficiency finally leads to cor pulmonale. Twenty percent to 50% of all children suffering from cystic fibrosis eventually develop focal

biliary cirrhosis. Possible additional symptoms of liver involvement are gallstones, obstructions of the intra- and extrahepatic bile ducts, cholestasis (possibly already at neonatal age), hepatopathy, and cirrhosis with portal hypertension.

Pancreatic involvement is typical. The thick glandular secretion leads to obstruction of the excretory ducts and eventually to exocrine pancreatic insufficiency. It appears soon after birth as copious, greasy, foul-smelling stools. Severe failure to thrive and vitamin insufficiency are the result. Sometimes, as a result of exocrine pancreatic insufficiency a distal intestinal obstruction syndrome is also present (meconium ileus equivalent, ileus symptoms due to poorly digested, concentrated intestinal contents; "DIOS"). The fibrotic changes in the pancreas in the course of the disease usually also causes endocrine pancreatic insufficiency with development of **diabetes mellitus**.

Fertility in men and women is compromised.

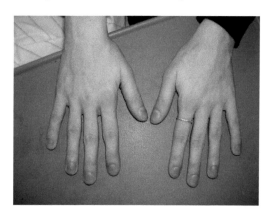

Clubbed fingers

Diagnostics: If the clinical picture justifies it, suspicion of cystic fibrosis is confirmed with a **sweat test**. After the sweating reaction is stimulated by pilocarpine iontophoresis, the sweat is collected in special containers. The chloride ion concentration is quantitatively determined by titration and the sodium ion concentration is determined photometrically. The test is positive if values for chloride > 60 mmol/L and for sodium > 70 mmol/L. A positive sweat test confirms the diagnosis. If the finding is positive, it is followed by **genetic testing**. In rare cases, the result of the sweat test is borderline or even negative, which makes it more difficult to establish the diagnosis.

The diagnosis can also be confirmed by measuring the **nasal potential difference** (NPD). The difference in ion distribution between the surface of the respiratory epithelium and the interstitium, chiefly caused by secretion of chloride and the reabsorption of sodium ions, leads to a measurable electrical tension, the transepithelial potential difference (PD). This potential difference can be particularly well measured at the respiratory epithelium of the lower nasal turbinate bone. Compared with a healthy individual, this tension is markedly more negative in a patient suffering from CF. The difference is intensified by administration of the sodium channel blocker amiloride.

It is already possible to establish a diagnosis in a newborn. The diagnosis can be established early, as part of newborn screening (3–10 days after birth) by determining the immunoreactive trypsin in dry blood (IRT test). This examination as part of general screening is controversial because it is highly sensitive and thus has a low specificity with a high number of false-positive results. Furthermore, it is not certain that early diagnosis has a positive effect on the course of the disease. The positive effect on the child's nutritional status is also controversial. On the other hand, as a result of early diagnosis, children are more likely to be in contact with other patients and are treated repeatedly and earlier with antibiotics and inhalation therapies. This leads to earlier infection with resistant microorganisms (e.g., *Pseudomonas aeruginosa*). Determination of pancreatic enzymes in the stool (Chymotrypsin activity, pancreatic elastase) and the lipid content of the stool provides information about the degree of exocrine pancreatic insufficiency.

Initial diagnostics should include a chest plate in two planes in order to determine the extent of pulmonary changes. Older children should also undergo complete pulmonary function tests. A deep throat swab or examination of the sputum will provide information about bacterial infestation of the respiratory tract. Liver changes, gallstones, and pancreatic changes can be determined with ultrasound. Blood inflammatory parameters (BSG, CRP, leukocytes), immunoglobulins, hepatic values, coagulation values, Vitamin A, D, and E levels as well as blood lipids, iron, ferritin, and renal values complete the diagnostic tests.

Monitoring of progress: Approximately every 3 months, patients should visit a CF outpatient department for monitoring of their overall health status and any problems, as well as for updates of the treatment plan. Every visit should include a history and a physical examination, measurement of height and weight, examination of the sputum or a throat smear, and pulmonary function tests. Every 6 months, a variety of laboratory tests should be done: (inflammation values, liver and coagulation parameters, iron, ferritin, renal values, albumen, blood sugar, and HbA_{1c}, Vitamins A, D, and E, immunoglobulins, and blood gas analysis). Once a year, body plethysmography, thoracic X-ray, upper abdominal sonography, and an oral glucose tolerance test should be performed (especially in children > 10 years).

Treatment: Causal treatment of cystic fibrosis has not yet been possible. The objective of treatment is to achieve a functional, normal condition and maintain it as long as possible. Early treatment, comprehensive training, care in specialized cystic fibrosis centers, and psychosocial care help to achieve the best possible quality of life for affected persons. Patients must be treated symptomatically all of their lives. This requires the collaboration of physicians, physical therapists, nutritionists, psychologists, and social workers with the patient and the parents. The primary objectives of treatment are to **maintain lung function and normal weight**. For this reason, the most important thing in treatment is **prevention and treatment of bronchopulmonary infections** by means of antibiotics (oral long-term treatment, additional [i.v.] therapy after an antibiogram), several times a day inhalation treatment (with inhaled antibiotics, bronchodilators, inhaled corticoids, and Dornase-α) and mobilization of secretions with breathing and physical therapy. Optimal hand hygiene should be maintained. The use of other people's inhalation devices must be avoided. Body contact should be limited and the inoculation status (incl. *Pneumococci*, *Haemophilus influenzae*) should always be up to date.

The objective of achieving a functional "normal" condition is easier to accomplish for the organs of the gastrointestinal tract than for the lungs. Of particular importance is a **diet high in calories** (the calorie requirement is chiefly determined by the respiratory situation; a poor respiratory situation calls for a higher calorie consumption because of increased respiratory effort) and **replacement of pancreatic enzymes, vitamins, iron, and trace elements**. It is also important to avoid additional organ complications such as formation of gallstones, e.g., by administration of ursodeoxycholic acid or treatment of the sequelae of liver cirrhosis and portal hypertension (e.g., sclerosing of bleeding esophageal varices).

Prognosis: The prognosis for cystic fibrosis is 90% determined by the extent of pulmonary involvement and the nutritional condition. The course of the disease is highly variable and also depends on environmental factors. Pseudomonas infections compromise the prognosis. The average survival time has improved drastically in recent years. The average life expectancy is between 42 and 50 years in the developed world. The individual course of the disease is not predictable. Therefore, it is important for the patient to complete the best education possible so as to have a chance on the labor market in spite of physical limitations.

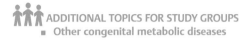 ADDITIONAL TOPICS FOR STUDY GROUPS
■ Other congenital metabolic diseases

63   Epileptic seizure

63.1 The emergency physician says: "That was certainly a seizure." What possible causes do you consider?
- **Syncope:** Unconsciousness caused by vasovagal, orthostatic, or cardiac factors, occasionally also with muscle clonus.
- **Event-induced seizure:** For example, in hypoglycemia, electrolyte disorder, alcohol/drug abuse, intoxication, lack of sleep, inflammatory disease of the CNS.
- Epileptic seizure.
- **Psychogenic attack:** Simulated attack, triggers are usually conflict or anxiety situations, usually before an audience, rhythmical twitching of the extremities, closed eyes, vocalization, crying during the attack, lack of postictal confusion, and subsequent sleep; also "arc of a circle": Opisthotonus when the head is reclined or in extreme convex ventral bending.
- **Hyperventilation tetany:** Tingling paresthesia in hands and periorally, hands in paw position (carpopedal spasms), possibly unconsciousness.
- **Respiratory affect seizure:** Usually in infants and toddlers, triggers are unexpected psychological or bodily stimuli such as rebukes, rage, fear, or pain; attacks make the impression of epileptic seizures, preceded by vigorous screaming: patients hold their breath, with cyanosis, stiffen their bodies, with individual contractions, and then wake up. Usually lasts less than 1 minute.

63.2 What is the most likely seizure type here? What do you look for in the physical examination?
- **Type of seizure: Grand mal seizure**; rationale: Initial screaming, sudden fall, tonic phase with extension of extremities, cyanosis caused by apnea, followed by a clonic phase with rhythmical twitches of extremities and postictal sleep; the patient does not react when addressed
- **General evaluation:** Overall condition, consciousness situation, orientation

- **Neurological examination:** Reflex status, meningism, pupillary reaction, motor function, sensory function, visuomotor coordination (isocoria, width of pupils, light reaction, mobility of eyes, coarse perimetry), speech disorders
- **Physical examination:** External signs of injury (e.g., bruises, hematomas, fractures caused by fall), indication of infection, noticeable smell (e.g., alcoholic fetor), bitten tongue, enuresis, encopresis

63.3 What further measures do you suggest?
- **Hospital admission with monitoring of vital signs** (heart rate, blood pressure, body temperature) to rule out event-determined seizures, syncope
- **Medical history:** Previous attacks, illnesses, skull trauma, medical history of early childhood (peripartal history, developmental milestones), familial seizures, or neurological diseases
- **Laboratory:** Complete blood count; inflammatory parameters (CRP, hematocrit), electrolytes (Na, K, ionized Ca); creatinine; hepatic values (GOT, GPT); CK (in tonic–clonic seizures, levels can be high from 24 to 48 hours following seizure); prolactin (level is high following general seizures); blood sugar (daily profile); blood gas analysis to rule out electrolyte imbalance; metabolic disorders; hyperventilation; inflammation
- **EEG and trigger EEG** (hyperventilation/flickering light/sleep deprivation): Epileptic potentials
- **Possibly lumbar puncture:** To rule out inflammatory CNS disease
- **Possibly cerebral imaging (MRI):** To rule out a space-occupying lesion with noticeable EEG changes (e.g., spike wave complexes, retardation, focus)
- **(Holter) ECG, Schellong test, tilt table test:** To rule out cardiac, vasovagal syncope
- In uncertainty, further examinations: For example, drug screening

Definition: An epileptic attack is a pathological form of reaction of the central nervous system in which abnormal and excessive discharges of neural connections in the brain take place.

Forms, etiology, and clinical aspects: A distinction is made between event-dependent seizures and epilepsy. *Note:* An epileptic seizure cannot be equated with epilepsy; under specific circumstances, any person can suffer a cerebral seizure. **Event-determined seizures** are epileptic reactions in acute inflammatory (e.g., meningitis, encephalitis), toxic (e.g., alcohol), metabolic (e.g., hypoglycemic, electrolyte disorders), and traumatic diseases or damage to the brain. The classical event-determined seizure in children is the fever seizure (see case 3).

Epilepsy is only present if two or more epileptic seizures occur that were not provoked by an immediate cause. Epilepsy in the strict sense can be genetically (hereditarily) determined. Epilepsy resulting from organic defects in the brain, e.g., after traumatic brain injury, brain damage in early childhood, or after inflammatory disease of the brain is called **residual** epilepsy. If the cause is not clear, the epilepsy is classified as **cryptogenic**. There is no uniform classification of epilepsies. There is a broad distinction between **generalized** and **focal** epilepsies.

Primary generalized seizures in which the neuronal discharge spreads primarily over both cerebral hemispheres include **grand mal attacks** (not age-related tonic–clonic, tonic, or clonic attacks) and **petit mal attacks** (age-related generalized attacks related to specific developmental stages of the brain, e.g., jackknife convulsions, Salaam spasms [series of lightning-fast myoclonic spasms with head bowing, throwing out of arms, and slow, tonic joining of hands as in a salaam greeting], absences [short loss of consciousness of a few seconds, usually with gaze movement], astatic [short loss of tone] or myoclonic attacks [short, suddenly occurring myocloni]). The tonic and motor components pass bilaterally. The seizure is accompanied by unconsciousness. This can be associated with autonomic symptoms (e.g.,

pupillary rigidity, apnea, encopresis, enuresis), biting the tongue, among other symptoms.

In **focal seizures** the discharges begin in a circumscribed neuronal system within one hemisphere. Information about the focus is provided by observation of the behavior during the seizure. A distinction is made between simple focal seizures (motor, sensory) that are not associated with loss of consciousness and complex focal seizures with impaired consciousness. It often happens that after a seizure begins as focal, it becomes generalized and is designated as a **secondarily generalized seizure**.

Sometimes a cerebral seizure is preceded by an aura, e.g., vegetative symptoms such as feeling unwell, feelings of heat, or sensory symptoms such as smell, taste, or acoustic hallucinations. If several cerebral seizures occur in a row and the patient does not regain consciousness between them, the condition is described as **status epilepticus**.

Differential diagnoses: Seizure in cardiac diseases (e.g., long QT syndrome), syncopes in circulatory regulation disorder, narcolepsy or other sleep disorders (e.g., night terrors), breath-holding spell with apnea caused by rage or pain, psychogenic seizures, hyperventilation tetany.

Diagnostics: See answer to question 63.3. When a seizure occurs for the first time, it is important to determine the precise circumstances (e.g., triggers) and symptoms through **observation** and **(third-party) history**. A careful **physical and neurological examination** follows.

Further diagnostics have the objective of finding possible inflammatory, toxic, or metabolic triggers: a part of the basic program is to draw **blood** and investigate the inflammatory parameters, electrolytes, blood sugar, and perform a blood gas analysis. To rule out an inflammatory disease of the CNS, a **spinal puncture** must be performed in case of doubt. If the clinical symptoms so indicate, a **toxicological examination** (drug screen, alcohol level) can be useful, but these studies are not generally recommended.

209

Case

63

Acute treatment of a generalized seizure

Medications	Posology	
	Infants	Toddlers and school-age children
Rectal diazepam	5 mg body weight < 10 kg	10 mg body weight > 10 kg
Diazepam i.v.	0.5 mg/kg body weight	0.3–0.5 mg/kg body weight
Midazolam p.o.	2.5 mg/kg body weight	5–7.5 mg/kg body weight
Clonazepam i.v.	0.01–0.1 mg/kg body weight	0.01–0.07 mg/kg body weight
Phenobarbital i.v.	6–15 mg/kg body weight	6–10 mg/kg body weight
Phenytoin i.v.	10–15 mg/kg body weight	10–15 mg/kg body weight

→ Cases 63 Page 64

The other underlying diseases possible in the differential diagnosis (see above) are ruled out by ECG (heart rhythm disorder), regular blood pressure measurement, and Schellong test or tilt table examination (circulatory regulation disorder), or a sleep laboratory study (night terrors). By recording EEG and provocation EEG (hyperventilation, flicker light, sleep deprivation), changes typical of epilepsy or suggestive of foci can be visualized. Pathological EEG changes can be generalized or located in foci. In addition, cerebral imaging is recommended, usually MRI, to rule out a cerebral cause, e.g., a space-occupying lesion.

Treatment: For **acute treatment** of a generalized attack to interrupt the attack, see Tab. Further measures serve to protect the patient from injuring himself: transfer to safe surroundings, wedge mouth guard between the teeth, etc.

Indication for **long-term treatment** with anticonvulsive agents is only made for relapsing or severe cerebral attacks. Various medications (carbamazepine, valproate, phenobarbital, etc.) are available, with selection determined by type of attack and EEG changes. Combination therapy using various antiepileptic agents may be necessary. A seizure log should be kept and treatment should be monitored by EEG and by regular determination of the serum-medication level, depending on the medication. Moreover, a careful watch must be kept over side effects of the drug therapy (for valproate, e.g., changes in the blood picture such as thrombocytopenia, hepatopathy with coagulation disorder, pancreatitis). Care by pediatricians and youth physicians experienced in pediatric neurology, or by a neuropediatric outpatient center,

is useful. In addition to drug therapy, it is important to maintain a regulated sleeping/waking rhythm with sufficient sleep, with no consumption of alcohol. In photosensitive epilepsy, triggers such as disco lights, television, and computer games should be avoided. Kindergarten and school personnel should be informed. In sports, limitations only apply to particularly dangerous sports such as swimming, climbing, and cycling in street traffic. Youths can only get a driver's license after 2 years without an attack. In choosing an occupation, only those occupations should be chosen that provide a regular waking/sleeping rhythm and do not endanger the patient or others (e.g., not roofer or truck driver).

Membership in a self-help group can be helpful in making daily life easier for people with epilepsy and people suffering from epilepsy and facilitating access to new information about the disease and possibilities for treatment.

Prognosis: Prognosis for epilepsy is highly dependent on the type of attacks and the response to medications. In uncomplicated epilepsy, attempts can usually be made to discontinue drug treatment after 2 years free of attacks, with unremarkable EEGs. Many patients remain free of attacks at this point. Epileptic syndromes such as West Syndrome or Lennox–Gastaut syndrome have a less favorable prognosis. The attacks are not stopped by drug treatment. Mental retardation is frequent.

👪 ADDITIONAL TOPICS FOR STUDY GROUPS
- Febrile seizure
- West syndrome
- Epilepsy syndrome

64   Salmonella enteritis

64.1 What information do you obtain from the fever curve? With what suspected diagnosis was the boy probably admitted?
- **Fever curve:** Septic fever can only be decreased for a short time by administration of antipyretics, copious watery stools, hypotension with tachycardia (BP 80/50, pulse 160/min), hypoxia (pO2 91%)
- **Diagnosis on admission: Salmonella enteritis**; rationale: high fever, bloody diarrhea, colicky abdominal pain

64.2 Interpret the laboratory values. What do you do next?
- **Laboratory results:** Massive rise in inflammation values (CRP from 6.6 mg/dL to 47.3 mg/dL),

hyponatremia, hypokalemia, differential blood picture: relative neutrophilia as proof of bacterial disease
- **Determination of the child's health status:** Septic shock (limited cardiovascular situation [tachycardia, tachypnea, hypotonia, cyanosis, prolonged recapillarization time, hypoxia]) in *Salmonella* disease
- **Further procedure:**
  - **Shock therapy:** Shock position (head down, legs up), i.v. fluid administration to stabilize the circulation (20 mL/kg body weight 0.9% NaCl or Ringer solution over 20 minutes), antipyretic measures (e.g., paracetamol orally 10–20 mg/kg body weight p.o. every 6 to 8 hours, ibuprofen 10 to 15 mg/kg body weight every 6 to 8 hours

→ Cases 64 Page 65

- **Intensive monitoring:** Blood pressure, heart rate, respiration, general condition, child's input/output
- Antibiotic treatment of the *Salmonella* infection because of the septic course (with ampicillin 100–300 mg/kg body weight in three individual doses i.v. or cefotaxim 100–200 mg/kg body weight in three individual doses i.v.) over 7 to 10 days.

64.3 Explain the epidemiology of the clinical picture.
- **Pathogens:** *Salmonella (S.) enterica* (2,000 Serovare), usually *S. typhimurium* or *S. enteritidis* in *Salmonella* enteritis
- **Pathogen reservoir:** Animals, especially chickens, swine, cattle
- **Transfer:** Usually by way of contaminated food stuffs such as meat from infected animals, egg-containing foods (e.g., mayonnaise), milk products (e.g., ice cream, pudding), drinking water; contamination in preparation (e.g., thawing poultry meat, interruption of cooling chain, insufficiently heated meat), rarely by direct contact with animals (reptiles kept as domestic animals, such as turtles, iguanas);

high-infectious doses necessary (10^5 microorganisms), an asymptomatic course is possible
- **Incubation time:** 5 to 72 hours
- Frequency depends on time of year (particularly warm months [pathogens have an easier time reproducing], but also during the time before Christmas [feasting on cookie dough]): Endemics associated with food (e.g., in kindergarten, senior housing) are possible

64.4 Is there a danger of contagion? What advice do you give the father?
- Transmission almost entirely through contaminated food; transmission from person to person is rare
- In high-risk patients (e.g., toddlers, old persons, persons with disturbed immunodeficiency / achlorhydria, undernourished persons, patients being treated with antacids) 10^2 microorganisms are sufficient to produce an infection
- Severe course in immunodeficiency
- **Recommendation:** Hygienic preventive measures such as protective gowns, the most careful hand disinfection, especially after contact with stool, diapers, etc., use of separate toilets

Comments

Definition: *Salmonella* are Gram-negative bacteria with peritrichous flagella, belonging to the family of Enterobacteriaceae. According to antigen patterns, *Salmonella* species are divided into over 2,000 different serovars.

Epidemiology: See answer to question 64.3.

Pathogenesis: A relatively high number of organisms (10^5 germs) must be taken in for an infection, since a large portion of the pathogens is killed by gastric acid. In high-risk patients (see answer to question 64.4) unspecific resistance can be lacking or reduced. In that case, smaller doses (10^2 organisms) are sufficient to cause infection. High-infectious doses are created by the fact that *Salmonella* multiply in nutrients before they are taken up by the body. The pathogens penetrate the intestinal mucosa and trigger increased elimination of fluid and electrolytes (= diarrhea). Usually, the infection remains localized but in high-risk patients sepsis and metastatic relocation to other organs (e.g., osteomyelitis, meningitis, endocarditis, pneumonia) can result from distribution of the pathogens in the blood.

Usually salmonella are excreted from a few days (to weeks) after an infection, and contagiousness persists during this period. Prolonged excretion is observed particularly in small children, but also after treatment with antibiotics.

Forms and clinical aspects: Depending on the clinical picture, a distinction is made between fresh,

asymptomatic infection, acute *Salmonella* enteritis, focal colonization resulting from bacteremia, septicemia, and chronic carrier status.

Acute Salmonella enteritis is the most frequently occurring form. Sudden onset is typical, with abdominal pain (colic-like, particularly before defecation), watery, often bloody diarrhea, and moderate-to-high fever. Usually the fever does not persist longer than 2 days, the diarrhea 1 week.

In about 20% of affected patients (especially in high-risk patients, see answer to question 64.4) there is **hematogenous spread** with sepsis (see sample case) or colonization of other organs.

Complication of septic shock: In bacteremia with excretion of endo- and exotoxins typical of the pathogen, marked vasodilation and damage to the vascular endothelium with extravasation of plasma and proteins can develop. This results in hypovolemia (and in the present example case, the pre-existing hypovolemia caused by gastroenteritis is even intensified). The outcome is septic shock. For pathogenesis and treatment principles of shock, see case 4. In septic shock, there should be additional anti-infections treatment (e.g., second- and third-generation cephalosporins. Possibly in combination with an aminoglycoside) or if necessary, surgical removal of foci in case of metastatic colonization.

Diagnostics: The diagnosis is established by **detection of pathogens**. This usually succeeds in the stool, but, e.g., also in the blood, for bacteremia.

→ Cases 64 Page 65

Differential diagnoses: Gastroenteritis (e.g., food poisoning by *Staphylococci*, other infectious pathogens, e.g., rotavirus) and sepsis of other origins, non-infectious diarrhea (e.g., cow milk protein intolerance).

Treatment: Uncomplicated *Salmonella* infection is treated symptomatically with fluid and electrolyte replacement as well as with diet (low-fat diet, slow buildup of diet). Antibiotic treatment is only indicated in a complicated course (bacteremia/sepsis, focal colonization, or in high-risk patients). Medications of choice are ampicillin or cotrimoxazol. Cephalosporins like cefotaxim and ceftriaxone are effective.

Prophylaxis: See answer to question 64.4. As long as diarrhea persists, children may not attend kindergarten or school. Asymptomatic children may return to community facilities, even if *Salmonella* is still being excreted in the stool (the disease is transmitted by contaminated food, not by excreta).

Mandatory reporting: There is an obligation to report suspicion, illness, pathogen excretion, and death.

The examining laboratory reports evidence of *Salmonella* to the Health Department. In addition, the treating physician is obligated to report suspicion and illness with *Salmonella* to the Health Department if the affected person works in a food-processing trade or if two or more similar diseases occur that suggest an epidemic connection.

Prognosis: The prognosis of the self-limiting gastroenteritis is very good. Especially in infants and toddlers, *Salmonella* are excreted for more than 3 months after an illness without occurrence of symptoms or need for treatment. If *Salmonella* can still be found in the stool 12 months after infection, the condition is called chronic excretion. The prognosis for the septic course depends on prompt start of treatment and complications that arise (metastasis). Meningitis and endocarditis caused by Salmonella are associated with a high degree of mortality.

ADDITIONAL TOPICS FOR STUDY GROUPS
- Gastroenteritis with other causes
- Shock (Clinical aspects, Diagnostics, Treatment)

Case
65

65　First care and first examination of a neonate

65.1　What is the meaning of the information the midwife gives you?
- II gravida = second pregnancy
- I para = the woman has already given birth to one child
- to term = 40 complete weeks of pregnancy
- Section with arrested labor, especially in case of disproportion = the pregnant woman is in the process of giving birth but no progress can be seen because the child is probably too large for the mother's pelvis
- CTG normal = cardiotocography unremarkable, i.e., the child's heart rate is normal, there is no sign of fetal hypoxia
- Section in 5 minutes = the operation begins in 5 minutes

65.2　What do you do next?
- After cutting the umbilical cord, start the APGAR clock and determine APGAR values (see Comments) at 1, 5, 10 minutes
- The child is laid on the heated resuscitation unit
- Suction is not necessarily required (see Comments)
- Dry the child, wrap it in a **heated** towel, auscultate heart sounds, check respiratory adaptation, rough clinical examination (five fingers, five toes, palate closed, anal opening present, abdomen soft, genitals normal, fontanelle in normal range) and then place

the child on the mother's breast or bring it to the parents (bonding)
- Acid-base status from the umbilical arterial blood (see answer to question 65.4 and Comments)
- First examination: search for (birth trauma) injuries, malformations, a repeated check of breathing and cardiovascular conditions, examination of abdominal organs, determination of neonatal maturity signs
- Vitamin K prophylaxis (see Comments)

65.3　What do you do next?
Breathing and cardiovascular system have not yet undergone postpartum adaptation: the child does not scream, the skin color is cyanotic, and it is limp in the midwife's arms. Resuscitation measures must be initiated swiftly, keeping in mind the importance
- Of **remaining calm oneself**
- Start APGAR clock
- Assign tasks (e.g., suction, drying, tactile stimulation)
- Basic measures: The most important thing is to **avoid loss of the child's heat**, i.e., dry the child and wrap in warm cloths. Hypothermia leads to an increased need for energy, excessive cooling makes the release of oxygen to the tissues more difficult, and there is a danger of hypoxia

- In resuscitating, strict maintenance of the formula in the box below

65.4 What is the purpose of the blood gas analysis on umbilical artery blood? How do you interpret the values?

- APGAR values are not sufficient to evaluate the newborn's condition. A reliable diagnosis of the condition is only possible in combination with blood gas analysis using umbilical artery blood, and thus the evaluation of the acid-base status (e.g., hypoxia, asphyxia, acidosis) is a reliable diagnosis of the neonate's condition.
- Blood should be taken from an umbilical artery before the placenta is delivered for examination of pH, pCO_2, and base excess (BE).
- BGA: pCO_2 ↑, pH ↓
- BE ↓ = combined metabolic-respiratory acidosis

A	Clear respiratory pathways
	Suction: first mouth, then nose (briefly and effectively, to avoid producing bradycardia by vagal irritation)
	↓
B	**Ventilation** (step-by-step plan)
	• Tactile stimulation of breathing (= rubbing soles of feet, intercostal muscles, back)
	• Possible oxygen administration through a mask (6–8 L/min O_2)
	• Possible distension with mask (see Comments)
	• Possible mask ventilation
	• Possible intubation and respiratory therapy
	• Possible administration of naloxone (anesthetizing the mother can lead to opiate-induced apnea in the child → antidote administration)
	↓
C	**Circulation**
	• Heart rate < 60: heart pressure massage
	• Check position of tube, evidence of pneumothorax
	• Fluid replacement: crystalline solutions (NaCl solution 0.9%, Ringer lactate) 10 to 20 mg/kg body weight or if necessary, blood (erythrocyte concentrate 0 Rh neg)
	↓
D	**Drugs**
	1 ampoule adrenaline diluted 1:1,000 with 9 mL NaCl 0.9%, dosage: 0.1 to 0.3 mL/kg body weight of this 1:10,000 diluted solution every 3–5 minutes intravenously (e.g., umbilical vein catheter) or by intraosseous access if i.v. or i.o. administration is not possible, then intratracheal administration of 1 mL/kg body weight

213

Case

65

Comments

First care by pediatrician: The responsibility to care for a healthy newborn is primarily with the obstetrician or midwife. This includes having a well-functioning resuscitation setup with all necessary equipment available. Naturally, the first care can be delegated to a pediatrician. Situations in which the presence of a pediatrician at the birth is recommended are:

- fetal emergency, such as hypoxia during birth (recognizable by pathological cardiotocography [late decelerations, severe variable decelerations]) or intrauterine acidosis (fetal blood gas analysis pH values < 7.25)
- green amniotic fluid
- umbilical cord prolapse
- amnion infection syndrome
- bleeding (especially placenta praevia)
- surgical delivery
- multiple birth
- premature birth, i.e., gestational age < 37 completed weeks of pregnancy (WP)

- estimated weight in ultrasound < 2,000 g
- mother's insulin-dependent diabetes mellitus
- protracted or complicated birth process
- child's position is abnormal
- child with deformities

Preparation: If you are called to the birth of a child as a pediatrician, it is important to have as much information as possible beforehand, so that you can provide the optimal first care for the child. This includes information about the degree of maturity, the condition of mother and child, abnormalities during pregnancy and if applicable, reasons for a surgical delivery, which you will have to learn from the obstetrician or midwife.

It is just as important to create optimal conditions for the first care and/or resuscitation of the newborn. For this purpose, the pediatrician has to know where all important equipment can be found: Where are the warm blankets? Where are

→ Cases 65 Page 66

the ventilation masks, ventilation bags, intubation equipment, umbilical clamps, medications, infusion needles, etc.? For this reason, before the first time on duty, it is vital to inspect the delivery suite and resuscitation unit (preferably after the work day and without a beeper) and become familiar with the instruments and medications located there. This will make the first "real" shift much easier. It is also possible to gain points and bolster team spirit by asking good questions of the midwives and delivery room staff.

Immediately before the first care, make sure the resuscitation unit is ready to go, as though with a check list.

- Is the heat lamp turned on?
- Are the doors closed (avoiding drafts)?
- Are there enough preheated cloths available to dry the child?
- Does the suction unit work?
- Is a suction catheter of the right size in place?
- Is the ventilation bag correctly assembled?
- Is the oxygen supply attached to the ventilation bag?
- Has the right size mask been selected?
- Does the ventilation apparatus work?
- Are the ventilation parameters and the oxygen concentration correctly set?
- Are the intubation instruments ready?
- Does the laryngoscope work?
- Has the right size spatula been selected?
- Is a tube of the right size ready?
- Is the APGAR clock set on 0?

First measures: When the child is born, it is usually brought by the midwife after the cord has been cut. Even the first look provides information about how the child is doing: A healthy, vigorous newborn has good tone (extremities flexed, screaming) and rosy skin (at least centrally). First the child is enveloped in warm cloths and dried, to protect him or her against heat loss.

Suction: After a normal vaginal birth with clear amniotic fluid, suction is not always necessary. Suction is stressful for the newborn, and in addition, deep and excessive suction can trigger bradycardia and apnea through vagus irritation. In any case, a newborn should be suctioned if it is breathing-impaired (obstruction of the respiratory pathways by amniotic fluid) or if the amniotic fluid was abnormal (green, bloody, or foul-smelling).

APGAR score: The APGAR score has proven useful for immediate evaluation of the postnatal condition of a (mature) newborn. It supports the decision as to whether resuscitation measures are necessary. If the child is not doing well, the resuscitation must naturally be started at once, even before the 1-minute APGAR value can be measured. A normal APGAR value after 10 minutes does not mean that further careful monitoring is unnecessary. This method is not as useful for children born prematurely because muscle tone, breathing, and reflex are closely dependent on gestational age.

APGAR score

Points	0	1	2
Skin color	Pale, blue	Centrally rosy, acrocyanosis	Rosy hands and feet
Heart rate	None	< 100/min	> 100/min
Reflexes when probing the nose	None	Grimaces	Coughing, sneezing, screaming
Muscle tone	Limp	Flexed extremities	Good, spontaneous movement
Breathing	None	Slow, irregular	Good, screaming

Evaluation: 7–10 vigorous, 4–6 slight depression, 0–3 severe depression

The APGAR clock is started when the umbilical cord is cut. At ages **1, 5,** and **10 minutes**, the skin color (Appearance), heart rate (Pulse), Reflexes when probing the nose (Grimace, coughing, resistance), muscle tone (Activity), and breathing (Respiration) are evaluated (see Tab. APGAR Score). The points for the individual categories are added to give the APGAR value. It must be kept in mind that the values are influenced to some extent by the partiality and experience of the examiner.

A normal newborn has a 1-minute APGAR score of 7–10; values of 4–6 indicate moderate

cardiorespiratory depression or "blue" asphyxia, and values of 0–3 indicate severe cardiorespiratory depression, the so-called "white" asphyxia. The child's prognosis for further development after complications at birth is most likely to correlate with APGAR value after 5 and 10 minutes.

Umbilical artery pH: See answer to question 65.4. A significant addition to the clinical evaluation of the newborn is determination of blood gases (pH, pCO_2, BE) in the umbilical artery blood. Normal pH values fall between 7.15 and 7.45. pH values under 7.15

→ Cases 65 Page 66

suggest hypoxia/asphyxia. Asphyxia is characterized by hypoxia, hypercapnia, and acidosis.

At first, the principal cause of acidosis is respiratory, due to increased CO_2 retention (pCO_2 normal values 35–45 mmHg); later, due to tissue hypoxia, increasing metabolic acidosis develops (BE becomes negative, normal values 0 ± 2 mmol/L).

Mother–Child–Father relations: As soon as possible after the first care, the healthy child, normally adapted postnatally, is warmly wrapped, shown to the mother or the parents, and left with them for a few minutes, possibly laid on the mother's breast. This is of particular importance for Mother–Child–Father bonding. As soon as possible (optimally 20–30 minutes postpartum), the child is positioned to breastfeed and the mother and child are left alone.

It is not particularly necessary to bathe the child in the delivery room (*caution:* heat loss). The vernix should not be removed completely. It protects the skin of the newborn from drying out.

First examination: This is followed by the first examination, in which the greatest attention is given to body measurements (weight, body length, head circumference), the maturity age (see Tab.), check for birth injuries (see case 20) and birth defects (e.g., esophageal atresia) as well as the child's postpartum adaptation.

The maturity age can be determined according to somatic (Dubowitz–Farr score) or neuromuscular

(Ballard score) criteria. A simplified schema for newborns > 30th week of pregnancy is the Petrussa index (see Tab. Petrussa index). In this index, points are assigned depending on development of the maturity markers and then added to 30. The sum gives the estimated maturity age in pregnancy weeks.

A thorough physical examination must be a component of the first examination. Particular attention must be given to the following:
- Breathing and lungs: Cyanosis, breath sounds (e.g., moaning), thoracic contractions, nostril flaring, respiratory rate (normal respiratory rate in a newborn is 40–60/min)
- Cardiovascular: Skin perfusion, heart sounds, pulse rate (normal 80–140/min) and rhythm, heart murmurs, peripheral pulses
- Abdomen: Enlarged organs, abdominal wall defects (see case 75), number of umbilical cord vessels (normal: two umbilical arteries [little knobs], one umbilical vein [wide, limp]), inner malformations are possible in case of deviations)
- Nervous system: Tone, neonatal reflexes, malformations such as meningocele or encephalocele
- Birth injuries: See case 20
- External malformations: For example, fissure formation, coloboma
- Extremities: Malformations, transverse palmar crease, malposition, and false posture of feet (e.g., pigeon toes, club foot), resistance to hip abduction
- Genitals: Testes descended, inguinal hernia, hypo- or epispadia, swollen testes (e.g., hydrocele), clitoris hypertrophy
- Anus: Deformities

Petrussa Index

	0	1	2
Skin	Light red, vulnerable, translucent	Rosy, veins visible	Firm, skin folds clearly recognizable
Nipples	Hardly any glandular tissue	Glandular tissue palpable, nipple recognizable	Mammary gland over the skin level
Ear cartilage	Hardly any cartilaginous tissue	Cartilage in tragus and antitragus palpable	Helix cartilage
Foot sole	Smooth, creases only in anterior third	Creases in anterior and middle third	Creases over the entire sole
Genitals:	Testicles not palpable, major labia do not cover minor labia	Testicles still inguinal, labia majora and minora approximately equal in size	Testes in scrotum, labia major cover labia minora

Vitamin K prophylaxis: For prophylaxis of a **Vitamin K deficiency hemorrhage**, the newborn receives 2 mg Vitamin K orally at the first examination. Vitamin K is only transferred to the placenta to a small extent. Therefore, the Vitamin K plasma level in newborns is low. Mother's milk contains only small amounts of Vitamin K, so that in breastfed infants, there is a risk of Vitamin K deficiency. There are three forms of Vitamin K deficiency bleeding:

Classical Vitamin K deficiency hemorrhage occurs in the first week of an infant's life and is the result of an

insufficient Vitamin K supply through the diet or an insufficient supply of nutrients.

Early Vitamin K deficiency hemorrhage with onset during the first 24 hours after birth, in practice occurs only in children of mothers who received drug treatment during pregnancy (e.g., anticoagulants, anticonvulsives, anti-tuberculostatics, antibiotics). It can be effectively prevented by regular Vitamin K replacement in the mother during the last month of pregnancy.

→ Cases 65   Page 66

Late Vitamin K deficiency hemorrhage occurs almost without exception in breastfed infants and children with cholestasis in the second to eighth week of an infant's life, seldom later. It is prevented by repeated administration of Vitamin K in examinations 1, 2, and 3.

Physiology of the postnatal period: The healthy newborn undergoes physiological changes after birth. Cold, touch, and changes in gases in the newborn's blood after clamping the cord ($pO_2\downarrow$, $pCO_2\uparrow$) are potent postnatal breathing stimuli. High negative intrathoracic pressures are necessary for expansion of the lungs. These are achieved by screaming, in part against the closed glottis. As a result, the vascular resistance of the pulmonary vessels falls rapidly. When the umbilical cord is clamped, the peripheral blood pressure increases, the vascular resistance increases abruptly, and the sympathetic nervous system is stimulated. The fetal circulation is transformed into a normal postnatal circulation, and the ductus arteriosus and the foramen ovale close.

Transfer from the delivery room: If the birth is spontaneous and without problems, and the mother wishes to give birth as an outpatient, she may go home with the baby as soon as the first examination has taken place. The entire stay in the delivery room should, however, last at least 1.5 to 3 hours to permit monitoring normal postpartum adaptation of the newborn.

In case of a cesarean section, a mature and postpartally well adapted child may be moved to the nursery after the first examination. After the stay in the recovery room, the mother is returned to the ward. If the newborn must be moved to the newborn ward or the newborn intensive care unit, this is usually done, depending on the newborn's condition, usually after the first examination and after the mother and/or father have seen it briefly, or, if possible, held it.

Cardiopulmonary resuscitation of the newborn: If there is a problem during the newborn's adaptation process, sufficient measures must be taken to prevent (additional) asphyxia for the child. The resuscitation is performed strictly according to the routine shown on p. ■■ (see answer to question 65.3).

The **basic measures for newborn resuscitation** include: suction, drying and tactile stimulation of breathing by massaging the soles of the feet, intercostal and paravertebral muscles, as well as administration of oxygen. With a lung recruitment maneuver (max. three times; put bag valve mask in place, compress bag with high pressure, may only be done by a neonatologist), the intra-alveolar fluid is pressed into the pulmonary lymph and circulatory system, thus improving the residual capacity.

During these measures, the child is carefully observed: can breathing movements be seen? Does the child become rosy? The heart rate is checked repeatedly by auscultation or palpation of the umbilical cord pulse.

Bradycardia in newborns is almost always caused by hypoxia, so it can almost always be eliminated by sufficient oxygenation. If the child continues to exhibit apnea or bradycardia, it is immediately intubated and ventilated.

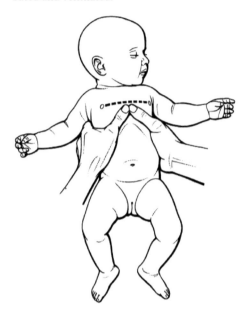

Extrathoracic heart pressure massage in newborn and infant

If sufficient ventilation does not increase the heart rate in the next 30 seconds to 80 to 100/min, supplementary heart pressure massage must be initiated. The ratio of compression to ventilation should be 3:1. In the newborn, the pressure point is the lower third of the sternum. Both hands grasp the thorax; pressure is exerted on the heart with both thumbs (see Fig.).

In addition, the position of the tube must be checked, to determine whether it is placed correctly or whether there is evidence of a pneumothorax.

Volume replacement can be administered through an umbilical vein catheter. Crystalline solutions such as physiological salt solution (NaCl 0.9%) or Ringer lactate are recommended. If a blood transfusion is needed (e.g., in case the child loses blood due to premature placental abruption), Rh-negative type O should be given. Albumin-containing solutions are no longer the medium of choice. If these measures do not provide visible success, administration of adrenaline intravenously (e.g., umbilical vein catheter) or intraosseously is indicated. If i.v.

or i.o. administration of adrenaline is not possible, adrenaline can also be administered endotracheally (100 µg/kg body weight). The use of sodium bicarbonate during cardiopulmonary resuscitation does not improve the outcome. It produces further increase of intracellular and central venous acidosis. If resuscitation lasts a long time and all other measures are unsuccessful, sodium bicarbonate can be administered.

The duration of resuscitation depends on the condition of the child, possible deformities, etc. Usually the resuscitation is interrupted after 30 minutes, since at that point, irreversible brain damage can be expected. If the child has died, the parents should decide whether they would like to see their child once more. They should then be allowed sufficient time and peace to make their farewells. If appropriate, you may offer to have a clergyman of their faith anoint the child and perform a post mortem baptism. It is important to offer the parents psychological care/support by a member of the clergy or a psychologist. A precise explanation of the cause(s) of death should only take place hours or days later, in quiet surroundings. The parents should have regained a little calm by this time and be better able to take the situation in. But even before this, one ought to be open to all questions.

ADDITIONAL TOPICS FOR STUDY GROUPS
- Injuries of birth trauma
- Other precautionary investigations

66   Influenza (the flu)

66.1 **What disease do you suspect as the source of the "epidemic"?**
Influenza; rationale: Accumulation of disease cases, illness in the patient's family, the "right" time of year (winter), unspecific respiratory symptoms (sore throat, dry, irritating cough), especially sudden onset with high fever, head and joint pains, severe malaise

66.2 **What do you know about the source of the clinical picture?**
– Droplet infection with influenza virus (different types [A, B, C])
– Type A is often responsible for epidemics and pandemics because of antigen shift/drift (see Comments)
– Influenza viruses colonize the respiratory tract and replicate in the respiratory epithelium
– Highly contagious, incubation time 2 to 3 days

66.3 **What complications of the disease are you familiar with?**
In particular high-risk patients (newborns, infants, pregnant women, patients with severe prior illnesses, persons > 60 years) are endangered:
- Bacterial superinfection (especially *Pneumococci, Haemophilus influenzae*) are possible
- Peri-/Myocarditis
- Encephalitis, myelitis
- Death

66.4 **What treatment seems useful to you?**
- **Symptomatic:** Antipyretic measures (e.g., paracetamol, leg wraps), large amounts of fluid, bed rest
- Neuraminidase inhibitors (see Comments)
- Prophylactic treatment of other family members with neuraminidase inhibitors

Comments

Definition: Influenza (Syn.: The flu) is an acute, serious infectious disease usually occurring in epidemics during the cold season of the year (the typical "flu season" lasts from December to April) which is different from an ordinary cold or grippe-like infection.

Etiopathogenesis and epidemiology: It is caused by influenza viruses of the Orthomyxovirus group. There are **three different types** (A, B, C). The genome is fragmented, so that new subtypes result from exchange of individual segments (Reassortment). For instance, erratic changes in antigen (antigen shift) arise through recombination of animal (reservoir: e.g., horse, swine, various bird species) and human influenza viruses. In large time intervals, about 15 to 20 years, an antigen shift leads to a worldwide pandemic. The most severe pandemic known today was the "Spanish Influenza" originating in Spain in 1918. Experts estimate that worldwide 500 million people were infected with the virus and 50 million people died as a result of it. Smaller changes of the surface antigens (point mutations; antigen drift) neuraminidase (N) and hemagglutinin (H) of type A influenza virus are responsible for the influenza epidemics that can be seen every year. The estimated influenza-associated deaths in the United States range from a low of 3,000 to a high of 49,000 people.

→ Cases 66 Page 67

The average **incubation time is 2 to 3 days**; the contagiosity is high. Influenza is transmitted by droplet contagion. The viruses colonize the mucosa of the upper respiratory tract. Since the body's resistance is subtype-specific, it is possible to contract influenza more than once.

Clinical aspects: The symptoms are unspecific and at the beginning of the illness they are difficult to distinguish from those of ordinary colds. The clinical picture depends on age. Thus, very young infants can exhibit clinical pictures similar to sepsis while older children have tracheitis, obstructive bronchitis, or bronchiolitis. Stenosing laryngotracheitis, exanthema, and gastrointestinal symptoms can develop in toddlers. The symptoms in school-age children and youths resemble those in adults. These are characterized by sudden onset with high fever, chills, head and joint pain, as well as severe malaise. Other symptoms are cough, hoarseness, and sore throat. In the group aged from 2 to 12, 30% of cases of influenza are accompanied by **otitis media**. A course with few symptoms is also possible.

Complications: Complications are chiefly caused by **bacterial superinfection**, and in high-risk patients (newborns, infants, pregnant women, older persons, children, and adults with prior diseases, e.g., chronic lung diseases such as bronchopulmonary dysplasia, bronchial asthma or cystic fibrosis, congenital or acquired heart disease, congenital or acquired immune defects, diabetes mellitus), often with a lethal outcome. Often there is pneumonia, caused by secondary bacterial superinfection with *Pneumococci, Staphylococci*, or *Haemophilus influenzae*. Rarely, but particularly feared, is fulminant influenza pneumonia, a necrotizing pulmonary infection with microabscesses caused by *Staphylococcus aureus*. Rarely, cardiac complications (myopericarditis) and cerebral complications (encephalitis, myelitis) occur.

Diagnostics: The diagnosis is not always easy to establish because of the unspecific symptoms in the early phase or in sporadic infection. The disease can only be diagnosed with sufficient probability in epidemics. For epidemiological reasons, at the start of an epidemic, it is useful to prove the presence of the virus (from gargling water or nose–throat secretions), especially when the course of the disease is severe. Rapid influenza A tests have a sensitivity of about 80% and are suitable for early diagnosis.

A weekly influenza surveillance report is prepared by the influenza division of the CDC. Activity estimates are reported by state and territorial epidemiologists. Knowledge of the disease's activity in one's own region facilitates diagnosis.

Treatment: Treatment is largely **symptomatic**. Antipyretic measures (e.g., paracetamol, ibuprofen, leg wraps), sufficient fluid intake, and rest are the basic components of treatment.

There are numerous medications that make it possible to treat influenza. This includes **neuraminidase inhibitors** (zanamivir, oseltamivir). They block the effect of the viral enzyme neuraminidase that is required for the release of new virus particles from infected cells and thus for the spread of the virus. However, neuraminidase inhibitors act only against influenza A and influenza B viruses, not against type C. Treatment should begin as early as possible, at the latest up to 48 hours after onset of symptoms. Oseltamivir is registered for children after the age of 1 year, zanamivir only after the age of 12.

If treatment with neuraminidase inhibitors is not possible, **amantadine**, an ion channel blocker (only efficacious in infections with type A influenza viruses) can be used. Amantadine inhibits replication of influenza viruses; the severe clinical symptoms are attenuated, and complications can usually be avoided. Here too, treatment must begin within the first 48 hours.

If an influenza patient also has a bacterial superinfection, the use of appropriate antibiotics is indicated.

Prophylaxis: Prophylaxis is advisable because the possible severe course, especially in high-risk patients (see complications) and persons in particular danger (e.g., medical staff).

It consists of **protective inoculation**, which must be renewed annually because of antigen shift/drift. The World Health Organization (WHO) has devised a central reporting system for this purpose, so that it can react immediately with a new vaccine if a new virus type appears. The recommended vaccines contain an antigen mixture that is efficacious against different influenza viruses. The inoculation should be administered before the start of the influenza season, that is, in October. The inoculation makes it possible to protect around 80% to 90% of those vaccinated from becoming ill or at least to achieve a mild, complication-free course.

If individuals have not been inoculated or if the vaccines do not correspond to the currently circulating viruses, prophylaxis can be carried out with neuraminidase inhibitors. Especially after contact with persons sick with influenza, preventive administration of neuraminidase inhibitors is advisable.

→ Cases 66 Page 67

A patient in whom influenza viruses have been directly detected must be reported to the Health Department within 24 hours.

Prognosis: If the course is free of complications, the prognosis is usually very good. However, it often takes weeks for complete convalescence. The prognosis for complicated influenza is, particularly in high-risk patients, very poor (often a lethal outcome).

ADDITIONAL TOPICS FOR STUDY GROUPS
- Simple infection/common colds (etiology, clinical aspects, diagnostics, treatment)

67 Hypospadia

67.1 Describe the finding. What is your diagnosis?
- **Finding:** Urethral opening at the corona penilis
- **Diagnosis:** Hypospadia

67.2 What do you look for in particular in the clinical examination?
- Urethral meatus recognizable: Distance from penile tip
- Meatal stenosis (only demonstrable during urination): Urination out of meatus possible?
- Urination: Direction of urine stream, complete bladder emptying possible?
- Bending (possibly during erection of penis): Does degenerate corpus spongiosum (= chorda) prevent erection?

- Palpation of testes: Elevation of testes?
- Thorough physical examination: Additional deformities (especially of kidneys/urinary bladder)

67.3 What further diagnostic measures are necessary?
- **Medical history of parents**: Hypospadia in the family
- **Ultrasound of kidneys/urinary tract**: Deformities

67.4 What therapy do you recommend? When should the treatment take place?
- Early elimination of possibly existing meatal stenosis by means of meatotomy (in infancy)
- Surgical correction of hypospadia up to 3 years of age, often necessary to perform surgery in several sessions

Comments

Definition and epidemiology: Hypospadia is incomplete closure of the urethra during the fetal period with **ventral** ectopic opening of the external urethral orifice. It is one of the **most frequently** occurring deformities in boys with an incidence of about 1:300. A familial increase is observed.

Etiopathogenesis: It can be **idiopathic** or caused by **hormonal** or **chromosomal** disorders. The basis of a hormonal cause is mostly an intrauterine androgen deficiency or a lack of androgen activity before the 14th week of pregnancy.

Clinical aspects: Hypospadia is characterized by a **defective opening of the urethra to the underside of the penis**, a dorsal foreskin apron (preputial apron), or a ventrally lacking fusion of the prepuce. Or the penile shaft can be bent to ventral (chorda) because of a degenerated corpus spongiosum. In urination, the urine stream is directed in a dorsal direction. In addition, there is often a meatal stenosis.

Classification of types of hypospadia is based on the position of the urethral opening (see Fig.).

Diagnostics: The diagnosis is clinical. Attention must be given to recognizing other deformities in the external genitalia. Deformities of the upper urinary tract are ruled out sonographically.

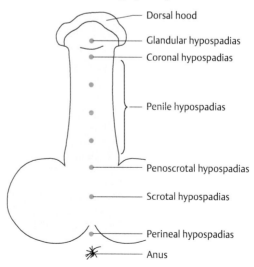

Schematic representation of types of hypospadia

→ Cases 67 Page 68

To rule out a **hormonal cause** (e.g., adrenogenital syndrome, very rare), a hormone assay should be performed (DHT, 17-OH-progesterone). Sometimes hypospadia is associated with syndromal diseases (e.g., Klinefelter syndrome, Smith–Lemli–Opitz syndrome). For this reason, it is important to screen for associated deformities in the clinical examination; in very severe forms of hypospadia, a chromosomal study is appropriate.

Differential diagnoses: In particular, in scrotal and perineal forms that resemble the female phenotype, male pseudohermaphroditism must be ruled out.

Treatment: The objective of surgical treatment is to straighten the penis shaft, achieve a correctly directed urinary stream and normal sexual function, as well as to create a cosmetically normal penis. Ideally, the operative correction should occur in the first 2 years of a child's life. If a meatus stenosis is present, it must also be corrected early. A large number of surgical techniques are available for the correction of hypospadia. The degree of severity and individual diagnostic constellations determine the method of choice. Glandular and coronal hypospadias with meatal stenosis usually require meatotomy and sometimes circumcision. In cases of severe deformities (e.g., scrotal hypospadias), creation of a new urethra out of penile shaft skin, foreskin, or transplantation of oral mucosa becomes necessary. For this reason, if there is a ventral apron prepuce, no circumcision, not even on religious grounds, should be done without consulting the pediatric surgeon.

Prognosis: The most frequent late complications are fistula formation, ureteral strictures, and residual bending. Their occurrence depends on the shape of the hypospadias and associated possibilities for correction (the closer the hypospadias is to the anus, the more difficult the reconstruction and the more severe the complications).

👨‍👦‍👦 ADDITIONAL TOPICS FOR STUDY GROUPS
- Other deformities of the external genitalia in boys (e.g., phimosis, epispadias, cryptorchidism)
- Development of the genitalia (embryology)

68   Normal and pathological development of puberty

68.1 What do you observe on examining the patient?
Swollen mammary glands bilaterally

68.2 What is the stage of puberty, according to the Tanner classification?
- **Breast:** The mammary gland is more enlarged than the areola = Tanner B3
- **Genital area:** Growth of individual, long, darkly pigmented hairs on the mons pubis = stage PH2

68.3 What diseases should you consider for differential diagnosis?
Based on the presence of secondary sex characteristics before the age of 8, the following diagnoses must be considered: **Precocious puberty** and **precocious pseudopuberty** (see Comments)

68.4 What further diagnostic measures are necessary?
- **Determination of body length/weight**, recording in percentiles; age-appropriate development of height/weight
- **Genital ultrasound:** Ovarian cysts, size of uterus
- **X-ray of left hand and wrist:** Determination of bone age
- **GnRH test:** In true precocious puberty, the LH/FSH can be stimulated; in precocious pseudopuberty, not

- **Several determinations of testosterone/estrogen:** Elevated over the prepubertal norm
- **Determination of TSH, fT3 fT4:** Hypothyroidism
- **Other hormone tests:** Prolactin, 17-hydroxy-progesterone, DHEA (Dehydroepiandrosterone), DHEAS (Dehydroepiandrosterone sulfate), β-HCG, to rule out diseases of the hypophysis (adenoma), the gonads and the adrenal cortex (e.g., adrenocortical adenoma, adrenogenital syndrome)
- **EEG, MRI, and ophthalmological examination:** Cerebral diseases (e.g., space occupying lesion)
- **Sonography/if indicated, abdominal CT and MRI:** Actively secreting adrenal cortex/gonadal tumors as cause of precocious pseudopubertas

68.5 What therapy is indicated?
- **Therapy of true precocious puberty:**
  – Observational approach (6 months): Progress of symptoms
  – If there is progress: Drug therapy with GnRH analogs (e.g., buserelin, triptorelin, leuprorelin) intranasal or i.m. to avoid a psychosocial burden/later substandard growth; slight side effects, symptoms completely reversible
- **Treatment of pseudopubertas praecox:** Treatment of the underlying disease, e.g., AGS, HCG-producing tumors, ovarian cyst, McCune–Albright syndrome

Normal pubertal development: In **girls**, puberty normally begins between the ages of 8 and 14. In boys, approximately 2 years later.

Characteristics of puberty in girls usually occur in the following order: Thelarche (development of the mammary glands), development of axillar hair and pubarche (development of pubic hair), growth spurt, menarche (onset of menstrual bleeding). The average age of menarche is 12.8 years.

In **boys**, the first sign of puberty is the increase of testicular volume from 1 to 2 mL before the age of 10 to 3 to 8 mL before appearance of the first pubic hair. This is followed by the development of the genitals and of the pubic and axillary hair growth. The pubertal growth spurt follows and reaches its maximum at the age of 14 or 15 years. Next is the change of voice. At the close of puberty, the final scrotal size is approximately 10 to 25 mL.

Norm variations of normal pubertal development: Norm variant of the physiological course of puberty is the isolated, premature occurrence of a sign of puberty. Such variations do not indicate an illness and have no effect on further development (bone/height development normal, hormone values age-appropriate). Further diagnostics should be undertaken to rule out puberty or pseudopubertas praecox. Treatment is not required.

Premature thelarche is isolated enlargement of mammary glands in girls. It usually occurs between the age of 6 months and 2 years. The cause is unclear. It is assumed that follicular cysts of different sizes produce enough estrogen to cause the growth of breasts without any other signs of puberty. No progress is observed.

In isolated **premature menarche**, cyclic vaginal bleeding occurs without other signs of pubertal development. Possible causes are transient ovarian follicular cysts. In differential diagnosis, vaginal foreign bodies must be considered. Treatment is not necessary (naturally, confirmed foreign bodies must be removed).

Premature pubarche is the early and isolated occurrence of pubic hair.

In **premature adrenarche**, there is an early development of axillary hair.

In **pubertal gynecomastia**, there is transient breast swelling on one or both sides in pubescent, and often also, in overweight boys. It is assumed that the cause is a transient imbalance between estrogen and androgen. The diagnosis is established clinically; additional examinations are usually unnecessary.

Premature development of puberty (pubertas praecox): This is the premature occurrence of secondary sex characteristics in **girls before the age of 8, and in boys before the age of 9** years. A distinction is made between true **precocious puberty** (pubertas praecox vera) triggered by premature hypothalamic and hypophyseal activity and **precocious pseudopuberty**, caused by adrenal, gonadal, or ectopic factors.

Pubertas praecox vera: It is estimated that the incidence of true precocious puberty lies between 1:5,000 and 1:10,000. Girls are affected in 80% of cases. The cause of the premature activation of the hypothalamic–hypophyseal–gonadal axis is unexplained in the majority of cases. Cerebral organic disorders such as tumors (astrocytoma, ependymoma, optic nerve glioma, or craniopharyngeoma), hydrocephalus, congenital deformities, a long-existing, untreated hypothyroidism, or status post trauma or cerebral infection are rarely triggers for premature development of puberty. Typical signs for true precocious puberty, in addition to the formation of typical secondary sex characteristics such as thelarche, pubarche, menarche, and premature sexual maturity often also include a growth spurt and acceleration of bone maturity. The epiphyseal plates close prematurely and children who started out as being of normal height remain short. Their final height seldom exceeds 155 cm. Psychological problems in the affected children and the parents' uncertainty can have a serious effect.

True precocious puberty: The concept of true precocious puberty includes all disorders that lead to premature development of puberty but not associated with activation of the hypothalamus–hypophysis–gonad axis. A distinction is made between isosexual (same-sex pubertal characteristics) and heterosexual (sexual characteristics of the other sex) forms.

The causes include hormone-producing ovarian cysts, ovarian tumors, congenital adrenogenital syndrome, tumors of the gonads or adrenal glands, or teratomas.

→ Cases 68 Page 69

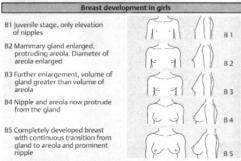

Development of pubic hair in boys and girls	
Stage 1 Juvenile stage, no pubic hair	Ph 1 Ph 2 Ph 3
Stage 2 Sparse, unpigmented hairs at the penile root or the labia majora	
Stage 3 Coarser, darker curly hair, extending to the symphysis	
Stage 4 Similar to adult picture, but not reaching to the thighs	Ph 4 Ph 5 Ph 6
Stage 5 Extent and density as in adults, reaching to the thighs	Ph 1 Ph 2 Ph 3
Stage 6 Hair extending along the linea alba toward the navel, in 80% of men, in 10% of women	Ph 4 Ph 5 Ph 6

Breast development in girls	
B1 Juvenile stage, only elevation of nipples	B 1
B2 Mammary gland enlarged, protruding areola. Diameter of areola enlarged	B 2
B3 Further enlargement, volume of gland greater than volume of areola	B 3
B4 Nipple and areola now protrude from the gland	B 4
B5 Completely developed breast with continuous transition from gland to areola and prominent nipple	B 5

Genital stages in boys

G1 Testicles, scrotum, and penis as in juvenile stage
G2 Testicular volume about 4 ml, scrotum larger, penis still in juvenile stage
G3 Testicular volume and scrotum larger, penis longer
G4 Testicular volume about 12 ml, scrotal pigmentation darker, penis longer and thicker
G5 Testicles, scrotum, and penis of adult size and appearance

Pubertal stages according to Tanner

Delayed development of puberty (Pubertas tarda): Pubertas tarda is a lack of secondary sexual characteristics in girls after the age of 14 and in boys after the age of 15. The causes are numerous. In addition to endocrine (e.g., hypothalamic or hypophyseal) and chromosomal disorders (e.g., Ullrich–Turner syndrome in girls) insufficient nutrition (e.g., anorexia nervosa), intense sport, and drug abuse (especially marijuana) lead to absence of puberty. The diagnosis is confirmed by measuring the sexual steroids in the peripheral blood. The determination of gonadotropins permits further subdivision into hypogonadotropic and hypergonadotropic forms. In differential diagnosis, the constitutional delay in development must be taken into account. Therapy includes replacement of the missing hormones, in case the underlying causes cannot be eliminated. Under this treatment, the secondary sexual characteristics mature and there is a positive effect on growth.

Diagnostics: See answer to question 68.4. Diagnostics are governed by the clinical aspects and should be

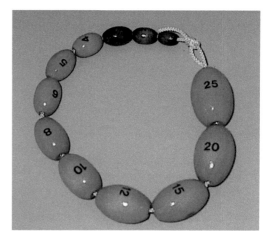

Orchidometer

restrained but purposeful. In the physical examination, the signs of puberty should be determined according to **Tanner's schema** (see Fig. Stages of puberty).

In boys, the scrotal size is determined with the **orchidometer** (see Fig. Orchidometer). **Sonographically,** a size increase of the gonads corresponding to the stage of puberty in boys and in girls, the increase in the size of the uterus, can be measured. Possibly, bilateral ovarian cysts can be confirmed. The bone age is found by an X-ray of the left hand and wrist. Hormonal analyses differentiate between normal and premature development of puberty or pubertas praecox vera and pseudopubertas praecox. EEG, MRI, and ophthalmological examination are recommended to rule out cerebral processes. If the bone age is not accelerated, hypothyroidism (determination of TSH and thyroid hormones) must be ruled out.

Treatment: See answer to question 68.5.

Prognosis: If therapy is begun on time, the prognosis for pubertas praecox vera and for pseudopubertas praecox is usually very good. No drawbacks of long-term effects of pharmaceutical treatment have been observed. After termination of treatment, pubertal hormone formation resumes, development of maturity is terminated, and a normal final size is attained. If therapy begins too late, secondary stunted growth must be expected.

ADDITIONAL TOPICS FOR STUDY GROUPS
■ Intersexuality

69.1 What do you do next?

- **Ensure breathing:** CPAP ventilation or intubation and respiratory therapy
- Infusion therapy with a glucose–electrolyte mixture for fluid replacement
- Circulatory stabilization: Crystalline solutions (NaCl 0.9% or Ringer-lactate 10–20 mL/kg body weight for 20 minutes), close monitoring of blood pressure
- **Laboratory:**
  - Blood/serum: Blood picture, differential blood count, CRP, electrolytes (Na, K), creatinine, liver values (GOT, GPT), blood gas analysis, blood sugar → signs of inflammation, evidence of metabolic disorder
  - Urine status, preferably on a sample obtained by bladder puncture: Urinary tract infection
  - Microbiological examination: Blood-, urine, spinal fluid culture → evidence of pathogen
  - Lumbar puncture: Meningitis
- **Antibiotic "blind" treatment** with broad-spectrum antibiotics i.v. (see Comments)

69.2 Interpret the laboratory values.

- **Blood/serum:**
  - Thrombocytopenia, leukocytopenia, and CRP elevation: Bacterial infection
  - Hyponatremia: Possible causes are dilution hyponatremia, dehydration, inadequate ADH secretion
  - Hyperkalemia: Possible causes are acidosis, excessively high parenteral feeding, hemolysis of the blood sample
  - Hypochloremia: Loss through vomiting
  - Clotting: Quick ↓, PTT ↑ → Use of clotting factors; Antithrombin ↓ → disseminated intravascular coagulation; fibrinogen ↑ → acute infection (acute-phase protein)
- **Spinal fluid:** Cell count ↑ ↑, spinal fluid sugar ↓, spinal fluid protein ↑ → purulent meningitis (see case 1)
- **Urine status:** No evidence of urinary tract infection, hyperosmolality as expression of dehydration or inadequate ADH secretion

69.3 Interpret the findings in the light of the clinical picture up to now. What do you know about this clinical picture?

- Clinical picture: **Neonatal sepsis** (= *Streptococcus* B sepsis; here: Late onset form, see below) with purulent meningitis; rationale: clinical and laboratory chemical signs of infection, consumption coagulopathy, evidence of germs in blood culture; distended fontanelle, vomiting
- Two forms:
  - **"Early onset" sepsis**: Occurrence first to third day of an infant's life; vertical infection (mother's recto-vaginal flora) especially with *Streptococcus* B, *E. coli*, *Staphylococcus aureus*, Klebsiella, Enterococci, Listeria; risk in newborns < 1%, in premature babies up to 20%, prognosis with prompt treatment is good
  - **"Late onset" sepsis**: Occurrence first to sixth week of an infant's life, especially horizontal (e.g., nosocomial) infection, e.g., with coagulase negative *Staphylococci* (*Staphylococcus epidermidis*), *Pseudomonas aeruginosa*, *Enterobacter*, rarely also fungi, viral infection (e.g., Herpes simplex virus); course usually with meningitis, prognosis worse than in early onset sepsis

69.4 In addition, the blood study shows hyponatremia. How do you interpret this electrolyte shift if you find out at the same time that the boy is gaining weight and excreting less?

- Especially **Schwartz–Batter syndrome** or **SIADH** (syndrome of inadequate ADH secretion): centrally governed pathologically elevated ADH secretion with water retention (causing weight gain) and dilution hyponatremia; occurs, among other things, in meningitis, cerebral bleeding, asphyxia, stress, opiate medication; treatment: fluid restriction, possibly diuretics (furosemide 1 mg/kg body weight), careful sodium replacement (control of Na level)
- Differential diagnosis: over-infusion, in that case polyuria

---

Comments

Classification: Bacterial infections can be divided into local and organ infections, systemic inflammatory reactions (=SIRS; clinical sepsis symptoms without identification of pathogens in the blood) and sepsis (clinical sepsis symptoms and evidence of pathogens in the blood).

Epidemiology: Bacterial infections are the most frequent diseases in the newborn period. Premature babies are at particular risk because early contractions and premature birth efforts are often triggered by amniotic infection syndrome (see below).

Etiology: The most important risk factor is an amniotic infection syndrome that often occurs after early rupture of the membranes and delivery > 18 hours. Additional risk factors are perinatal asphyxia, protracted birth, and meconium aspiration.

223

Case

69

→ Cases 69 Page 70

Clinical aspects: The clinical picture is very variable and extends from asymptomatic to a foudroyant course with lethal outcome. The less mature the newborn, the more frequently the clinical picture becomes septic.

The clinical symptoms of an infection are very unspecific in early and newborn babies as well as young infants (< 6 months). Muscle hypotension, decreased reactions or hyperreactivity, sensitivity to touch, restlessness, unwillingness to drink, sudden or frequent pauses in breathing and/or bradycardia, sighing, tachypnea, dyspnea, elevated oxygen requirement, tachycardia, arterial hypotension, temperature instability, impaired skin perfusion with protracted recapillarization time (> 3 s), pale and marbled skin all can be early evidence that the child has a severe infection.

In mature newborns, the infection often takes the form of pneumonia and the symptoms resemble a respiratory distress syndrome (see case 55). *Caution:* Never be satisfied with a diagnosis of respiratory distress syndrome in a mature newborn; always rule out sepsis.

In late onset sepsis, there is often sepsis with symptoms such as distended fontanelle, fever, lethargy extending to coma and cerebral seizures.

Diagnostics: The mother's fever and/or elevated signs of inflammation (CRP > 2.0 mg/dL [> 20 mg/L], leukocytosis > 16,000/μL), green, fetid amniotic fluid, and fetal tachycardia are evidence of amniotic infection syndrome. A cervical and vagal smear taken from the mother should already be carried out prenatally for identification of the pathogen. In the newborn, the germs of the mother's rectovaginal flora can be found in the auditory canal or gastric juice. If there is suspicion of infection, ear or gastric juice should be taken immediately after the birth from the newborn and examined.

Observation of the healthcare staff or the parents ("The child doesn't look good to me/us at all") must always be taken seriously. If there is the slightest reason for expecting an infection, the inflammatory parameters (CRP, blood picture [leukocytes, differentiation of leukocytes, platelets], blood sugar, BGA) in the blood should be determined, and blood, urine, and spinal fluid should be microbiologically examined under the microscope. The proof of a *Streptococcus B* infection is the only proof of the pathogen in the blood or spinal fluid culture. Throat, ear, skin, or navel smears are only a proof the germ is colonizing, i.e., in spite of everything: If the child shows signs of newborn sepsis and if there is *Streptococcus B* in the smear, the child is treated as for *Streptococcus B* sepsis until the blood culture result is received.

Note: If there is a suspicion of sepsis, a lumber puncture is always part of a newborn's examination.

Laboratory changes that indicate a bacterial infection are leukocytopenia (< 6,000/μL, a leukocyte plunge is highly suggestive of an infection) or leukocytosis (> 30,000/μL). *Caution:* Erythroblasts must be subtracted from the number of leukocytes. In immature children, the differential blood count often shows erythroblasts/normoblasts, which are incorrectly included with leukocytes when the cells are counted by machine; left shift in differential blood picture (increased occurrence of rod nuclei and juvenile granulocytes in the white blood picture), thrombocytopenia (< 100,000/μL; cause: increased use) and elevation of the CRP value > 2 mg/dL (*caution:* diagnostic window → CRP does not rise until 12–24 hours after infection). Other inflammatory indicators that are developed earlier as part of an infectious event are cytokines such as interleukin 6 and 8. However, their assay is not yet routinely possible in every laboratory.

Other unspecific proofs of bacterial infection are hypo- or hyperglycemia, glycosuria, hyponatremia, hypocalcemia, and metabolic acidosis.

Differential diagnoses: In differential diagnosis in a septic clinical picture of the newborn, a metabolic error (metabolic emergency) in a congenital metabolic defect must be kept in mind. Evidence is obtained by blood gas analysis (marked metabolic acidosis) and determination of the blood sugar (usually hypoglycemia).

Treatment: The indication for **antibiotic treatment** is broadly established since early start is decisive for the success of the treatment. Antibiotic must first be calculated ("blind") and is always i.v. Conclusions about the pathogen can be made from the time of the infection (see answer to question 69.3). The selected antibiotic combination should cover the broadest germ spectrum possible. The CDC has been pessimistic for some time about administration of antibiotic prophylaxis against Group B *Streptococcus* infection because of the unnecessary danger of creating super-bugs. However, studies dating from 2015 show a 40-fold variation in practice in US NICUs across the 50 states. The recommendations for antibiotic treatment of newborn infection from the German Association for Pediatric Infectious Diseases read as follows:

- **"Early onset" sepsis**: Ampicillin (150–200 mg/kg body weight/d to 300–400 mg/kg body weight for meningitis) + cephalosporins (e.g., cefotaxim 100–200 mg/kg body weight/d) + aminoglycoside (e.g., gentamycin 5 mg/kg body weight/d)

■ **"Late onset" sepsis:** Ceftazidime (100 mg/kg body weight/d) + aminoglycoside (e.g., netilmicin 5 mg/kg body weight/d) or glycopeptide antibiotics (e.g., vancomycin 15 mg/kg body weight/d)

After the antibiogram has been received, it may be necessary to modify the antibiotic treatment. If the clinical suspicion is not confirmed and no pathogens could be found in the blood cultures, the antibiotics should be discontinued. In a clinically mild course without evidence of a pathogen, treatment over a period of 5 to7 days is recommended. If the evidence of bacteria in the blood culture is positive, the treatment should be carried out for a period of at least 7, but preferably 10 days. In meningitis, the treatment should be continued for 2 to 3 weeks. In addition, supportive measures such as intense monitoring, stabilization of circulation, if necessary, treatment of seizures and protection of breathing. If there are marked pauses in breathing or oxygen need ($FiO_2 > 0.4$) CPAP (= continuous positive airway pressure) ventilation can become necessary. Positive pressure is built up in the respiratory pathways, over a tube that is inserted into the throat (throat CPAP) or through nasal cannulas (nose CPAP), with a ventilation machine (high flow, PEEP). This reopens atelectatic lung areas, the functional residual capacity is elevated, and gas exchange is improved. If this does not overcome the breathing pauses, or if the oxygen need continues to increase, intubation and ventilation may become essential.

Prophylaxis: In case of colonization with *Streptococcus B*, early rupture of the membranes, or clinical or blood evidence of infection, treatment of the mother with penicillin during the delivery process can effectively prevent early onset sepsis in the child. However, prophylactic antibiotic treatment during pregnancy is not useful since colonization usually resumes after termination of the treatment. There are only a few possibilities for prophylaxis of late onset sepsis. Meticulous hygiene (e.g., careful disinfection of the hands, no jewelry on the hands of nursing staff/ physicians, disinfection of stethoscopes, disinfection of surfaces) is a basic prerequisite. Foreign materials (e.g., indwelling venous cannulas, central venous catheters, and bladder catheters) are often the point of entry for a pathogen. Therefore, they should only be left in place as long as absolutely necessary.

Prognosis: With adequate treatment and monitoring of early onset sepsis, the lethality, even in small premature babies, is less than 1%. Late onset sepsis, especially with meningitis, has a poor prognosis. Cerebral late damage, such as motor disorders, hydrocephalus, and mental retardation, is observed in many cases. The lethality of meningitis in late onset sepsis is high because of the associated cerebral edema. It lies at approximately 25%.

 ADDITIONAL TOPICS FOR STUDY GROUPS
■ Other infections of new and premature babies (e.g., herpes simplex, lues, Listeria)

225

Case

70

70 Adenoid hyperplasia

70.1 What do you observe on examining the patient? What additional information from the medical history do you find interesting?
■ **Inspection:** Adenoid face (= characteristic "simple minded" facial expression with open mouth and mouth breathing)
■ **Medical history:**
  – Does the little girl snore at night? → adenoidal hyperplasia
  – Have breathing pauses during sleep been observed?→short, complete displacement of the respiratory pathways
  – Does the child often have a cold? → mouth breathing
  – Does the child suffer from relapsing middle ear inflammation?→Displacement of the Eustachian tubes by adenoids leads to insufficient aeration of the middle ear with resulting middle ear inflammations
  – Is there evidence of decreased hearing?

70.2 Make a suspected diagnosis. How do you confirm the diagnosis?
■ **Obstructive sleep apnea syndrome with adenoid vegetation**; rationale: Adenoid face, night sweats, fatigue, and daytime difficulty concentrating
■ **Confirmation of diagnosis:** Detailed physical examination including
  – Palpation of cervical lymph nodes
  – **ENT status:** Inspection of the throat and nasal cavity (foreign bodies), evaluation of teeth (malalignment of teeth), posterior rhinoscopy (hyperplasia of the adenoids/palatal tonsils), inspection of the auditory pathways (eardrum secretions, otitis media), hearing test (tympanometry, audiogram), if necessary, digital examination of the gums (submucous cleft palate)

→ Cases 70 Page 71

- **Obstructive sleep apnea syndrome:** The shift of the upper respiratory pathways leads to unsuccessful breathing motions and longer breathing pauses (> 10 seconds); this leads to hypoxia and rising CO_2 which in turn lead to a waking reaction (arousal) and increased breathing. The results are night sweats, daytime tiredness, difficulty concentrating, apathy

- **Adenoid vegetation:** Hyperplasia of the adenoids, interfering with nose breathing; the result is frequent infections of the respiratory pathways, relapsing otitides, snoring, obstructive sleep apnea syndrome, failure to thrive

70.4 What therapy is required?

Surgical treatment by adenotomy

Comments

Definition: Adenoid vegetation is an enlargement of the adenoids (tonsilla pharyngealis) as an expression of a particularly active immune defense in childhood. In colloquial speech, they are incorrectly called "polyps."

Anatomy: The adenoids, as a part of the lymphatic tonsillar ring (Waldeyer throat ring), are at the transition from the nasal cavity to the throat in the nasopharynx (see Fig.). Like the palatine tonsils, it is responsible in that location for defense against pathogens. Other components of the Waldeyer tonsillar ring are the tonsillae tubariae, tonsillae lingualis, the lateral strands (plicae tubopharyngiae), and lymphoepithelial collections at the Morgagni ventricle of the larynx.

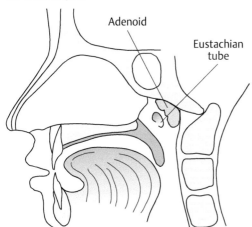

Schematic representation of the position of the adenoids

Pathogenesis and clinical aspects: See answer to question 70.3. The enlarged adenoids hinder nose breathing, i.e., children breathe loud through their mouths. They sniff constantly. Their speech is unclear. They develop a typical **adenoid face** with open mouth, a stupid, almost dull-witted facial expression (see Fig. example case). If the symptoms persist for a long time, tooth malalignments develop because of the lacking contact between lower and upper jaw. Patients snore because of impaired nose breathing; often they develop obstructive apnea (extended breathing pauses because of obstruction of respiratory pathways) with hypoxia and increased CO_2 retention. Their sleep is restless. For this reason, the children are sleepy and in a bad mood during the day. Difficulty concentrating, unwilling to participate, and poor performance are the consequence of the obstructive **sleep apnea syndrome**. Immediately next to the adenoids lies the entrance to the middle ear, the Eustachian tube (see Fig.). If this is covered by the adenoids, fluid collects in the middle ear and an eardrum effusion (serous otitis media) is formed. Increasing infections lead to relapsing middle ear inflammations and infections of the respiratory pathways. Impairment of sound conduction with decrease in hearing and delay of speech development can be the result. In addition, children suffer frequently from lack of appetite and failure to thrive; the impaired nose breathing makes eating difficult. Food doesn't taste good because the smell is missing.

Differential diagnoses: Choanal atresia and other malformations of the nasopharynx (e.g., submucosal cleft formations, cysts) must be ruled out, foreign bodies in the nose and other causes for chronic prevention of nose breathing (e.g., allergies, lymphomas, or other space-occupying lesions).

Diagnostics: Classical medical history and typical facial expression can already lead to a suspected diagnosis of adenoid vegetation. A thorough physical examination must follow. Particular attention should be given to the ENT area (see answer to question 70.2). For this purpose, request an **ENT consult**. For diagnosis of sleep apnea syndrome, a sleep laboratory study (polysomnography) may become necessary. For this purpose the patient spends up to three nights in a special **sleep laboratory**. The patient's sleep is monitored by video. Noises, such as snoring, heartbeat, and respiration rate are continually recorded. The oxygen saturation is measured by pulse-oximetry and the breathing movements are captured by special sensors. Breath flow probes register the breathing flow through mouth and nose. Sleep depth can be determined by EEG leads and waking reactions can be recorded. This study provides information about the extent of the obstructive apnea. The indication for surgical treatment can thus be more easily established, especially for toddlers.

Treatment: The indication for surgical intervention, adenotomy, is established clinically. Until the operation, treatment is symptomatic with decongestant nose drops, mucolytic agents (e.g., ambroxol 7.5–15 mg/d in 2–3 individual doses), and where there are signs of bacterial infection, antibiotics (e.g., amoxicillin 50–100 mg/kg body weight). Any symptomatic adenoidal hyperplasia that does not regress after 2 to 3 months should be surgically treated, and in particular if complications or a sleep apnea syndrome is present. In case of serous otitis media, paracentesis is performed and, if necessary, ear tubes are inserted.

Prognosis: In 85% of cases, the symptoms improve after adenotomy.

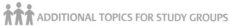
ADDITIONAL TOPICS FOR STUDY GROUPS
- Otitis media
- Tonsillar hyperplasia

---

71 Counseling of parents of screaming child, breastfeeding, and nutrition

71.1 How do you evaluate the parents' situation? What advice would you give the parents?
- **Evaluation of the situation:**
  - The child's clearly unspecific screaming
  - Intense insecurity of the parents, who looked for many suggestions and tips and tried them out
  - Stress for the parents because of absence of the child's rhythm, lack of sleep, worry about the child, neighbors' annoyance
- **Information and counseling for parents:**
  - First calm the parents.
  - Unspecific crying is a frequent problem in many families; it reaches its peak around the sixth to eighth week and is usually limited to the first 3 months of an infant's life.
  - This is not a matter of the parents' mistakes but represents a phase of adaptation and learning for both parents and child.
- **Recommendations for the parents:** Improvement often comes from
  - Structuring the day's regimen (e.g., fixed feeding times, since screaming does not always mean hunger)
  - A great deal of attention, speaking to the child, picking up and holding the child often, rocking it in their arms and carrying it around
  - Alternating "time off" for each parent, to provide relief
  - Quiet and consistent behavior of the parents (no panic when the child is screaming. Do not jump right away at the first cry. Do not constantly change the feeding plan, day's schedule, etc. Speak with the child quietly when it screams)
  - If necessary, offer inpatient treatment, to provide quiet and support for parents and child (child and mother are admitted to the hospital. Treatment: A structured daily schedule, psychological care, support for a screaming child is given by the nursing staff)

71.2 What are the advantages of nursing? How long should the baby be exclusively breastfed? Are there situations in which the mother should be advised not to breastfeed?
- **Advantages of breastfeeding:** Economical; constantly available; always at the right temperature; low bacterial content; contains biologically valuable, easily digestible protein (high whey protein content facilitates digestion) and special fatty acid structure, especially long-chain, polyunsaturated fatty acids (easier to absorb); low mineral content (protects the still-immature kidneys); contains protective and immune factors (IgA), atopia and obesity prophylaxis; lactose in the mother's milk encourages formation of intestinal bifidus flora, which also gives it an anti-infectious effect (inhibition of Gram-negative bacteria and fungi); vitamin content (except Vitamins D and K) covers the infant's needs; sufficient trace elements; encourages mother–child bonding; decreases the risk of sudden child death; promotes uterine shrinkage in the mother by secretion of oxytocin during nursing.
- **Duration of breastfeeding:** Exclusively until the fifth/sixth month of an infant's life, then gradual addition of food.
- **The child should not be breastfed** in case of
  - **HIV infection:** High risk of vertical infection through the mother's milk; no breastfeeding under any circumstances.
  - **Hepatitis B infection:** Child may be breastfed after receiving both the vaccine and hepatitis B immune globulin.
  - **Hepatitis C infection:** Relative contraindication; infection risk probably exists only where there is a high viral load.
  - Open tuberculosis: Danger of droplet infection.
  - **CMV infection:** Only applies to premature births < 32nd week of pregnancy; since in these babies, the diaplacental transfer of protective antibodies

→ Cases 71 Page 72

has not yet occurred, they can be infected with CMV through the mother's milk. In that case, a severe course of the disease is possible. Pasteurizing the mother's milk is possible.

- **Consuming diseases** and **neoplasms:** The stress is too high for the mother.
- Taking **certain medicines** (e.g., cytostatics, thyreostatic agents, immunosuppressants, certain antibiotics, ergotamine preparations, valproic acid derivatives): Possible damage to the child through passage of the medication into the mother's milk.
- **Alcohol dependency:** Quantitatively and qualitatively insufficient milk, passage of the alcohol into the mother's milk, possible damage to the child.
- **Drug dependency:** Possible damage to the child through passage of addictive substances into the mother's milk.
- **Galactosemia:** normally first detected through newborn screening: A firm contraindication for breastfeeding (or for feeding with galactose-containing infant formula).

228

Case

71

71.3 **What is meant by early stage, stage 1, and stage 2 food? How do these infant foods differ from each other? How do you evaluate the development of the child's diet up to now? What do you recommend to the family?**

- **"Early stage, stage 1, and stage 2 food":** Industrially prepared infant food based on cow's milk
- **"Early stage":** Infant starter food; as thin and liquid as mother's milk; contains lactose as the only carbohydrate; can be fed unhesitatingly during the entire first year
- **Stage 1 food:** Infant starter food; a fluid thicker than mother's milk; in addition to lactose contains a small proportion of starch [2%] and other carbohydrates, more filling
- **Stage 2 food:** The next food; contains other carbohydrates besides lactose, especially starch, a higher protein/mineral content; feeding from the age of 5 months possible (nutritionally not necessarily needed)
- **Determining the child's nutritional buildup:** The infant is only 8 weeks old and the diet has been changed several times in this short period. This is a sign of the parents' serious insecurity and the bad advice they have received. Stage 2 food is not suitable for infants under 6 months because, through their composition, they exert excessive stress on the child's still immature kidneys

71.4 **What should a nutrition plan for the first year of a child's life normally look like? (see Fig.)**
- **First 4 to 6 months:** Feed only milk
  - Ideal: Only breastfeed
  - Or partial breastfeeding and additional feeding of industrially prepared infant milk
  - Or exclusive feeding with industrially prepared infant milk
- **From the fifth to seventh month:** Introduction of solid food by replacing one-milk meal at 4-week intervals
  - Puree of vegetables, potatoes, and meat
  - then puree of whole milk and grain
  - then puree of grain and fruit
- **From the 10th month:** Introduction of the family's diet, being careful:
  - No small, solid food that could be aspirated, such as nuts, bits of carrot, pieces of apple
  - No very fatty food
  - Slow habituation to food that is hard to digest, such as legumes

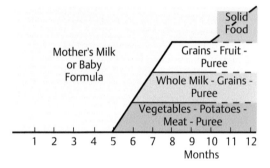

Schematic dietary plan

71.5 **Do infants need nutritional supplements in addition to mother's milk or formula?**
- Independently of the type of milk or solid food, the recommendation is:
- **Vitamin K:** Prophylaxis for Vitamin K deficiency hemorrhage (see case 65), is administered at the first examination—third health screening, Vitamin K 2 mg p.o.
- **Vitamin D:** Rickets prophylaxis, Vitamin D_3 400–500 IU/d p.o. during the first year of a child's life
- **Fluoride:** Caries prophylaxis (0.25 mg/d), usually combined with Vitamin D in tablet form
- **Iodine:** Risk of iodine deficiency, especially in breast-fed infants, therefore, consistent supplementing of iodine for pregnant and breastfeeding women (200 µg/d)

Comments

Consultation for screaming child: In the first trimester, important maturation and adaptation processes affecting nutrient uptake, digestion, immune defense, thermoregulation, and organization of a sleep–wake rhythm take place. In this process, the infant, whose self-regulation abilities are limited, must be adequately supported by its parents. If this does not happen, **regulation disorders**, such as excessive screaming, sleep disorders, feeding and thriving disorders, set in. These behavioral abnormalities are extreme expressions of otherwise normal behavioral patterns and represent crises in a normal development. Fifteen percent to 30% of all parents experience the same thing as the parents in the example case: the child screams—often without an obvious reason—and simply cannot be calmed down. This can lead to insecurity and excessive demands on the parents. Therefore, it is important to educate the parents about the screaming. On the one hand, a child screams in order to communicate physical needs, such as hunger and such problems as pain, boredom, overtiredness, and too much stimulation. Often the type and intensity of the screaming provides information about the cause (e.g., hunger, pain, or simply just boredom).

On the other hand, screaming can be observed without any clear reason, called **unspecific screaming**, which is blamed on a disturbance of the sleep–wake rhythm (difficulty falling asleep, lack of sleep, overtiredness). Unspecific screaming has a characteristic course: It increases from week to week, reaching its peak around the sixth to eighth week of an infant's life. Usually, it does not last longer than 3 weeks. The screaming period takes place largely in the afternoon and evening. However, the parents are often unsure, and look for the cause in their own incorrect behavior. Often, they assume that some food is not tolerated or ascribe the screaming to stomach colic (3-month colic). But one must ask: Does the child scream because it has an abdominal pain or does it have an abdominal pain because it is crying? When the child is screaming, it swallows large amounts of air. The mother stops nursing, the feeding routine is changed, advice is requested from friends, relatives, and experts.

It is important in dealing with these matters to **calm down the parents** by explaining what is involved in unspecific screaming, and that this screaming only lasts for a limited time. The infant's day should be structured; this means firmly fixed feeding times. Nursing or the baby bottle should not be the response to every screaming episode. The parents should pay attention to the child, try to quiet it down by speaking to it, singing, playing, or carrying it around. Increased attention and carrying the child around at times when the child is not screaming decreases the intensity and frequency of the screaming intervals.

If necessary, it can be helpful to admit to the hospital (together with the mother), to bring some tranquility into the situation. The parents must be told that food intolerance is usually not the problem. On the contrary, constant modification of the diet leads to stress on the juvenile organism especially when the infant is fed foods that, as in the example case, are not yet appropriate for the infant.

The infant's nutrient requirement: Current recommendations for infant nutrition take into account: 1. The increased energy and nutrient requirement due to growth and development. 2. The fact that digestion, metabolism, and the immune system, at least in the first year of a child's life, are in the development stage.

The infant's daily requirement is approximately **100 to 120 kcal/kg body weight**. To satisfy this, the diet should consist of 45% fat and carbohydrate, respectively, and 10% of protein. Infants regulate their own appetite if they are being breastfed or fed age-appropriate infant starter food (= feeding on demand or ad libitum; a fixed schedule is only necessary for a screaming child). It can be seen that the child is receiving enough food if he or she is thriving normally. In the first year of a child's life, a weight gain of 150 to 200 g per week is desirable.

Mother's milk: A diet consisting **exclusively of mother's milk in the first (4 to) 6 months** is recommended. On the basis of its composition, mother's milk is particularly easy to digest and precisely adapted to the child's needs (see answer to question 71.2). The composition of the mother's milk changes, particularly with regard to the protein and fat content of the immunoglobulin-rich colostrum (so-called premilk), that is produced by the mother in the first week of the newborn's life, to a so-called transitional milk (second week of the newborn's life) and to mature mother's milk (from the third week, richer in energy, i.e., more fat and lactose). The composition even changes during the feeding process (first low fat, then richer milk) and during the course of the day.

The differences in the composition, compared to cow's milk, are shown in the table (see Tab.). Mother's milk is easier to digest, since the protein content with less casein, the lipid content with the high lipase content contained in mother's milk, and the higher carbohydrate are optimally adapted to the infant's nutritional needs. Mother's milk, moreover, is richer in unsaturated fatty acids, immunoglobulins, minerals, and lactose.

Nursing: For advantages of breastfeeding and duration of breastfeeding, see answer to question 71.2. But the discussion returns to breastfeeding again and again: The greatest concern is that mother's milk is contaminated with chlororganic compounds such as plant protective substances, PCB, dioxins among other things that enter the mother's milk through the food chain. It has not yet been possible

→ Cases 71 Page 72

to find evidence of damage to breastfed infants. Please see note. No limitations of the recommendation to breastfeed have been necessary up to now.

Breastfeeding must be learned. The mother already receives detailed training in breastfeeding technique in childbirth preparation classes, so she will understand the conditions that create a good outcome and provide satisfaction for her and her baby. The child should be placed in a comfortable position and be offered both breasts at every meal. Nursing time should be limited to 10 or 15 minutes, to prevent sore nipples and rhagades. The breast should be kept clean and dried after nursing. Normally nursing happens on the principle of self-demand feeding (ad libitum), i.e., the child "announces" that it is mealtime, usually at 2 to 4 hour intervals. The nursing mother should eat a healthy diet (plenty of fruit and vegetables, avoiding foods that cause flatulence).

In breastfeeding, demand controls supply, i.e., frequently placing the baby to the breast can increase milk production. With formula-feeding, portions are increased according to the needs of the child and in increments according to the formula package instructions.

Breastfeeding problems: There are situations in which feeding mother's milk or breastfeeding is contraindicated (see answer to question 71.2). The mother's **smoking** is not a contraindication for breastfeeding. It is true that nicotine passes into the mother's milk in significant amounts, but there is no evidence for damage to the child. But the child should under no circumstances be exposed to cigarette smoke (increased risk of SIDS, see case 42).

	Mother's milk	Cow milk
Energy content kcal/100 mL	67–70	66
Albumen g/100 mL	1.0	3.3
Fat g/100 mL	3.5–4.0	3.5
Carbohydrate g/100 mL	7.0	4.8
Whey protein: Casein	2:1	1:4
Saturated fatty acids:unsaturated fatty acids	50:50	65:35
Minerals g/100 mL	0.2	0.7
Fat soluble vitamins	+++	+
Water-soluble vitamins	+	+++
IgA, lysozyme	+	0

Other impediments to breastfeeding on the part of the mother are flat or concave nipples, which make it difficult to position the child at the breast. Nipple shields (= cap for the nipple, made of rubber or silicone) can be helpful here. In agalactia or hypogalactia, frequently offering the child the breast and large amounts of fluid for the mother can help the mother. Mastitis caused by milk stasis must be treated with antibiotics. The milk stasis is treated by regularly pressing out the painful concretion and frequently offering the breast to the baby or pumping the milk. If the bacterial count is too high (bacteria > 10^5 mL), offering the affected breast must be temporarily interrupted; the milk is then pumped and discarded. Often the milk coming in is accompanied by intense pain, which keeps the mother from breastfeeding. Warm compresses can be helpful here as well as a temporary limitation of the amount of fluid the mother drinks. Sore or bleeding nipples are often only caused when the baby licks them instead of latching onto the breast. If possible, the baby should put their mouth around both the nipple

and the areola, not just the nipple. Here too, nipple shields can offer temporary relief.

For the child's part, the inability to suck in very immature premature babies, severe illness (e.g., congenital heart defect, connatal pneumonia), metabolic disorder (e.g., congenital lactose intolerance, galactosemia), surgery, deformities of the jaw or the digestive tract, can make it difficult or impossible to breastfeed.

Taboos or incorrect ideas, a lack of information and preparation, anxiety, inexperience, lack of support from the partner are frequent reasons why a mother does not want, or no longer wants to breastfeed.

Mother's milk substitute: If the mother is not breastfeeding, many commercially produced infant foods are available (see answer to question 71.3). The permitted protein sources are modified cow milk products and soy protein isolates (for special cow's milk-free diets). In atopic dispositions, non-breastfed infants should be fed with HA foods based on protein hydrolysates. For vegetarian diets or cow's milk-free diets, cow's milk-free soy foods are available. They do not prevent allergies and are only suitable for treatment of cow's milk protein allergies to a limited extent (*caution:* cow's milk protein allergy is often associated with a soy protein allergy). There are also other special foods, such as anti-reflux food (with an additive of carob seed meal as a thickener), that (should) prevent the infant from "spitting" or special foods that prevent mild digestive problems (constipation, flatulence).

There is also the possibility of preparing the infant's formula oneself. However, this cannot achieve the hygienic and nutritive quality of commercially prepared infant formula. To prepare it, pasteurized whole milk (e.g., 100 mL) is mixed with water 1:1, thickened with 5 g starch, with the addition of 3 g oil (rape seed, soy, sunflower, or corn germ oil). From the age of 6 months, 5 g carrot puree (Vitamin A) and 20 g fruit juice (Vitamin C) must be added.

Solid food: At the age of 5 to 7 months, mother's milk or mother's milk substitute are no longer sufficient as the only food. Protein and energy content as well as zinc and iron concentration no longer cover the infant's needs. For this reason, from this age onward, addition of a solid food is recommended. Premature introduction, before the fifth month increases the risk of allergy development. Month for month, the solid food replaces one-milk meal with a puree (see answer to question 71.4). As a result, the water content of the diet is reduced, and an additional 200 mL/d of fluid is recommended. The most suitable liquid for this purpose is boiled tap water in the form of unsugared tea. Boiled tap water is also suitable for preparation of the bottle and the puree; it is not necessary to use mineral water or special commercially available water for preparation of infant food. The drinking water satisfies the requirements; concentrations of nitrite, nitrate, and sodium are constantly monitored. Toward the end of the first year, whole milk may be consumed. It is not suitable earlier as the only drink fed from the bottle because

of the stress exerted on the child's kidneys by proteins and minerals.

Toward the end of the first year (after the 10th month) the food should be gradually adapted to the family's diet. It should consist of a healthy mixture of foods with a moderate proportion of fat. Children should gradually become accustomed to foods that cause flatulence; spices should be moderately used. Care should be taken with small, hard foods such as nuts, pieces of carrot, and berries. These entail the danger of aspiration.

Prophylaxis: See answer to question 71.4.

Fluoride prophylaxis: Fluorides protect the tooth enamel from plaque by forming calcium fluoride precipitates. The effect of locally used fluoride-containing toothpaste, rinses, and D-fluorettes is more important than the systemic effect. However, many parents are concerned at the moment about the fluoride content because recently the media have had a great deal to say about the carcinogenic effect of excessive fluoride replacement. It is possible to convince the parents that fluoride replacement is not dangerous by informing them of the state-sponsored fluoride replacement in drinking water, carried out in most European countries, e.g., Sweden. In Sweden, an elevated cancer rate has not been detected. In addition, one should explain to the parents that it is not possible to provide children with sufficient calcium and fluorides through the mother's milk or with balanced solid food. This means that bone and tooth development are potentially always in danger. This means that with fluorettes, it will later be possible to save many dentist, orthopedist, and physiotherapist costs. If the parents do not wish their child to receive fluoride replacement, pure Vitamin D replacement can be prescribed.

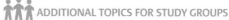 ADDITIONAL TOPICS FOR STUDY GROUPS
- Nutrition for toddlers, preschoolers, and school children
- Tooth development and caries prophylaxis
- Counseling for breastfeeding

---

72 Tuberculosis

72.1 What are your next steps in establishing a diagnosis?
- **Physical examination:**
  - Taking and recording body measurements in percentiles (age-appropriate body development)

- Evaluation of the overall condition (impairments, skin color/turgor)
- Lungs: Auscultation (crackles, side different or weakened breath sounds, obstruction)
- Heart: Auscultation (heart sounds, frequency, rhythm), palpation of the pulse, signs of cardiac insufficiency (edema)

→ Cases 72 Page 73

- Abdomen: Organ enlargement, resistances, intestinal sounds (increased, decreased)
    - Lymph node status (local or generalized lymph node swelling)
    - Palpation of the fontanelles (tense [in cerebral pressure/meningitis], sunken [in dehydration])
    - Measuring fever: Elevated temperature
- **Laboratory:** Blood picture, CRP, sedimentation rate, electrolytes, blood sugar, blood gas analysis, urine status
- **Throat smear:** Identification of pathogens
- **Abdominal ultrasound:** Evidence of gastroesophageal reflux, organ enlargement, space-occupying lesions
- **Echocardiography:** Ruling out a cardiac defect
- **Thoracic X-ray:** Pneumonic infiltrates, evidence of foreign body aspiration, heart size

72.2 Describe what you notice on the thoracic X-ray. What is your suspected diagnosis, in light of the medical history, and how can you confirm it?

- **Thoracic X-ray:** Soft infiltrate in the left lower field with connection to the pulmonary hilus
- **Suspected diagnosis: Tuberculosis**; rationale: medical history and clinical aspects (patient from Eastern Europe, persistent cough, fatigue, tiredness, night sweats), thoracic X-ray (suspicion of a primary focus)
- **Confirmation of diagnosis:**
    - **Tuberculin skin test:** Mendel–Mantoux skin test 1 unit tuberculin (see Comments)
    - **Examination of empty stomach secretion** (on 3 consecutive days): Microscopy after Ziehl–Neelsen staining (acid-fast bacilli?, succeeds less frequently in childhood than in adults because of a lower bacterial count and density), **PCR** (yields rapidly accessible evidence), **culture** (Gold standard, necessary for determination of resistance, but results only after 4–6 weeks)
    - With negative bacteriological results and continued clinical suspicion: Bronchoscopy with bronchoalveolar lavage (BAL) and bacteriological examination of the BAL fluid

72.3 Give a brief picture of the course of this disease.

- **Pathogens:** Immobile, acid-fast bacilli of the mycobacterium tuberculosis complex
- **Infectious pathway:** Droplet infection, low infectiousness
- **Incubation time:** 4 to 12 weeks
- **Course:** See also Comments
    - **Primary tuberculosis:** Usually pulmonary manifestation; if resistance is good, unnoticeable course

with formation of a primary complex and encapsulation/calcification of the infectious focus (however this can still contain viable mycobacteria)
    - **Postprimary tuberculosis (early form):** With poor resistance, there is hematogenous/lymphogenous dissemination from the primary focus; manifestation forms: caseous pneumonia, minimal lesions, disseminated seeding (miliary tuberculosis), tuberculous meningitis
    - **Postprimary tuberculosis (late form):** Through reactivation of old tubercular foci; manifestation sites: lymph node tuberculosis, kidney, bone, or joint tuberculosis

72.4 What do you know about the treatment of this disease?

- **Latent infection/tuberculin conversion** (see Comments): Isoniazid for 9 months
- **Tuberculosis treatment** with a combination of three or four different tuberculostatics (isoniazid, rifampicin, pyrazinamide, ethambutol, streptomycin). Combination therapy is necessary to prevent the development of resistances. Choice of medication and duration of treatment depend on the degree of severity (see Comments). If necessary, the treatment is modified according to the antibiogram.

72.5 What inoculation does the mother mean? Will you inoculate the child? What are the general recommendations for prophylaxis of this disease?

- **BCG inoculation** (**B**acille–**C**almette–**G**uerin); designation for attenuated live *Mycobacterium bovis* vaccine as a protective inoculation against tuberculosis
- The inoculation has not been recommended since 1998 because of a low benefit-risk ratio and therefore the mother's request of an inoculation is not granted
- Report to responsible health department office: When the mother's information is confirmed, chemical prevention is initiated
- Chemical prevention for 3 months with isoniazid in confirmed cases of tuberculosis exposure or latent tuberculosis infection
- **General prophylaxis suggestions:** Specific tuberculin testing in suspicion of Tuberculosis (chronic cough, failure to thrive, night sweats) and contact with persons who have tuberculosis, long stay in a country where the prevalence of tuberculosis is high (developing countries [Asia, Africa], Eastern Europe/Russia) or emigrants from countries where the prevalence is high, in children with HIV infections and immune deficiency

Comments

Definition: Tuberculosis is a **chronic, bacterial infectious disease** caused by pathogens of the *Mycobacterium tuberculosis* complex and characterized by granuloma

formation in infected tissue and cell-mediated hypersensitivity. The chief site of manifestation is the lungs.

Epidemiology: It is diffused throughout the world. Incidence and lethality are particularly high in developing countries. In recent decades, tuberculosis has become less important in industrialized countries because of improved social and hygienic conditions as well as efficacious treatment methods. But as a result of migration from countries with a high prevalence of tuberculosis as well as the spread of AIDS, the public has again become more conscious of the disease in recent years.

The incidence of tuberculosis in the United States in 2014 was 2.96 cases per 100,000 persons. In addition to children, the populations most at risk are immune suppressed persons (e.g., HIV infected persons, drug addicts, alcoholics, and the malnourished).

Etiopathogenesis: *Mycobacteria* are **immobile bacilli**. They grow aerobically and have a low rate of division. Because of their particular wall structure (glycolipids, waxes), they are **acid fast** and especially resistant to noxa.

The pathogens enter the alveoli and are there phagocytized by alveolar macrophages. These represent the antigen structures on their cellular surfaces and in this way activate the T-lymphocytes and thus the specific, cellular immune response. The cytokines formed by the T-helper cells attract more macrophages that are transformed into giant cells at the infection site. The histiocytic at the site differentiate into epithelioid cells. This group of cells aggregates to a compact structure around which a fibrin border wall is formed by activation of the fibroblasts. Subsequently necrosis sets in (= caseous degeneration), fibrosis and calcification inside the granuloma. A prerequisite for granuloma formation and thus isolation of the inflammatory process is an intact cellular immune system. If resistance is weak, the process cannot be isolated, and the infection spreads.

Tuberculosis is largely spread from person to person by **droplet infection**. The source of infection is usually infected adults with open pulmonary tuberculosis who spread the pathogen by coughing or sneezing. The tuberculosis bacteria can remain suspended in the air for hours. Thus, contagion can even take place when the patient has long since left the room. Whether or not contagion occurs depends on the frequency and intensity of the contact, the number and virulence of the inhaled pathogens, and the resistance status of the exposed person. Extrapulmonary tuberculosis (lymph nodes, urogenital system, bones, joints, digestive organs) only presents a risk of infection if the disease focus has a contact to the outside through a fistula. Other infectious pathways, e.g., through milk contaminated with *M. bovis*, have grown very rare in the industrialized countries. The incubation time is 4 to 12 weeks; the infectiousness is low.

There are different **stages of tuberculosis** (see Tab. Stages of illness with tuberculosis) and differences between open and closed tuberculosis. Open pulmonary tuberculosis occurs through liquefaction of necrotic pulmonary foci with formation of caverns. If connections are created between the caverns and the bronchial system, the patient becomes "open," i.e., tubercle bacilli can enter the outside world through coughing or sneezing. Then the patient is contagious. In closed tuberculosis, on the other hand, there is no danger of infection.

Course of the illness and clinical symptoms: The point of entry for the tubercle bacilli is usually the respiratory pathways; the **primary infection or the primary tuberculosis** therefore often develops in the lungs. Very rarely, it manifests outside the lungs, in the intestines, cervical lymph nodes, or the skin. The primary infection usually has a subclinical course, especially in older children. Sometimes there are a few days of coughing and subfebrile temperatures. Infants and toddlers exhibit unspecific symptoms such as coughing, fever, lack of appetite, failure to thrive, and night sweats. The first contact with the mycobacteria, after a latency of 4 to 6 weeks, creates the **primary focus** that can be located anywhere in the lungs. Association with lymphangitis and lymphadenitis is called a **primary complex**. Many primary foci are located close to the pleura, and there can be an associated pleural reaction (e.g., pleuritis, pleural effusion).

In some children, there can be a progression of this uncomplicated tuberculosis (early form) or a reactivation of the endogenous tuberculosis infection (late form often after years). The disease is then called **postprimary tuberculosis**. The most frequently affected are children with weak immunity, infants, and toddlers, or children after pertussis or virus infections. Caseous pneumonia can spread through the blood or along anatomical structures (early form), with symptoms such as coughing, fever, dyspnea, and lack of appetite. If the foci fuse, caverns can develop, thus creating an open tuberculosis (see above). In a few cases, the primary complex seeds into the blood or the lymph and creates little lesions, the so-called minimal lesions (early form) in the lungs (e.g., Simon focus) or other organs.

Stages of illness with tuberculosis	
Exposure to tuberculosis	Contact with an infectious person
(Latent) tuberculosis infection	Positive tuberculin test without manifest signs of illness or radiological changes
Falling ill with tuberculosis	Primary infection or primary tuberculosis
	Postprimary tuberculosis
	Late sequelae of tuberculosis such as fibrotic lesions, calcifications, scars

If all the organs of people with weakened immune systems (HIV patients, alcoholics, etc.), infants, and toddlers cannot isolate the tuberculosis infection to the point of infection, there is a disseminated seeding of pathogens with formation of tubercles in all organs (**miliary tuberculosis**, early form), most frequently in the lungs, meninges, liver, spleen, kidneys, adrenal glands, and choroid. Next to tuberculous meningitis, this is the form of tuberculosis with the most severe course and has a high lethality. The affected organs are shot through with multiple millet-seed like (milium = millet seed) granulomas. The symptoms resemble sepsis. **Tuberculous meningitis** (early form) is the most feared extrapulmonary manifestation of tuberculosis. It begins gradually with uncharacteristic symptoms, such as headache, tiredness, personality change, loss of energy, and fever. After a few days or weeks, symptoms resembling meningoencephalitis set in (seizures, paralysis, consciousness impairment, and even coma). In infants and toddlers, the course is foudroyant. The meningeal inflammation affects especially the brainstem. It is associated with a gelatinous, fibrous exudate that eventually surrounds cerebral nerves and arteries.

Abdominal tuberculosis (early form) develops through dissemination in the blood or the swallowing of infectious material. It is most often localized in the jejunum, ileum, the ileocecal region, and the appendix. The symptoms are abdominal pain, diarrhea, and weight loss. Lymph node enlargement can lead to obstructions. **Peritonitis tuberculosa** is another complication (migratory peritonitis).

Examples of late forms of postprimary tuberculosis are **Lymph node tuberculosis** (slow enlargement of cervical and submandibular lymph nodes with little clinical impairment of the overall condition), **tuberculous pleuritis** (penetration of subpleural tuberculous foci into the pleural space, causing unilateral exudative pleuritis, fever, chest pain, shortness of breath), **urogenital tuberculosis** (rare in children, usually not detectable clinically; untreated, it leads to pyelonephritis, renal failure, epididymitis or adnexitis, and thus to sterility), **bone tuberculosis** (usually in older patients, especially affects thoracic spine), and **joint tuberculosis** (swelling, pain, limited movement in large joints, also in small joints in children).

Diagnostics: In addition to a detailed **medical history**, which should concern itself especially with such risk factors as contact with persons infected with tuberculosis or persons with chronic cough, members of risk groups (e.g., asylum seekers, after a stay abroad, recent infections), a thorough physical examination is also important. **Laboratory tests** only show unspecific changes such as a slight elevation of the inflammation parameters (sedimentation rate, CRP, leukocytes), lymphopenia, or anemia.

If there is a suspicion of a tuberculosis infection, a **tuberculin skin test** is indicated. The method of choice is the Mendel–Mantoux intracutaneous test. Widely used tests such as the tine test are no longer recommended because of their low sensitivity and specificity. The tuberculin skin test checks whether the organism has dealt immunologically with mycobacteria (late type immune reaction). The immune reaction can be confirmed by a local injection of a highly purified *M. tuberculosis* extract (TPPD = tuberculin purified protein derivative). The test becomes positive 6 to 12 weeks after a primary infection (*caution:* diagnostic window). Usually, a standard dose of 10 units (= 0.1 mL injection solution) is injected into the inner side of a lower arm, strictly intracutaneously (see Fig.). In suspicion of active tuberculosis, an initial test dose of only 1 unit (see answer to question 72.2) is used, in order to avoid overshoot of the immune response. The injection is performed with a tuberculin syringe and a fine, short, beveled needle. The opening must point upward.

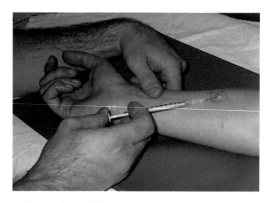

Application of a Mendel–Mantoux test

→ Cases 72 Page 73

The injection must cause a white welt that disappears spontaneously in a few minutes. Seventy-two hours (late type reaction) after the injection, the result (diameter of the papule in mm) can be read. The test is considered positive if the diameter of the **palpable induration is more than 5 mm**. Redness alone has no diagnostic value. If the reaction is positive, the epidemiological situation (tuberculosis incidence in the region, contact with or membership in a risk population) must be considered. If the induration is greater than 10 mm, it must be assumed that a tuberculosis infection is present. *Caution:* Even though an infection is found, the test **result can be a false negative** (anergia), e.g., after live vaccine inoculations, virus infections (especially measles), with congenital/acquired immune deficiencies, malignancies, miliary tuberculosis, meningitis tuberculosa. On the other hand, false-positive results are possible in cases of infection with non-tuberculous mycobacteria or because of a BCG vaccination. A significant change in the diameter of the induration compared to an earlier test (increase > 9 mm) is called a tuberculin conversion. This indicates an interim infection with mycobacteria. A first positive test result is indication for a **thoracic radiograph** in two planes to rule out or confirm a pulmonary manifestation. A primary focus will appear as a soft infiltrate. If the primary focus heals, only enlarged, calcified hilar lymph nodes will be seen radiologically.

In suspicion of tuberculous meningitis, the **spinal fluid** must be examined (see Tab. Spinal fluid findings in meningitis tuberculosa). In evidence of urogenital tuberculosis, the urine must be examined (sterile pyuria, asymptomatic hematuria).

The diagnosis is confirmed by detection of mycobacteria. This can be done by microscopic examination with Ziehl–Neelsen or auramine staining. *Caution:* This can only prove the presence of acid-fast bacilli; whether they are really tubercle bacilli must be determined by further testing (culture, PCR). If acid-fast bacilli are found microscopically, suspicion of a probably contagious tuberculosis must be established, and appropriate measures (isolation of the patient, tuberculostatic therapy) must be initiated. Proof by culture takes a very long time, 4 to 6 weeks, because of the slow division rate of tuberculosis bacteria. However, this proof is absolutely required for confirmation of diagnosis and determination of resistance. A rapid proof of *M. tuberculosis* is possible with PCR. Usually sputum, gastric juice, or puncture material in an extrapulmonary form is used to prove the presence of bacteria. Detection of germs from gastric juice only succeeds in 40% to 50% of cases. To increase the likelihood of verification,

especially in young patients who are not yet able to produce sputum, on three successive mornings on an empty stomach, gastric juice is obtained with a stomach tube (instill 20–50 mL distilled water and aspirate into a sterile syringe).

It is particularly important to find the source of infection by active search for cases (see prophylaxis) among contact persons. This can prevent further dissemination of the disease.

Spinal fluid findings in meningitis tuberculosa	
Microscopy	Pleocytosis (20–500 cells/µL), especially lymphocytes
Appearance and color	clear to xanthochrome, spider web clotting (only arises after long standing and falls apart when it is moved)
Spinal fluid sugar	↓ (< 40 mg/dL)
Albumen	↑ (> 400 mg/dL)
Bacteriology	Low bacterial count, Ziehl–Neelsen stain not sensitive, proof through culture, PCR

Differential diagnoses: Heart defect, gastroesophageal reflux with relapsing pneumonia, foreign body aspiration, cystic fibrosis.

Treatment: Rapid discovery of ill and infectious persons and rapidly initiated, efficacious combination therapy with different tuberculostatics is decisive for effective tuberculosis control. Selection of medications is determined by the antibiogram. First-line antitubercular drugs are isoniazid (INH), rifampicin (RMP), pyrazinamide (PZA), ethambutol (EMB), and streptomycin (SM); second-line drugs (reserve medications in case of resistance or incompatibility) are prothionamide (PTH), *para*-aminosalicylic acid (PAS), terizidone, amikacin, capreomycin (CM), or ciprofloxacin. The treatment always lasts several months, as determined by the degree of severity and course of the tuberculosis (see Tab. Drug treatment of tuberculosis). Patients with sensitive strains are usually no longer infectious after 2 to 3 weeks of treatment.

The side-effect rate of tuberculostatic therapy is very low in children. UNH and RMP can lead to a transient elevation of transaminases. PZA leads to a transient elevation of uric acid that can make therapy with allopurinol necessary. Because of the possibility of (reversible) vision disorders (neuritis of the optic nerve, early symptom impaired color vision), children who receive ethambutol must be regularly examined by an ophthalmologist. Streptomycin is ototoxic, and therefore hearing must be tested before, during, and after therapy.

235

Case

72

→ Cases 72 Page 73

Tuberculosis stage	Recommended treatment	Duration of treatment
Exposure to tuberculosis (e.g., contact with an infectious person)	INH	3 months
Latent tuberculosis infection, i.e., tuberculin conversion without clinical or radiological signs	INH	9 months
Uncomplicated pulmonary tuberculosis	INH + RMP + PZA	2 months
	INH + RMP	4 months
Complicated primary tuberculosis (e.g., with lymph node penetration and/or ventilation disorder through bronchial lymph node compression)	INH + RMP + PZA	2 months
	INH + RPM	7 months
Severe forms such as miliary tuberculosis and meningitis tuberculosa	INH + RMP + PZA + SM	2 months
	INH + RMP	10 months
	+ prednisolone (initial)	6 weeks

Prognosis: With consistent and prompt treatment, tuberculosis can be cured. Tuberculous meningitis can only heal with early diagnosis and initiation of optimal therapy; untreated, it usually leads to death. In many cases, defects are healed with paralysis, seizures, cognitive defects, and hydrocephalus.

Prophylaxis: BCG inoculation is not generally recommended for use in the United States because of the low risk of infection with *Mycobacterium tuberculosis*, the variable effectiveness of the vaccine against adult pulmonary TB, and the vaccine's potential interference with tuberculin skin test reactivity. Instead, targeted tuberculin testing (active search for cases), especially in children with tuberculosis contact or membership in a risk group, in order to be able to diagnose a primary infection as early as possible and treat it. Widespread annual testing and radiographic monitoring are also no longer recommended because the resources involved and the radiation load are greater than the benefit (only a small number of cases detected). Permission to visit community facilities is only granted after three negative sputum or gastric juice samples, collected on different days, visible clinical improvement (symptom-free interval must be at least 2 weeks long), after generally accepted treatment, and radiologically confirmed improvement. A doctor's certificate is required.

Mandatory reporting: The active disease, requiring treatment, and death due to tuberculosis must be reported.

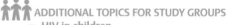 ADDITIONAL TOPICS FOR STUDY GROUPS
- HIV in children
- Immune deficiency syndrome

73.1 What do you ask the patient?

- **Onset of symptoms:** Original onset, situation-specific connection, time of day (only in the daytime or at night as well), stress-dependent (during school/leisure time, physical activity), related to meals/defecation/urination
- **Pain intensity** (possibly using pain scale, see Fig.), type of pain (dull, sharp, penetrating, colic-like, persistent), pain duration (minutes, hours, days)
- **Location of the pains:** Where, alternating, radiation
- **Accompanying symptoms:** Vomiting and diarrhea (quality of the vomitus/stool), lack of appetite, lassitude, reduced capacity for stress, decreased performance, lack of weight gain/weight loss

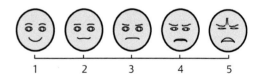

Pain scale for young children

- **Previous illnesses:** Acute diseases requiring treatment, urinary tract infection, abdominal surgery, anemia, hypothyroidism, joint diseases, seizures, diabetes mellitus, cholelithiasis

- **Use of medications:** For example, antibiotics, iron preparations, non-steroidal antirheumatic agents, antiepileptic agents
- **Diet:** Meals, foods (fruit, vegetables, sweets [see Comments]), beverages, amount of liquid consumed
- **Stool history:** Regular/irregular, consistency, color, odor, blood deposits
- **Urination:** Dysuria, pollakisuria, urine color, abnormal odor
- **Gynecological medical history:** Menarche, menstruation disorders, dysmenorrhea
- **Social history:** Psychosocial stress factors, e.g., parents' divorce, school problems, severe illness or death in the family/among friends
- **Family history:** Especially "familial abdominal pain stress," chronic inflammatory intestinal disease, functional disorders (e.g., irritable colon [irritable bowel syndrome], migraine, hypochondria), depression, other diseases (e.g., acute gastrointestinal infections, *Helicobacter pylori* gastritis, ulcers, diabetes mellitus, cholelithiasis, lipid metabolism disorder)

73.2 What do you look for in the physical examination?
- **Evaluation of the general and nutritional condition:** Somatogram/percentile, BMI (age-appropriate body development, over-/underweight)
- **Patient's posture:** Impairment by pain, depressive/suffering posture
- **Physical examination:**
  - Skin color: Yellow, pale, sallow
  - ENT area: Inspection of mucosa, tongue, tonsils, eardrums
  - Lymph nodes: Enlarged, painful
  - Heart: Heart sounds/ -murmurs/-frequency
  - Lungs: Tachypnea, dyspnea, crackles, bronchial obstruction
  - **Abdomen:** Inspection (bloated, concave), auscultation (peristalsis), palpation (pain on pressure, defensive tension, pain on percussion, resistances, organ enlargement, renal bed painful on percussion)
  - **Rectal examination:** Inspection of the anus (eczema, mucosal changes, fistular tracts) and always, rectal-digital examination (width of ampulla, sphincter tonus, stool/blood on the finger stall)
  - Genitals: Stages of puberty (age-appropriate body development)
  - Inguinal region: Inguinal hernia
  - Skin and skin adnexa: Skin color/surface, hematomas, efflorescences, blood supply; hair (shaggy/shiny); nails (changes in nails, hippocratic nails)
  - Measurement of blood pressure, pulse, and temperature (e.g., axillorectal temperature difference in appendicitis)

73.3 What are the possible causes of the patient's complaints?
For chronic abdominal pain (Def.: abdominal pain more than one time per week over a period of at least 2 months), there are:
- **Functional causes:** About 75% of the relapsing abdominal pains do not have a primary organic cause; they often occur in ambitious, sensitive children in stress situations in the form of navel colic, irritable colon, chronic gastritis, chronic constipation, spastic colon
- **Organic causes:**
  - **Abdominal:** For example, relapsing enteritides, urinary tract infections, relapsing incarceration of hernias, postenteritis syndrome, food intolerance, carbohydrate malabsorption (e.g., lactose intolerance), dysmenorrhea, ovarian cysts, ovarian torsion, chronic inflammatory intestinal diseases (Crohn's disease, ulcerative colitis), Meulengracht disease, gastritis, chole-/urolithiasis, relapsing pancreatitis, inflammatory diseases of the internal genitals
  - **Extra-abdominal:** For example, transmitted pain in involvement of the diaphragmatic pleura and heart, radiating pain from the spine

73.4 What further tests do you consider necessary "basic tests" to differentiate between the causes of the complaints?
- **Laboratory:**
  - Blood/serum: (Differential-) blood picture (Hb, leukocytes, platelets), inflammatory parameters (CRP, sedimentation rate), electrolytes (Na, K), blood sugar, blood gas analysis, liver enzymes (γ-GT, GOT, GPT, LDH, aP), total bilirubin, pancreatic enzymes (lipase, amylase), renal retention values (creatinine, urea)
  - Urine: Albumen, leukocytes, erythrocytes, nitrite, glucose, possibly bacteriology
  - Stool: Pathogen diagnosis (among others Giardia, worm eggs)
  - Abdominal ultrasound: Concrements, invagination, abnormal intestinal dystopia, abnormalities of intestinal wall, free fluid, meteorism, constipation, organ enlargement, lymphoma, urinary retention, gynecological ultrasound (ovaries, uterine size)

73.5 This time, you can again not find an organic cause for the complaints. What recommendations do you give the patient now?
- Conversation to explain that the symptoms are not dangerous
- Nutritional advice: Healthy, varied diet with plentiful fruit and vegetables, plentiful fluid
- Usefulness of keeping a record of abdominal pains
- Stress reduction
- Physical activity, recreational sport
- If necessary, care by a child psychologist

237

Case

73

General: Abdominal pain is a **frequent symptom** in children of all ages (incidence 15%–20%). The cause is not necessarily located in the stomach. The younger the child, the less specific the information they can give about the type, duration, and especially location of the pain. Small children will locate even ear and throat pain in the abdominal region. A thorough and complete physical examination of the patient is therefore obligatory.

Acute abdominal pain (etiology, clinical aspects, treatment): It is characterized by a sudden onset without prior complaint of abdominal pain and must always be taken seriously. A quick decision must be made as to whether this is an **acute abdomen**, which requires immediate, often surgical, treatment: Abdominal pain and defensive tension are usually within a circumscribed location, persistent, and intense and are often accompanied by nausea and vomiting. Often the symptoms are progressive. The causes of the acute pain are abdominal (gastrointestinal, urogenital, gynecological [see Tab.]) and extra-abdominal (symptoms associated with respiratory pathway disease, see case 53, general diseases [e.g., diabetes mellitus see case 54, blood and blood vessel diseases such as purpura Schoenlein–Henoch see case 8, hemolytic crises, e.g., in sickle cell anemia]).

The **diagnostics must be carried out swiftly**. In addition to laboratory parameters (inflammatory values, lipase, amylase, GOT, GPT, urinalysis), abdominal sonography is performed (e.g., free fluid as evidence of an acute inflammatory event, perforated appendicitis, intra-abdominal bleeding after abdominal trauma; urinary retention with kidney stone, evidence of pyelonephritis, invagination, volvulus). In addition, an overview of the abdomen (ileus, free air) and the thorax (pneumonia with abdominal involvement) can be necessary in order to explain the cause of the acute abdomen. A surgeon and, for girls, a gynecologist should be called in early so that the appropriate treatment can be initiated.

The **treatment** of acute abdominal pain is determined by the cause. It is useful to admit the patient for monitoring and to order fasting at first, and to initiate infusion therapy (Ringer solution or glucose electrolyte mixture) until the cause of the symptoms becomes clear. An enema can also be helpful to stimulate intestinal peristalsis and eliminate possibly existing constipation. *Caution:* If there are signs of peritoneal inflammation, suspicion of

appendicitis or mechanical ileus, an enema is contraindicated (danger of perforation).

Chronic abdominal pain (etiology, clinical aspects, treatment): **Chronic abdominal pain** exists when the symptoms occur more than one time per week over a period of at least two months. Diagnosis is difficult because of the many possible differential diagnoses (see answer to question 73.3). In chronic abdominal pain, it is important first to distinguish between organically caused abdominal pain and function abdominal pain.

Organic causes of chronic abdominal pain are suggested by reduced overall condition, weight loss, growth retardation, paleness, persistent fever, vomiting, blood in the stool, persistent diarrhea, abdominal pain and defensive tension, locally circumscribed but distant from the navel, as well as nighttime awakening because of the abdominal pain. For possible causes, see answer to question 73.3. The most important will be discussed below in greater detail.

Carbohydrate malabsorption includes lactose intolerance, fructose and sorbitol malabsorption. In lactose intolerance, a distinction is made between the rare, congenital absolute lack of lactase and hypolactasia. In hypolactasia, for reasons that are not yet understood, the activity of lactase in the intestinal mucosa is reduced. Consuming large quantities of milk products and lactose-containing foods (many instant and ready-made products such as baked goods and sausage contain lactose) leads to diarrhea with stomach cramps. Approximately 30% of adults suffer from symptoms of hypolactasia. In **fructose malabsorption**, the consumption of fruit, fruit juice, and sweets that are rich in fructose leads to abdominal pain and diarrhea. The cause is not known. The diagnosis is confirmed by a pathological H_2 breath test after administration of the relevant carbohydrate. Treatment of both disorders is based on reduced consumption of the carbohydrate in question. Complete abstinence is usually unnecessary because residual activity of the enzyme is still present. In lactose intolerance, the enzyme lactase can be added to milk products, which improves tolerance. In fructose malabsorption, fruits with high glucose and low fructose content (e.g., bananas) are usually well tolerated. The presence of glucose facilitates the diffusion of fructose through the intestinal mucosa. For this reason, fruit in the form of fruit salad is usually tolerated.

The most frequent abdominal causes of acute abdominal pain

Newborns	Infants and toddlers	Older children and youths
• Malformations of the gastrointestinal tract	• "Three-month colic"	• Gastroenteritis
• Volvulus	• Gastroenteritis	• Acute appendicitis (Case 50)
• Meconium ileus	• Invagination (Case 5)	• Constipation (Case 56)
• Necrotizing enterocolitis (Case 55)	• Constipation (Case 56)	• Urinary tract infection (Case 44)
• Incarcerated inguinal hernia (Case 58)	• Hirschsprung disease	• Chole-/urolithiasis
	• Incarcerated inguinal hernia (Case 58)	• Gynecological diseases (e.g., ovarian cysts with twisted stems)
	• Scrotal torsion (Case 17)	

In **postenteritis syndrome** (Syn.: Postenteritis malabsorption syndrome) a previous enteritis or prolonged diet in gastrointestinal infection led to mucosal damage, and as a result, overall enzyme activity was decreased. Pre- (e.g., oligosaccharides) and probiotics (e.g., *Lactobacilli, Bifidobacteria*) are used to normalize the intestinal flora and milk products are reintroduced. Soured milk in yogurt, buttermilk, etc. are best tolerated. (Allergic) food intolerances such as cow's milk protein intolerance or celiac disease (see case 19) can also lead to chronic abdominal pain. Diagnostics include serological examination, elimination test on the food in question and, if necessary, biopsy and histology of the changed intestinal mucosa. The treatment consists of a special diet that in cow's milk protein intolerance is maintained for a specific time period and in celiac disease must be maintained for a lifetime.

Peptic gastrointestinal diseases and ***Helicobacter pylori* infections** are characterized by epigastric pain, bloody vomitus or evidence of blood in the stool, awakening during the night because of abdominal pain, and pain with an empty stomach or pain during eating. The diagnosis is confirmed with an esophagogastroduodenoscopy with biopsies for histological examination and a urease quick test (*Helicobacter pylori* confirmation). In case of confirmed, symptomatic *Helicobacter pylori* infection, eradication therapy (triple therapy for 7 days: proton pump inhibitor [omeprazole + clarithromycin [Klacid] or metronidazole [Klont] + amoxicillin]) should be administered. Ulcers or evidence of *Helicobacter pylori* are treated with H$_2$ antagonists (e.g., ranitidin) or proton pump inhibitor (e.g., omeprazole).

If the abdominal pain is colic-like, gallstones or kidney stones must be ruled out. This is best done sonographically. If stones are found, drug, surgical, or lithotriptic treatment must be initiated. If the pains occur after meals or especially after high-fat meals and if they radiate into the back or along the belt line, the possibility of chronic or relapsing pancreatitis must be considered. The cause of this could be cystic fibrosis, deformities (pancreas anulare/divisum), autoimmune processes (lupus erythematosus, sarcoidosis). Evidence is provided by laboratory tests (amylase, lipase, trypsin) and upper abdominal ultrasound. Treatment consists of pancreatic enzyme replacement, pain therapy if necessary, and avoidance of flatulent foods.

In case of chronic diarrhea with bloody stools, chronic inflammatory intestinal diseases such as Crohn's disease and ulcerative colitis must be considered. The diagnosis is established histologically, which requires endoscopy with biopsies. Drug treatment (e.g., with glucocorticoids, 5-aminosalicylic acid, azathioprine) and often also surgical treatment (in case of fistulas, abscesses, fissures, perforation, stenosis) are required. In addition, among others, diseases such as epilepsy (abdominal epilepsy), migraine (abdominal migraine), Meulengracht disease (intermittent icterus and abdominal pain after a period of hunger and stress), and urine transport disorders can cause chronic abdominal pain.

Functional abdominal pain includes irritable bowel syndrome or navel colic. Irritable bowel syndrome is defined as relapsing abdominal pain that improves after defecation. Often the symptoms are accompanied by irregular bowel movements (with regard to frequency and consistency as well as excretion of mucus and gas formation). Typically the symptoms only occur during the day, periumbilically. Sometimes constipation is the chief symptom.

In children between the ages of 8 months and 5 years, unspecific, chronic diarrhea (large amounts of malodorous, watery and slimy diarrhea, often undigested) is observed, without a failure to thrive. This is also called "toddlers' diarrhea" or "peas and carrots syndrome."

The diagnosis of functional gastrointestinal disorders is a diagnosis by exclusion. In addition to the thorough physical examination, medical history, and basic diagnosis (see answers to questions 73.1, 73.2, and 73.4), it is particularly important to listen to the patient carefully. Often there is evidence of psychological stress factors in the school or family environment. The children and youth coming to the doctor are usually particularly sensitive and fearful, while the parents are often over-anxious. Young people in the process of puberty tend to be

239

Case

73

→ Cases 73 Page 74

markedly self-involved. Self-observation and anxiety are of major importance and can, among other things, cause "abdominal pain" (see case 78).

The most important **therapeutic approach to functional abdominal pain** is attentive listening and taking the individual complaints seriously. Emphasizing the fact that the symptoms are not dangerous can already soften them. Changing the diet to healthy, varied foods, drinking in sufficient quantity, and changing the life style (stress reduction, recreational sports, autogenic training) also help. A hot water bottle and herbal tea sometimes work wonders. It can also be useful to keep a record of abdominal pain episodes, including their frequency and the circumstances under which they occurred. Drug treatment is possible with spasmolytics (butylscopolamine 0.3–0.6 mg/kg body weight), prokinetics (metoclopramide 0.1 mg/kg body weight), and also placebo. The support of a child and adolescent psychologist can be helpful.

General abdominal pain diagnostics: The diagnostic procedure for abdominal pain begins with a thorough medical history that should include not only the current complaints but also the earlier medical history and family history (see answer to question 73.1). While taking the history, observe the patient and the level of their stress, and the interaction with their parents. This is followed by a complete physical examination (see answer to question 73.2). In palpating the abdomen, the examiner must somehow cleverly distract the patient (e.g., have them tell a story about kindergarten, school, favorite activity, while carefully palpating the abdomen with warm hands) in order to evaluate the abdominal pain correctly when pressure is applied. The examination is completed by a basic diagnosis (see answer to

question 73.4). The findings and clinical suspicion must be complemented with:

- **Special laboratory diagnostics:** For example, gliadin and endomysium antibodies and antibodies against transglutaminase (*Caution:* Rule out a lack of IgA, otherwise the antibody test will give a false negative) (celiac disease), IgE-RAST (food allergy), iron, ferritin (iron absorption disorder, anemia diagnostics)
- **Breathing tests:** H_2 breathing tests (for carbohydrate malabsorption see above) with lactose, saccharose, fructose, glucose, sorbitol; C_{13} urea breathing test (therapy monitoring after *Helicobacter pylori* eradication therapy)
- **Endoscopy with biopsies for histological or microbiological examination:** Esophagogastroduodenoscopy (esophagitis, ulcers, gastritis, celiac disease [with biopsy of small intestine mucosa]), colonoscopy (chronic inflammatory intestinal disease, polyps)
- **pH measurement:** Gastroesophageal reflux
- **X-ray:** Abdominal survey radiography (free air [perforation of a hollow organ], ileus, shadow-producing concrements [gall-/kidney stones], atypical air distribution pattern [e.g., massive over-bloating]); thoracic radiograph (pneumonia)
- **Colon contrast enema or small intestine contrast imaging (Sellink):** Fistulas, stenoses in chronic inflammatory intestinal diseases
- **Sweat test:** Cystic fibrosis

ADDITIONAL TOPICS FOR STUDY GROUPS
- Additional symptoms in gastrointestinal diseases (e.g., nausea, vomiting, urge to vomit, diarrhea, constipation) and their etiology, diagnostics, and treatment
- Gastroenteritis
- Appendicitis

---

74   Overweight and obesity

74.1 **Describe what you observe in the appearance of the 15-year-old boy (see Fig.).**
Gynecomasty, marked fat deposits, hypogenitalism, genu valgum

74.2 **What do you find particularly interesting in the medical history?**
- **Patient's history:** How long has the patient been obese, prior illnesses, sleep behavior, physical impairments, medications, nutritional history (see below), leisure activities (see below), performance in school, social environment, physical development to the present (patient's health screening documentation with body dimensions/percentiles; birth weight

and physical development in the first years of the child's life), in addition, for girls, menarche and menses (duration, frequency), stress (e.g., teasing, fear of gym class, or leisure activities with friends)
- **Nutritional history:** Number and type of meals, sweets and snacks (which ones, how many, how often), beverages (which ones, how many)
- **Leisure behavior:** Favorite activities, physical activity (sports), endurance, TV watching/video games, smartphone, etc.
- **Family history:** Risk factors (arterial hypertension, diabetes mellitus, fat metabolism disorders, gout, cholecystolithiasis), height/weight of parents/siblings

- **Social history:** Family structure (e.g., parents divorced, single parent, employed, siblings), friends, neglect, patient's relationship to parents/siblings, what school does the patient go to (favorite subject), friends (size, bonding)

74.3 Calculate the BMI (Body Mass Index). How do you evaluate the result (see Appendix BMI tables)?
- BMI = (body weight [kg]/height [m])2 = 94 kg/(1.80 m)^2 = 29 kg/m^2
- Evaluation: Thus the BMI > 97% over the age and sex normal value; this represents obesity

74.4 What do you particularly look for in the physical examination? What further tests would you consider useful?
- **Physical examination:**
  - Fat distribution pattern (abdominal obesity), morphological abnormalities such as short fingers and toes, high palate, polydactyly, to rule out syndromal diseases (e.g., Prader–Willi syndrome, Klinefelter syndrome)
  - Determination of puberty stages according to Tanner (see case 68)
  - Screening for diseases associated with obesity: arterial hypertension (24-hour blood pressure measurement), orthopedic examination (poor posture, excessive stress on joints, spinal diseases)
  - Skin: Striae, acne, skin infections (skin folds), acanthosis nigrans (in type II diabetes mellitus), hair growth, pseudogynecomastia (enlargement of the male breast without participation of the glandular tissue, frequently by lipid deposits in overweight)
- **Laboratory:**
  - Triglycerides, cholesterol, lipoproteins (VLDL, LDL, HDL): Lipid metabolism disorder

- Blood sugar/oral glucose tolerance test: Diabetes mellitus, pathological glucose tolerance
- Uric acid: Hyperuricemia (gout)
- Thyroid gland values (TSH, fT3 fT4): Hypothyroidism
- **Further tests if necessary:** Abdominal sonography especially in case of abdominal pain (to rule out cholelithiasis, fatty liver), 24-hour blood pressure measurement, determination of bone age (radiograph: Left hand and wrist; accelerated e.g., in nutritional obesity, decreased in syndromal diseases), hormonal analysis (e.g., cortisone in suspected Cushing syndrome), chromosomal analysis (e.g., to rule out Prader–Willi–Labhardt syndrome, Down syndrome) with morphological evidence

74.5 What is the most probable cause for the fact that puberty has not yet begun?
The cause of apparently delayed puberty is probably the obesity; growth is increased, resulting in adiposogenital pubertal obesity with apparent hypogenitalism; onset of puberty in males is somewhat delayed due to decreased secretion of gonadotropin.

74.6 What advice do you give the patient and his parents? What are the possibilities for planning therapy in the most efficacious way?
- Reassurance about lacking signs of puberty and explanation that the reason is probably obesity
- Recommendation: **Weight loss** because of the risk of sequelae (see Comments) and psychological stress (teasing by schoolmates)
  - Reducing energy intake by changing the diet and increasing energy consumption through exercise
  - Best chance of success: Joining an outpatient obesity therapy group and participation of the family in the patient's treatment

Comments

Definition: Overweight and obesity are characterized by **increased body fat**. For adults, overweight can be quantified by calculating the body mass index (BMI):

$$BMI\ [kg/m^2] = \frac{Body\ mass\ [kg]}{Body\ height\ [m]^2}$$

In children and adolescents the absolute value of the BMI is not a sufficient parameter because of its physiological age and sex-dependent variability. For this reason, the relative BMI (related to the age- and sex-specific 50th percentile) is used. Children whose relative BMI is between the 90th and 97th percentile are classified as "overweight"; if the value is above the 97th percentile, they are considered to be obese.

Epidemiology: The prevalence of overweight and obesity in children and adolescents has increased significantly in the past 20 years. According to the Centers for Disease Control and Prevention, childhood obesity has more than doubled in children and quadrupled in adolescents in the past 30 years. In 2012, more than one-third of children and adolescents were overweight or obese. The cause of the rapid increase in prevalence is not absolutely clear, but an important factor is surely the increasing lack of exercise among children.

Etiopathogenesis: Overweight occurs when over a long period, more energy is taken in than consumed. Energy consumption is determined by basal metabolism, thermogenesis, and activity. The unused energy is stored in the form of fat tissue.

A distinction is made between the much more frequent multifactorially determined **primary obesity** and the very rare **secondary obesity** that is the result or a symptom of other diseases (see below). In many children and their families, diet and eating behavior have changed: the choice of tasty but calorie-rich foods is large. Fast foods and ready-made products are regularly found on the menu of many families. Increasing inactivity of children and adolescents as a result of long hours of TV and computer games, as well as increasing motorization are another important factor. Examination of families and research with twins also document a genetic component in the cause of obesity: the basal metabolism of children with obese parents is approximately 20% below that of children with the same weight and normal-weight parents. Predisposing factors can already be found during pregnancy and the nursing period. Children of diabetic and obese mothers have an increased birth weight and an elevated risk of becoming obese themselves. Even low-birth weight babies, who quickly catch up in weight, are later more often overweight than other children. Infants who were breastfed are significantly less often obese, depending on how long they were breastfed, than children who were not. Other factors are eating disorders of the mother, such as anorexia or bulimia nervosa and the psychosocial environment. Children with little challenge or support have a higher risk of obesity and there is a negative correlation between the parents' level of education and children's overweight. Obesity is seldom a symptom or consequence of another disease (secondary obesity). This includes syndromally caused obesity (e.g., Prader–Willi–Labhardt syndrome, Laurence–Moon–Bardet–Biedl syndrome), endocrinological (e.g., Cushing's disease, growth hormone deficiency, hypothyroidism), as a result of CNS diseases (e.g., craniopharyngioma, radiation sequelae), and pharmacological (e.g., steroids, thyreostatics, valproic acid). Very rarely there are genetic causes such as leptin deficiency or a mutation of the melanocortin receptor.

Clinical aspects: In addition to overweight and excessive fat deposits, patients are usually noticeable for their above-average height (obesity gigantism). Boys often exhibit (see example case) pseudogynecomastia ("pseudo" because it is not caused by glandular tissue but by fat deposits). The fat deposits give the false impression of hypogenitalism. The start of puberty can be late in boys and early in girls. Moreover, girls have a tendency to hirsutism.

Usually there are striae distensae in the upper arms, chest, thighs, abdomen, and hips. Often, there are skin infections, especially in skin folds.

Complications: It has become well known that overweight and obesity **are serious risk factors** for **cardiovascular diseases** in old age. But it is only now being understood that they are also a disease in themselves. It is more difficult for pediatrics to accept this disease because most of its effects are only seen in adults. In contrast to adults with years of obesity, children and adolescents generally only exhibit discrete symptoms and findings of obesity-related diseases such as metabolic syndrome with hypertension, dyslipoproteinemia, impaired glucose tolerance and hyperuricemia, cardiovascular diseases with arterial hypertension and atherosclerosis, cholelithiasis and fatty liver, orthopedic diseases with incorrect posture, incorrect positioning, and epiphysiolysis, as well as obstructive sleep apnea syndrome. Psychosocial consequences are low self-esteem, depression, isolation, and eating disorders with increase in obesity.

Diagnostics: It begins with a detailed medical history (see answer to question 74.2) and a thorough physical examination. The parents are asked to leave the room and the examination should, if possible, be conducted by a physician of the same sex, to be respectful of the increased modesty of adolescents. In the examination, particular attention is given to the extent of the obesity; weight and height are determined, recorded in percentiles, and the BMI (see answer to question 74.3) is calculated. The stage of puberty is determined, e.g., by the Tanner criteria (see case 68). In addition, there is screening for evidence (see answer to question 74.4) for associated health disorders (see Complications) such as arterial hypertension (blood pressure measurement) or abnormal posture. Laboratory tests should find causes of underlying disease as well as medical sequelae of the obesity. Elevated resting blood pressure readings make a 24-hour blood pressure study necessary. If there is a suspicion of gallstones, abdominal sonography will provide a confirmation. An oral glucose tolerance test reveals a pathological glucose tolerance or type II diabetes mellitus. Moreover, it is necessary to recognize sighs of a serious underlying psychiatric illness such as depression, bulimia, or craving for food so that, if necessary, a child psychologist or psychiatrist can be called in.

If there are suggestions (e.g., delayed growth, retardation of psychomotor development) of a secondary obesity, further studies are required, such as chromosomal analysis, hormone analyses, or radiography to determine bone age.

Treatment: The objectives of obesity therapy are to reduce energy intake and increase energy consumption. In the long term, this can only be achieved by

→ Cases 74 Page 75

changing the nutritional and exercise habits of the patient and their family (!), ideally through interdisciplinary collaboration with dieticians, behavioral and physical therapists, or sport clubs. Forming therapy groups and educating the family is helpful here. The goal of the therapy is not only weight reduction but particularly also stabilization of the reduced weight. The basis for this is a healthy, balanced, low-fat mixed diet with plentiful fruit and vegetables. None or hypocaloric weight loss diets can indeed promote rapid weight loss but they are not helpful for long-term weight stabilization (yoyo effect). Physical activity should be increased; child-appropriate endurance sports such as bicycle riding and swimming are particularly recommended.

Prognosis: The prognosis is only good over the course of years with consistently maintained therapy. Only 30% of children can be permanently cured. The later the obesity begins, the greater is the probability that the affected person will also be obese as an adult. The severe, chronic sequelae of overweight are extensively known in adult medicine. They are associated with elevated morbidity and mortality. Preventive measures and education are necessary.

🏃🏃🏃 ADDITIONAL TOPICS FOR STUDY GROUPS
- Anorexia nervosa
- Bulimia nervosa
- Prader–Willi syndrome
- Bardet–Biedl syndrome

75 Falling from the changing table (craniocerebral trauma, child abuse)

75.1 What do you look out for during the examination?
- Undress the child completely
- **Screening for external signs of injury:** For example, bruises (also in the hair of the head), palpable steps in the skull cap, hematomas, swollen points, limited range of motion, pain on active/passive joint movement, pain on being touched
- **Physical examination:** Particularly
  - Auscultation of the lungs (breath sounds the same bilaterally): Rule out chest injuries, pneumothorax
  - Abdominal palpation (pain on pressure, defensive tension): Rule out injuries of internal organs
  - Inspection of auditory pathways (otorrhea): Rule out petrous bone fracture
  - Inspection of ear drums (ear drum hematoma): Rule out petrous bone fracture
  - Inspection of nose (rhinorrhea): Rule out fracture of base of skull, spinal fluid fistula
  - Palpation of fontanelles (tension, bulging): Rule out intracerebral bleeding
- **Neurological examination:** Reflex status (intrinsic muscle reflexes, pupillary reaction, polysynaptic reflexes, pyramidal tract sign) tone, spontaneous motor activity, sensory system

75.2 Your examination does not uncover any abnormalities. What do you explain to the parents? What do you recommend?
- **Reassuring the parents:** Falls from the changing table are very frequent; up to now there are no signs of craniocerebral trauma (impairment of consciousness, vegetative symptoms, neurological abnormalities, etc.); Probably this is just a cranial bruise
- **Tips for avoiding accidents:** Change diapers on the floor; do not leave child unwatched

- **Hospital admission:** To monitor vital signs (pulse, breathing, blood pressure, pupillary reaction) for 24 to 48 hours necessary, since there is still always the danger of cerebral hemorrhage and it is difficult to monitor an infant at home

75.3 Is it possible to monitor the child at home? What are the grounds for your decision? What do you have to inform the parents about if they want to monitor the child at home?
- Yes, with sufficient care, monitoring is possible (here, the mother is a nurse) at home because after his fall into the laundry basket the 5-month old infant exhibited neither associated vegetative symptoms nor impairment of consciousness. Presumably, he "only" suffered a bruise to the skull (= blunt head trauma without other symptoms).
- In spite of everything, careful observation of the infant (especially while he is sleeping) is necessary to rule out intracerebral hemorrhage:
  - Vigilance: Increased tiredness, sleepiness, lack of reaction to awakening stimuli when he is sleeping
  - Vegetative symptoms: For example, paleness, vomiting, poor eating and drinking, restlessness
- If the infant exhibits any abnormalities, immediate return to the doctor.

75.4 What is disturbing about this case?
- Unclear course of events in the accident: How, exactly, did the child come to fall?
- Why did the mother only bring the child in hours after the trauma?
- What is the explanation for the bruise at the back of the child's head if he fell on his stomach?
- The red skin on the belly suggests the mark of a hand: Violence?

→ Cases 75 Page 76

- What caused the older hematomas on the buttocks: relapsing effect of violence?
  → Suspicion of child abuse

75.5 **What do you do next?**

- Careful, detailed history, do not mention suspicion of abuse at first
- Meticulous documentation (possibly photograph the injury)
- Thorough physical examination, search for other injuries, e.g., hematomas, scars, fractures, abnormal posture
- Admission of the child for monitoring in case of concussion (clinical: increased tiredness, rapid falling asleep, vomiting), for further diagnostics (see below) to clarify provisional diagnosis of child abuse and possibly take further measures (treatment strategy, parenting counselor, family help, or even placing the child in a home)
- Further diagnostics:
  - Cerebral ultrasound: Indication of cerebral hemorrhage
  - Abdominal ultrasound: Injury to intra-abdominal organs
  - Laboratory: Blood picture (Hb, platelets), clotting
  - Fundoscopy: Retinal bleeding frequent in CNS injuries not caused by accidents
  - If necessary, skeletal X-ray: Fractures

Comments

Craniocerebral trauma: Craniocerebral trauma means functional impairment of the brain caused by external violence. The degree of severity of craniocerebral trauma in infants and children is classified according to the expanded **Glasgow Coma Scale** (according to Ritz) (see Tab.).

Cardinal symptoms of all craniocerebral traumas is **posttraumatic impairment of consciousness**. Retro- and anterograde amnesia, paleness, nausea, vomiting, headaches, or vertigo can also occur. In substantial brain injuries, there are location-related neurological deficits ranging to serious circulatory and respiratory functional impairment in severe craniocerebral trauma. Because of the lacking symptoms (see above), cranial bruising is not considered a craniocerebral trauma in the narrow sense. Diagnosis and Treatment depend on the severity of the craniocerebral trauma (see case 23). Even in cranial bruising and mild craniocerebral trauma,

even a two-stage intracerebral hemorrhage can develop. The danger is greatest during the first 24 to 48 hours. For this reason, careful monitoring of the vital signs for at least 24 to 48 hours after the trauma is recommended. If there is no impairment of consciousness, this monitoring can take place at home after the appropriate urgent description to the parents of the symptoms to watch for in case of complications (see answer to question 75.3). If it is not clear how the accident happened or there was definitely a trauma, the monitoring should in any case take place in the hospital. If the parents refuse to have the child admitted, careful instruction about possible consequences (as drastic as death) in case of inadequate monitoring should be provided to them, and documentation of the informational conversation is also required.

		Points for the finding	
		< 24 months	> 24 months
Verbal answer	5	Fixates, recognizes, follows, laughs	Speaks understandably, completely oriented
	4	Fixates, follows inconsistently, does not recognize with certainty	Confused, disoriented, incoherent speech
	3	Can sometimes be awakened, does not eat or drink	Answers are inadequate, a jumble of words
	2	Motor restlessness, cannot be awakened	Incomprehensible sounds
	1	No response can be triggered to visual, acoustic, or sensory motor stimuli	No verbal utterances
Opening eyes	4	Spontaneous opening of eyes	
	3	Opens eyes when called	
	2	Opens eyes in response to pain stimulus	
	1	Does not open eyes for any stimulus	
Motor response	6	Targeted grasp when commanded, obeys other motor commands promptly	
	5	Targeted defense against pain stimulus	
	4	Untargeted flexion in response to pain stimulus	
	3	Untargeted flexion in response to pain stimulus to arms, extension tendency in legs	
	2	Extension of all four extremities in response to pain stimulus	
	1	No motor response to pain stimulus	
Oculomotor behavior	4	Conjugated eye movements; pupillary light reaction can be triggered	
	3	Doll eye phenomenon with conjugated bulbous movements	
	2	Divergent position of bulbi	
	1	No reaction, pupillary reaction to light extinct	
Evaluation:			
Slight craniocerebral trauma		17–19 points	
Moderate craniocerebral trauma		12–16 points	
Severe craniocerebral trauma		≤ 11 points	

245

Case
75

Child abuse: The second part of the example case seems quite similar to the first. Nevertheless, there are discrepancies that with attentive history taking raise the possibility that the event was not an accident.

If a child is brought to the doctor with an injury, the doctor must ask whether the type of injury can be consistent with the facts presented in the history, be typical for the accident, whether the location of the injury matches with the accident event, and whether there is evidence of numerous traumatic events. Overlooking child abuse can have fatal consequences for the child and possibly for the child's siblings since, usually, abuse is a **repeated crime**.

On the other hand, erroneous accusation of the parents or guardians must by all means be avoided. The following guidelines should sharpen the doctor's discrimination:

- **Abnormal behavior on the part of parents or guardians:** Delay in calling on the doctor; self-contradiction in description of the event; frequent changes of doctor
- **Abnormal behavior on the part of the child:** Failure to laugh; lack of emotional detachment, contact disorder, tolerance of even painful examination without reaction
- **Typical physical findings:** Reduced overall condition, lack of grooming, underweight, small stature
- **Type of injury:** Sharp force (stab wounds, cuts), blunt force (welts, finger marks, signs of grabbing, shaking trauma fractures), heat trauma (burning/scalding, cigarette burns), chemical trauma (especially alcohol, sedatives, acids, and alkali)

Hematomas are frequent in children and must not be given excessive weight. But there are typical distribution patterns that probably point to abuse (see Fig. Distribution patterns of hematomas).

→ Cases 75   Page 76

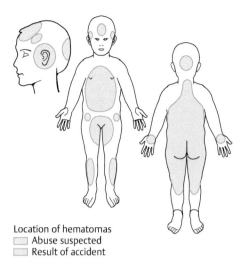

Location of hematomas
☐ Abuse suspected
☐ Result of accident

Typical distribution patterns of hematomas in child abuse and after accidents

Shaking trauma, known as **shaken baby syndrome**, is particularly important for infants. This is the associated occurrence of subdural hematomas, retinal bleeding, and diffuse cerebral injury caused by severe shaking of the infant. Occasionally there are also humerus, rib, or metaphyseal fractures. The head of the child, who is usually grabbed by the thorax or upper arms, rolls back and forth without control (see Fig. Shaking an infant). Shear forces separate the brain from the dura mater that fits closely against the bone. This leads to tears in the bridging veins and a subdural hematoma. The symptoms can be unspecific and resemble sepsis. This form of child abuse is found particularly with screaming babies and over-stressed parents.

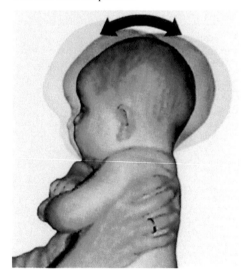

"Shaking" an infant: the head rolls back and forth uncontrollably

→ Cases 75 Page 76

If the suspicion of abuse increases, it is important to **document the injuries** as exactly as possible and even to photograph them. One must always consider and perhaps rule out differential diagnoses such as coagulation disorders or osteopathy.

To recognize additional acute or older injuries, the completely undressed child must be carefully examined. The anogenital area must also be examined to rule out sexual abuse.

Further diagnostics include the growth parameters for an objective inquiry into a possible failure to thrive, that can give important evidence of abuse and neglect. For infants and toddlers, a screening skeletal survey to look for old and new fractures is recommended (strict indication because of radiation load). Another important component of the diagnostics is fundoscopy to rule out retinal bleeding, which exhibits a high correlation with CNS injuries not caused by accidents. Further instrumental diagnostic tests are dictated by the acute symptoms and the child's clinical condition. Necessary laboratory tests in addition to a blood panel include, in particular, the coagulation status and possibly bleeding time. If appropriate, liver and pancreas tests, as well as urinalysis, should be performed to detect possible organ damage.

In addition to the **problems of establishing a diagnosis**—is this an accident or abuse?—there is the question of further procedure. In addition to treatment of acute injuries and their effect, the question of short- and long-term protection of the child is the most important consideration in determining future procedure. The suspicion of abuse must **never** be expressed in the admission interview. Expression of this suspicion would entail the risk that the parents or guardian would take the child away again, thus defeating the possibility of an intervention. Rather, a careful attempt is made to learn as much as possible about the child's situation, the present event, and the family and its social situation. It may even be possible to win the family's trust. It is also useful to collect additional, important information by speaking with the treating pediatrician, surrounding hospitals, kindergarten, or school.

After confirmation of the diagnosis, careful documentation, and exclusion of relevant differential diagnoses, it is time to confront the parents or guardian with the suspicion of abuse and to clarify the situation. The guiding principle should be "Help before Punishment." Inpatient treatment of the child can achieve crisis intervention and defusing of the family situation; this can prevent repetition of the event. The collaboration of pediatrician, psychologist, child protective services, and social workers with the parents is important. Working together, they should establish a treatment strategy. Educational guidance, parenting counseling, family support, or education of the child in a daytime group, supervised living and possibly placement in a care home are possible forms of treatment. Early contact with public institutions such as child protective services or child protective association can provide monitoring possibilities. These public institutions have the right, among other things, to inspect the apartment and to investigate siblings. This also reveals possibilities to change social conditions, e.g., by providing a different apartment, job, etc. If the parents refuse to cooperate or if the abuse has resulted in severe injuries, a report must be made to the investigative authority.

From the legal point of view, **abuse constitutes a bodily injury**. There is no obligation to report, either for the physician or for laymen. The physician is obligated by confidentiality, which prevents him from revealing the information he was entrusted with or the findings he uncovered. At the same time he takes responsibility for the health of the little patient, who cannot protect himself. To avoid danger to the patient's body, life, and freedom, the physician can make a report on the grounds of a "justifying emergency."

ADDITIONAL TOPICS FOR STUDY GROUPS
- Sexual abuse
- Neglect

---

76 Omphalocele and laparoschisis

76.1 What is your diagnosis? What is involved in this deformity?
- **Non-ruptured omphalocele**
- **Definition:** Umbilical cord hernia; hernial sac consists of umbilical cord membrane (amnion) and peritoneum. Contents of the hernia are usually small and large intestine and possibly parts of the liver.

76.2 What steps do you take next? What does the postpartum care of the child require?
- Cover the defect with sterile, warmed, moist (0.9% NaCl) compresses to avoid injury to the hernial sac and infection.
- Attachment of a urine drainage bag because the urine has a caustic effect and can damage the prolapsed organs.
- Pack the child's lower body in a sterile plastic sack to avoid cooling/infection.
- Insertion of a large-lumen gastric tube to prevent bloating of the intestinal loops.
- Starting a peripheral i.v. for volume therapy.
- Intubation and ventilation to avoid filling the intestinal loops with air and causing bloating.
- Antibiotic treatment (e.g., ampicillin + cefotaxim + aminoglycoside) because of the high risk of infection.
- Transfer of the child in a transport incubator (in lateral recumbent position to ensure better circulation to the prolapsed organs) to a pediatric surgery center for operative therapy. Obtain prior written authorization for surgery from the parents and send it with the child or have the parents accompany the transfer.
- Surgical closure of the abdominal wall defect. There may be no correlation between the size of the abdominal cavity and the prolapsed abdominal organs. In that case, a one-step closure with sudden increase of intra-abdominal pressure can lead to

necrosis of liver and intestines. For this reason, the closure is done in two stages—temporary closure with an interposition graft of amniotic membrane, dura, pericardium, or prosthetic material. In the following days, the hernial contents "slide" back into the abdominal cavity, the temporary grafts are made smaller every 2 or 3 days and completely removed after approximately 10 days. The final closure of the abdominal wall is made by suture.
- Introduction of new food is often protracted; long-term parenteral nutrition is often necessary.

! 76.3 This deformity often occurs with a specific syndromal clinical picture. Name and explain this clinical picture.
- **Wiedemann–Beckwith syndrome** (Syn.: EMG syndrome): **E**xomphalos (= omphalocele), **M**acroglossia (= large tongue), **G**igantism (pre- and postnatal excessive growth)
- Additional symptoms/clinical factors: Coarse facial features, hypoplasia of mid-face, notched ears, organ enlargement (liver, kidneys, heart, etc.), hemihypertrophy, hyperinsulinism with hypoglycemia, elevated risk of premature birth (in 30% of cases associated with polyhydramnion)
- Etiology: Usually unclear, rarely a duplication of 11 p15 or uniparental paternal disomy
- Frequency: 1:12,000 to 1:15,000 births
- Prognosis: Normal psychomotor development, elevated risk of neoplasms (e.g., Wilms tumor, adrenal cortex carcinoma, hepatoblastoma)

76.4 List other deformities in the same spectrum.
Laparoschisis (Syn.: Gastroschisis): Abdominal wall defect; median gastroschisis usually to the right of the navel with prolapse of the abdominal organs (stomach, intestines, liver, spleen, internal genitalia, etc.)

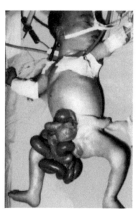

Laparoschisis

Comments

General: Omphalocele and Laparoschisis are congenital abdominal wall defects. Children with abdominal wall defects are mostly born by cesarean section since the diagnosis is usually made prepartally by ultrasound.

Omphalocele: Definition: See answer to question 76.1. It occurs with a frequency of 1:3,000 births. The cause is an embryonic developmental disorder with incomplete regression of the physiological umbilical hernia. In this condition, abdominal organs remain outside the abdominal cavity in a hernial sac that consists of umbilical cord membranes and peritoneum. The size of the omphalocele is very variable (cherry to child's head size). Very small omphaloceles can be overlooked at birth so that when the umbilical cord is tied off, intestinal loops can be injured. In large omphaloceles, the prolapsed organs are easily recognized in the hernial sac. Usually the affected organs are sections of small and large intestine, but part of the liver can also be found in the hernial sac. If the hernial sac already ruptures in the uterus or peripartally, it can be difficult to distinguish this defect from a gastroschisis (see below). There is then a high risk of infection (peritonitis) and intestinal injury. For treatment, see answer to question 76.2. In **50% of cases**, there are **more defects** present, e.g., heart defects, deformities of the urogenital tract, chromosomal disorders (trisomy 13, 18, and 21), Wiedemann–Beckwith

syndrome (see answer to question 76.3). The prognosis for omphalocele is definitely affected by these associated deformities.

Gastroschisis: Definition: See answer to question 76.4. It occurs with a frequency of 1–2:10,000 births.

The etiology is not known to the present day. Because of the abdominal wall defect, the abdominal organs (intestine, stomach, liver, spleen, internal genitalia) prolapse but there is no hernial sac. The umbilical cord inserts normally. Additional malformations are rare. Because of the missing hernial sac, the portions of the intestine that were previously floating in the amniotic fluid are edematous, swollen, and bloated, covered with fibrin and meconium, and frequently stuck to each other. The intestine is often twisted (*Caution:* in that case, immediate untwisting is required). Treatment is similar to the treatment for omphalocele (see answer to question 76.2). The prognosis for gastroschisis is relatively good when there are no associated malformations. There may be intra-abdominal adhesion postoperatively and there is a risk (20% of cases) of developing necrotizing enterocolitis (see case 55).

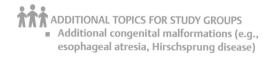

ADDITIONAL TOPICS FOR STUDY GROUPS
- Additional congenital malformations (e.g., esophageal atresia, Hirschsprung disease)

77.1 **Enter the measured values in the percentile curve. Interpret the findings.**

All values lie far below the 10th percentile. This birth is classified as "small for gestational age" (SGA).

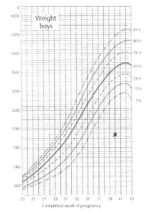
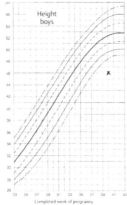
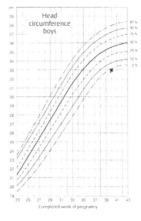

77.2 **What do you ask the mother? What do you look for in the pregnancy log?**

- **Mother's medical history:**
  - Acute diseases (For example, rubella, first herpes infection, "influenza" symptoms) during pregnancy
  - Chronic diseases, For example, diabetes mellitus Type I, arterial hypertension
  - Medications during pregnancy: For example, anti-epileptic agents, anti-hypertensive agents
  - Nicotine/alcohol/drug abuse during pregnancy
  - Course of pregnancy
- **Pregnancy log:** Rubella titer, blood pressure values, intrauterine growth course, course of pregnancy, abnormal ultrasound findings, placental morphology
- If necessary, consultation with the gynecologist overseeing the pregnancy

77.3 **What do you think of that?**

- Every cigarette smoked during pregnancy harms the unborn child. For this reason, there should be no smoking during pregnancy.

- Smoking during pregnancy raises the risk of premature birth, perinatal mortality and morbidity, and causes postpartum withdrawal symptoms in the infant.
- Giving up smoking during pregnancy has no negative effects on the unborn child; there are no withdrawal symptoms.

77.4 **What problems related to nicotine abuse could arise in the child postpartum?**

Symptoms of nicotine withdrawal (For example, shakiness, irritability, difficulty drinking), breathing impairment, hypoglycemia and tendency to hypothermia, polyglobulia, hyperbilirubinemia, intracerebral hemorrhaging.

77.5 **Name the chief connatal infections, their pathogens, and the typical clinical symptoms in newborns.**

Case
77

→ Cases 77 Page 78

Prenatal diseases of the so-called TORCH complex

Disease; Pathogen	Typical symptoms
Toxoplasmosis; Toxoplasma gondii	Hypotrophy; triad encephalitis, chorioretinitis, hepatitis; in a severe course: maculopapulous exanthema, thrombocytopenia, hepatosplenomegaly
Rubella; rubella virus	Rubella embryopathy (Gregg syndrome: hypotrophy, inner ear deafness, heart defect, cataract, microcephaly, etc.), rubella fetopathy (hepatitis, hepatosplenomegaly, thrombocytopenia with purpura, petechiae, extramedullary blood formation, hemolytic anemia, meningoencephalitis)
Cytomegaly (CMV); CMV virus	Hypotrophy, hepatitis, encephalitis with intracerebral calcification, microcephaly, inner ear deafness, eye involvement, thrombocytopenia
Herpes simplex; herpes simplex virus type 1 or 2	Hypotrophy, bullous exanthema, microcephaly, chorioretinitis, microphthalmus
Others (HIV, hepatitis B, measles, parvovirus B19, chicken pox, lues, listeria infection)	

Comments

Small for gestational age (Definition and epidemiology): If weight and length of a newborn are below the 10th percentile determined for the gestational age, the child is classified as Small for Gestational Age (SGA). The overall percentage of children born SGA, as reported by the U.S. National Vital Statistics System for 2005, is 10%.

Classification of growth retardation: Disorders (e.g., chromosomal aberrations, virus infection, nicotine and drug abuse) within the first 16 weeks of pregnancy lead to **symmetrical retardation**. Body weight, body length, and head circumference are equally affected. **Asymmetrical retardation** usually only affects body weight and develops in the last trimester of pregnancy. It is due either to decreased oxygen or nutrient availability to the fetus because of placental insufficiency or the result of the fetus' increased oxygen and nutrient requirement (e.g., in infections), which cannot be met by the normal supply.

Etiology: There are various causes for retardation of intrauterine growth (see Tab. Possible causes of retardation in intrauterine growth). In a good one-third of cases, the cause of the growth retardation remains unclear.

Problems and findings: Children born too small have particular perinatal problems. Perinatal mortality and morbidity is elevated. A decreased maternofetal oxygen supply (placental insufficiency) can lead to fetal acidosis and peripartal asphyxia with postpartal shortness of breath syndrome. Increased peripartal stress increases the risk of intracerebral hemorrhage. Moreover, hypotrophic children tend to hypothermia (lack of subcutaneous fatty tissue) and hypoglycemia (lack of substrate). Sixty percent to 80% of children born too small show signs of catch-up growth—an accelerated rate of growth— in the first 2 years.

Drug and nicotine abuse during pregnancy: Starting within a period from the first 24 hours up to 10 days, the mother's nicotine or drug abuse leads to more or less intense withdrawal symptoms in the newborn. Frequent symptoms are irritability, tremor, shaking, skin scaling (caused by rubbing), elevated muscle tone, short sleep phases, shrill screaming, and excessive sucking. Sometimes poor ability to drink, vomiting, diarrhea, sneezing, tachypnea, and sweating occur. Postpartal breathing disorders can be expected especially if the mother was still using drugs shortly before the birth (heroin, methadone, etc.), which have a respiratory depressant effect. The severity of the withdrawal symptoms can be estimated with the Finnegan score (Neonatal drug withdrawal score with which 20 symptoms, including tremors, screaming, sleep phases, breathing are evaluated).

→ Cases 77 Page 78

Various causes for retardation of intrauterine growth

Maternal causes	Fetal causes	Placental diseases
• Nicotine/alcohol/drug abuse	• Chromosomal disorders	• Placental insufficiency
• Medications (antiepileptic drugs, antihypertonic drugs)	• Multiple pregnancy	• Placental infarct
• Severe underlying diseases (e.g., arterial hypertension, type I Diabetes mellitus severe pulmonary, cardiac, and renal systemic diseases)	• Congenital deformities	
	• Metabolic diseases	
• Severe undernourishment (especially in the last trimester), young age of the mother, low social status	• Prenatal infection with the TORCH complex (see answer to question 77.4)	

Newborns should be monitored in the hospital after drug or nicotine abuse in pregnancy. Pronounced withdrawal symptoms require treatment with medications, e.g., with phenobarbital, chloral hydrate, or tincture of opium.

Prenatal diseases of the TORCH complex Toxoplasmosis:
■ **Toxoplasmosis** is caused by the parasite *Toxoplasma gondii*. The primary host is the cat and the secondary host is human beings. The infection takes place through oral uptake of oocytes from cat feces (smear infection, soil/garden work, insufficiently washed vegetables or fruit) or consumption of undercooked meat containing cysts (e.g., steak, raw ham, salami). The incubation time is 4 to 21 days. Postnatal infection usually has a symptom-free course in immunocompetent people. If the first infection occurs in pregnancy (incidence 0.5%), the parasites reach the fetus via the placenta. The infection risk for the fetus depends on the stage of pregnancy. It rises from about 15% in the first semester to about 70% in the third trimester. The extent of the clinical symptoms correlates with the age of the pregnancy and the degree of parasitemia. The later the fetus is infected, the less severe is the clinical picture. The classical triad of encephalitis (with formation of intracerebral calcifications, hydrocephalus), chorioretinitis, and hepatitis is found in only 3% of infected fetuses. Underweight, hepatomegaly, prolonged icterus, weak suck, or cerebral seizures. The diagnosis is established serologically through the presence of antibodies. Proving the presence of toxoplasma PCR; direct microscopic demonstration of the pathogen is also possible. Diagnostics to confirm congenital toxoplasmosis, in addition to a detailed examination of the entire body status and a thorough neurological examination, also include an examination of the ocular fundus (chorioretinitis), skull ultrasound (intracerebral calcification), and hearing test (decrease of hearing). If abnormalities are found, a lumbar puncture should be performed. The cell count, protein, and glucose are measured, and a toxoplasma PCR confirmation should be attempted. If a fresh infection of the pregnant woman is confirmed, treatment must be initiated immediately, even if this cannot always prevent infection of the child. Up to the 16th week of pregnancy, spiramycin,

then sulfadiazine, pyrimethamine + folic acid for 4 weeks.
■ **Rubella** is transmitted by droplet infection; the pathogen is the rubella virus. The incubation time is 14 to 21 days. A first infection in the first 3 months of pregnancy results in miscarriage, premature birth, and rubella embryopathy. Even infection after the third month of pregnancy can lead to fetal damage (rubella fetopathy). The frequency of damage to embryo or fetus is 1:6,000–10,000 live births. The clinical symptoms of **rubella embryopathy** (Gregg syndrome) is characterized by hearing impairment, heart defects (especially pulmonary artery or pulmonary valve stenosis, open ductus arteriosus Botalli, ventricular septum defect), cataract, microphthalmus, and the typical pepper and salt retinopathy, microcephaly, and hypotrophy. In an infection after the third month of pregnancy the **rubella fetopathy** develops with (possibly in the course of the disease) hepatitis, hepatosplenomegaly, thrombocytopenia, extramedullary blood formation, hemolytic anemia, and meningoencephalitis. The diagnosis is confirmed by positive verification of Rubella-IgM antibodies in the child's serum. There is no specific treatment. For prevention of rubella embryo and rubella fetopathy, rubella immunization is administered to all girls, at the latest before onset of puberty. The rubella titer is checked during pregnancy care. When a pregnant woman who is not immune is exposed to rubella, immunoglobulin administration can be considered. The efficacy of this measure has not yet been confirmed.
■ In a first infection with **cytomegaly** virus (CMV) during pregnancy, the unborn child develops a connatal cytomegaly infection in 3% to 4% of cases. Sources of infection are body fluids (vaginal secretions, sperm, urine, saliva, mother's milk) as well as blood and blood products. The incubation time is 4 to 8 weeks. Ten percent to 15% of infected fetuses become ill and then usually also exhibit long-term damages. Premature birth is frequent. The earlier in the pregnancy the infection takes place, the more severe the clinical picture. Symptoms of connatal cytomegaly infection are pronounced hepatosplenomegaly, thrombocytopenia, hemolytic anemia with extramedullary blood formation, encephalitis with impaired brain development, formation of

intracerebral calcification and microcephaly, eye involvement (e.g., chorioretinitis, cataract, micro-phthalmus) and inner ear hearing impairment. The diagnosis is established by detection of the virus in the urine (and saliva) (CMV early antigen); IgM and IgG antibodies are only of secondary importance in diagnosis. Treatment with ganciclovir for 6 weeks is recommended because it is well tolerated. (However, the efficacy is unclear; pre-existing damage is not improved. The incidence of hearing damage is reduced.) No certain prevention of cytomegaly is known. In newborns and prematurely born children, only CMV-negative banked blood should be trans-fused; mother's milk should only be fed to small, prematurely born infants if the mother's CMV status is negative or after pasteurization of the milk. In case of professional exposure (e.g., pediatric nurses, kindergarten teachers), women who hope to have children should give particular care to hygiene in handling stool or urine (i.e., careful hand washing or use of gloves after/during changing diapers).

- Primary infection of a pregnant woman with **herpes simplex** (types 1 + 2) very rarely harms the fetus. The incubation time is between 1 and 42 days. The greatest fear is related to neonatal infection (see case 39). In the rare connatal infection, there are symptoms such as hypotrophy, hydrocephalus, chorioretinitis, and microphthalmus. The prognosis for this infection is not favorable.

The O in TORCH stands for **Others**, e.g., HIV, hepatitis B, measles, parvovirus B19, chicken pox, lues, Listeria infection.

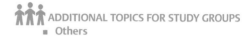 ADDITIONAL TOPICS FOR STUDY GROUPS
  ■ Others

78　Somatization syndrome

78.1　Summarize the boy's complaints. What else interests you in the medical history?
- **Summary of symptoms:** Subjective decrease in efficiency for the past 5 weeks, palpitations, relapsing chest pain, shortness of breath, tingling paresthesia, nausea
- **Medical history to objectify the symptoms:**
  - Decrease in efficiency: Sports achievement (difference compared to schoolmates), increased tiredness, changes in school performance, problems falling/staying asleep, night sweats, nycturia
  - Palpitations: Onset of symptoms at rest, sudden onset of symptoms, maximal heart rate, arrhythmia, caffeine (coffee, soft drinks)/alcohol/nicotine/drug abuse
  - Chest pain: Situation-dependent onset of symptoms (at night, at rest, under stress [specify], type of pain, dependent on ex-/inspiration)
  - Shortness of breath: Sudden onset, situation-dependent onset, shortness of breath associated with anxiety, interference with breathing in or out
  - Tingling paresthesia in hands: Associated with shortness of breath, limitation of motor ability in the hands, bilateral onset, onset at other points in the body
  - Nausea: Urge to vomit, vomiting

78.2　What could be the organic causes of these complaints? What do you do next to rule out these organic causes?
- Take the complaints seriously and do not shrug them off. Listen.
- Possible organic causes: Anemia, hyperthyroidism, paroxysmal tachycardia, myocarditis, pneumothorax, pneumonia, stress asthma, heart failure, neoplasia
- Further procedure:
  - Thorough physical examination: Especially auscultation of the heart (heart sounds, rhythm, heart rate), palpation of peripheral pulse (pulse deficit), signs of heart failure (hepatomegaly, venous obstruction, peripheral edema), auscultation of lungs (crackles, asymmetrical respiratory sounds, percussion sounds), palpation of the thyroid gland (goiter), inspection and palpation of the spine and the musculoskeletal system (myalgia, scoliosis, pressure or compression pain over spinal nerve roots)
  - Consultation with primary doctor (prior diagnostics)
  - Instrumental examination: ECG, stress ECG, long-term ECG, echocardiography, repeated blood pressure measurement, pulmonary function test, thoracic X-ray (pneumothorax, heart failure)
  - Laboratory tests: blood picture, sedimentation rate, CRP, CK-MB, GOT, GPT, γ-GT, TSH, if necessary, additional tests, e.g., virus serology (coxsackie virus, influenza, enterovirus)

78.3　How do you evaluate the boy's complaints?
- It is most likely that the complaints are innocuous and not organic in nature.
- The cause is probably the increased self-observation of puberty.
- Shortness of breath, nausea, and tingling paresthesia as symptoms of hyperventilation, e.g., out of fear of a serious illness.
- *But:* In spite of everything, take the complaints seriously and rule out possible organic causes.

- To reassure the youth: Careful diagnostics were able to rule out an organic cause for the symptoms; the patient is organically healthy.
- Explain that puberty is a developmental phase in which the body changes decisively (the youth

becomes a man); these changes make many young people insecure and are observed with particular attention. This insecurity can intensify anxiety.
- Recommend regular sports activity; diversion, for example, listening to music, relaxation techniques (e.g., autogenic training).
- Invite him to come to your office at any time if anxiety or symptoms recur.
- If the symptoms persist, offer psychological support.

Comments

Puberty: Puberty is a phase of **increased self-awareness**. Adolescents are unusually preoccupied with themselves. Their bodies go through truly dramatic changes from child to adult and they are thus regarded with more attention. Externals are considered very important, and many adolescents are dissatisfied with themselves.

In this phase of development, adolescents become increasingly **anxious.** In addition to overall anxiety about the future (e.g., anxiety about war, environmental destruction), there are personal fears, with special emphasis on fear of unemployment and sickness. However, in comparison to other age groups, young people are only rarely affected by serious diseases; typical adolescent diseases are acne, goiter, or diseases of the ligaments and skeletal system. Typical **psychosomatic complaints** are headaches, stomach, and lower abdominal pain, often in connection with the onset of menstruation. Girls are more likely to complain of such symptoms than boys. Feelings of stress, loneliness and meaninglessness, anxiety, and excessive demands are often the basis of psychosomatic symptoms. Intensive self-observation can make the complaints seem overly important; the fear of illness can take on the features of panic. A frequent reaction is hyperventilation, which leads to tingling paresthesia around the mouth and in the hands. Because the feelings are so labile, there is a high risk in puberty of developing neurotic and psychotic behaviors.

There is a high readiness to take drugs. Young people take drugs for a great variety of reasons: It is a demonstrative imitation of adult behavior (especially smoking and drinking alcohol) and a conscious breaking of parents' rules. Often drugs give adolescents access to friends who are considered particularly cool. But drugs can also be a way to overcome frustration and dissatisfaction. Drugs manipulate the psychosomatic state of mind; psychotropic substances improve the mood and provide an escape into a better experience.

Typical psychiatric diseases that start in puberty are anorexia nervosa (see case 27), bulimia nervosa, and psychogenic obesity.

Diagnosis and Treatment: In speaking with the adolescent, it is important to know about the developments that are particular to this phase in life. If the young person is accompanied by his parents, it can be helpful to speak with the patient alone first. The patient is given complete attention. Disturbances during the conversation, even just taking notes, should be avoided. The patient is allowed to tell his story; by thoughtfully summarizing what the patient has said, it is made clear that the young person's problems are being taken seriously. It may be possible to create a trusting relationship.

When the patient describes anxiety states, it is important to differentiate between normal and pathological anxiety. Pathological anxiety is "free-floating," i.e., it is not proportional to the situation and does not let itself be dispelled by sensible arguments, so as to avoid the situations that trigger it.

The conversation is followed by a physical examination. This too should take place without the parents, unless the patient wishes otherwise. The patient's modesty should be particularly respected. Possible organic causes for the complaints must be carefully ruled out. In addition to confirming the diagnosis, this gives the young person and the worried parents a sense of security. If organic causes of the symptoms are ruled out with certainty, there must be a truthful conversation with the young person to explain the psychosomatic origin and the "normality" of such symptoms in certain developmental stages. Often this kind of informational talk can already have a therapeutic effect. Diversion, active sport, relaxation techniques, and an offer of further conversations are other useful therapeutic approaches. If the symptoms do not improve or are even intensified, psychological advice and support should be offered.

253

Case

78

→ Cases 78 Page 80

79.1 What do you do next to find out why, in spite of multiple attempts at therapy, there has been no improvement?
- **Detailed medical history:** Start of the illness, course to the present, known triggers, prior treatment (with what and how long was the patient treated?), family history (atopy?)
- **Determine triggers:** Allergy diagnostics (food, aeroallergens by means of RAST), superinfection (skin smear), irritating factors (history: cigarette smoke, clothing, washing habits, hard water), stress

79.2 What therapy do you recommend to your acquaintances?
- **Recognizing and avoiding triggers**
- **Acute treatment:**
  - Local anti-irritant treatment, e.g., cortisone cream, possibly pimecrolimus
  - In superinfection, additionally antibiotic therapy (after antibiogram) and local antiseptic measures

(e.g., dyes or antiseptics like chlorhexidine or triclosan)
- **Wearing hypoallergenic clothing:** Breathable, soft, easily washable (e.g., cotton fabrics, silk, microfiber, soft linen fabrics)
- **Systematic basic skin care:** Use of oil and fat-containing creams and moisturizing bath salts to increase the moisture and fat content of the skin
- **Parent and patient training:** Explanation of atopic diseases and especially neurodermitis; recognition and avoidance of triggers, systematic basic skin care, a diet appropriate for children and neurodermitis, psychological workup of conflict and stress situations, exchange with other affected families

79.3 The parents are afraid of cortisone side effects. What is your opinion of using cortisone-containing medications?
Fear of cortisone is unfounded with targeted application. Cortisone preparations are very effective medications that cut through the vicious circle of "itching-scratching-skin damage-healing-itching."

Comments

Definition and epidemiology: Neurodermitis (syn.: atopic eczema, atopic dermatitis, endogenous eczema) is the most frequent chronic skin disease in children. It is on the spectrum of the atopic diseases (bronchial asthma, allergic rhinoconjunctivitis, neurodermitis).

Atopia (= tendency to allergy) is an elevated sensitivity of skin and mucosa to environmental materials. Usually the family history is positive; blood IgE concentrations are elevated.

In recent years, the incidence of atopic diseases has increased. The prevalence atopic disease in children in the United States is 10% overall, with a range of 8.7% to 18.1%.

Etiology and pathogenesis: A genetic disposition is decisive in the onset of the disease. In order for neurodermitis to manifest, other factors must also be present (e.g., food allergy, house dust mites, mold formation, pollen, animal epithelium, cigarette smoke, not breastfeeding, acute and chronic stress situations).

Symptoms of neurodermitis are based on **IgE-mediated type I reaction** (allergic reaction of immediate type). In addition to a disordered immune response of the skin, the **barrier function of the skin is impaired**. There are fewer skin oils, or their composition is incorrect. As a result, the ability to bind water is decreased and more water is lost. The skin is dry and therefore particularly sensitive to irritation and pathogens.

Clinical aspects: The severity of clinical symptoms, triggers, and course are very different, individually. Neurodermitis is characterized by chronic relapsing, severely itchy eczema with age-dependent distribution. In addition to marked skin dryness, the complete picture of neurodermitis includes red, weeping eczema foci with formation of little blisters and nodes, crusts, and flaking. The skin manifestations heal or persist with lichenification.

In infants, the first skin changes (cradle cap = crusta lactea), especially on the scalp, at the hairline and on the forehead. The changes are large surfaces of skin reddening with flakes and weeping areas (see Fig. Cradle cap).

→ Cases 79 Page 80

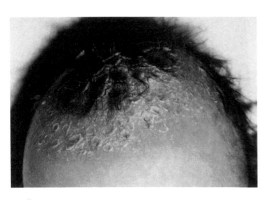

Cradle cap

The changes can spread to the whole body. It is notable that the diaper area is almost always free of the rash. In older children, the clinical distribution pattern of the skin changes is different (see Fig. Distribution pattern). The most frequently affected locations are the flexor surfaces of the elbow and knee joints. Eczema can also appear on the eyelids, hands, and feet. The skin is chronically inflamed and thickened. This is called lichenification. Neurodermitis can be complicated by superinfection, especially with *Staphylococcus aureus* (= impetiginized neurodermitis), but also with viruses such as herpes simplex (= eczema herpeticum).

Diagnostics: The diagnosis is made on the basis of **objective signs of illness** (skin changes), course (relapsing occurrence), and **subjective complaints** (itching). In speaking with the patient, an attempt is made to identify possible **triggers**. In addition, an attempt should be made to **identify allergies**: in children up to 6 years old, the **CAP-RAST test** is the method of choice for finding type I sensitization. In addition, the total **IgE** should be determined. In older children, the **prick test** is used to reveal sensitization. The test can only be performed if the condition of the skin permits and in the last 2 weeks before the test the patient has neither taken antihistamines nor applied topical immunosuppressants. It serves as a screening test in patients with moderate sensitization and is highly sensitive to pollen, house dust mites, and pet dander. Foods can also be tested. After the inner side of the lower arm has been cleaned and oil has been removed with alcohol, two rows of a maximum of 10 marks are drawn on the

skin with an indelible pencil. The distance between test points should be at least 2 cm. Then one drop of allergen-containing material is dropped onto the marked locations. The skin is then superficially pricked through the drop with a prick lancet (no bleeding) and slightly raised at the side. After each prick, the lancet is discarded and a new lancet is used for the next prick so that there is no mixing of the allergens. In addition, a negative control (physiological saline) and a positive control (histamine solution 0.1%) are applied and also pricked. The exposure time should be at least 5 minutes; if the reaction is intense, it must be interrupted by wiping off the allergen solution. The test result is read after 20 minutes and evaluated according to the extent of the erythema and the weal (Ø = no reaction (+) = weak reaction, + = significantly weaker than histamine reaction, ++ = weaker than histamine reaction, +++ = equal to histamine reaction, ++++ = stronger than histamine reaction). In addition, a **skin smear** should be used to determine whether there is a bacterial colonization of the skin.

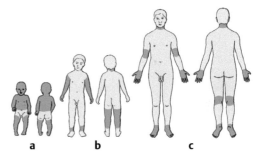

Distribution pattern of the neurodermitis according to age (a) infants, (b) toddlers, (c) youths and adults

Treatment: See answer to question 79.2. The basis of the long-term neurodermitis treatment is careful and, most importantly, consistent **basic skin care** with **fat-containing creams** and baths with moisturizing, itch-calming, and anti-inflammatory supplements. This improves the skin condition, strengthens the skin barrier, and reduces the frequency of acute flare-ups. Supplements to basic creams such as urea or D-panthenol intensify the desired action. Systemic **antihistamines** can be used to calm itching (e.g., dimetindene maleate [fenistil]). Medical radiation of the skin with light produces improvement of the skin condition in many

→ Cases 79 Page 80

patients with neurodermitis. In an acute flare-up, a skin smear must be examined to determine whether there is a superinfection. If germs are detected, treatment with antibiotics, determined by an antibiogram (skin smear), and additional application of local antiseptics is required. Concurrently, local anti-inflammatory treatment is applied, e.g., with cortisone-containing preparations. Cortisone preparations should only be used in the short term. Use on the face, skin folds, and genital area is not recommended because the skin in these areas is highly permeable to externally applied corticosteroids. This makes the risk for cortisone side effects particularly high. There are very efficacious new medications for these locations, such as pimecrolimus or tacrolimus. However, these immunomodulators may only be used from the age of 2 for treatment of neurodermitis. Evening primrose oil can also be efficacious because it has a positive effect on the lipid metabolism of the skin. Numerous alternative methods, e.g., Bach flower remedies, autologous blood treatment, bioresonance procedures, are available for the treatment of neurodermitis. Up to the present, there are no unbiased studies confirming the efficacy of these therapies.

Prophylaxis: If there is a positive family history, the child should be exclusively breastfed for the first 4 months after birth. If breastfeeding is not possible, the child should be fed a hypoallergenic infant formula in the first 4 months after birth. Breastfeeding or formula feeding should continue following the introduction of solid foods. Feeding with solid foods should begin at the earliest at 5 months and at the latest at 7 months of age (see case 71).

Prognosis: The course of neurodermitis is unpredictable. In 60% of children the disease disappears by the end of puberty; in 40% the symptoms persist to varying extent up to adulthood. In most cases, neurodermitis can be adequately treated by avoiding triggers and systematic treatment.

ADDITIONAL TOPICS FOR STUDY GROUPS
- Allergy
- Bronchial asthma

80 Anomalies in pediatric examination; neonatal reflexes

80.1 What do you do next?
- **Create trust.** Since little children do not yet understand the significance or necessity of a medical examination, they react with anxiety/rejection/resistance. For this reason, the child should be given sufficient time to become familiar with the situation, i.e., for the examiner: approaching the child carefully and gently.
- The examiner should introduce themselves and greet the mother and especially the child, speaking with the child on their own level and not patronizingly, ask the child's name, admire their toy, etc.
- Then the medical history conversation with the mother can begin, while observing the child and establishing eye contact.
- Make contact with the child, e.g., through the doll.
- During the examination, the child stays in the mother's arms.
- Have the mother undress the child.
- Let the child play with the examination instruments (see Fig.).

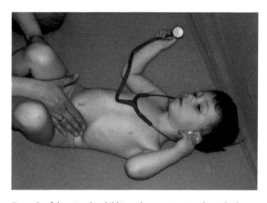

Example of drawing the child into the examination through play

80.2 Describe how you examine the child. What do you look for in particular?
- **In general the following applies:**
  - The child can be examined in the arms of the person who brought them.

- Try to distract the child with a stuffed animal, keys, etc. or to include the child in the examination through play (e.g., let them "telephone" with the stethoscope; examine the doll or stuffed animal first).
- The examination does not follow a strict order of events; it should be adapted to the child's collaboration.
- Perform unpleasant examinations like inspection of the eardrum/throat last.

■ **Observing the child while taking the medical history:** Evaluation of overall and nutritional condition, state of consciousness, tone, movement, protective posture, skin, interaction with the child's responsible person, abnormal behavior.

■ **Observation/inspection of the child as the responsible person completely undresses them:** For example, skin, tonus, movement, conspicuous thorax shape, chest wall depressions.

■ **Examination process:** The same examination techniques are used as in adult medicine, but not according to a strict order of events; they should be adapted to the child's collaboration. No organ system may be left out.
- Inspection of skin: Color, turgor, blood supply, exanthema, petechiae, injuries, traces of scratching, signs of abuse (see case 75)
- Auscultation of heart: Heart sounds, frequency, rhythm
- Auscultation of the lungs: Comparing breathing sounds on the two sides, crackle, obstruction
- Palpation, auscultation, and percussion of abdomen (for a screaming child, when they pause for breath): Organ enlargement, pathological resistances, protective tension, intestinal sounds, meteorism
- Palpation of lymph nodes: Enlargement (local or generalized)
- Neurological status: Signs of meningism (see case 1), reflex status
- Inspection of genitals and anus: Skin changes, deformities
- Instrumental examination of throat and ears: Evaluation of tonsillar ring, tonsils (size, coating), inspection of auditory canals, eardrums, pressure on tragus (pain?)

▍80.3 What tips for taking blood can you give your colleague?

■ **Every prick inflicted on a child should be well considered:** Is the blood draw really necessary? Can the blood draw be combined with the insertion of an indwelling venous cannula? Might a capillary blood draw be sufficient?

■ In anxious children and if it is not an emergency, a "magic band aid" (anesthetizing cream on a band aid for 30–45 minutes) can be applied to the puncture site. Then the prick will not hurt as much.

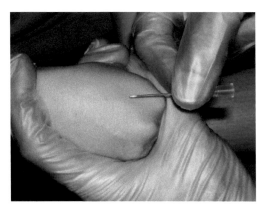

Venous puncture

■ Everything should be well prepared; an experienced nurse holds the child and passes materials.

■ A tourniquet is usually not necessary; if the puncture site is on the back of the hand, one can squeeze the child's hand in one's own (see Fig. Venous puncture); or the nurse clamps off the upper arm or calf manually, thus also holding the extremity still. It is important not to squeeze too long because this is painful.

■ Parents can console or distract the child during the procedure but sometimes, it can be helpful for the parents to leave the room, since the child does not necessarily understand that the parents allow anyone to hurt them.

▍80.4 Describe the chief reflexes.

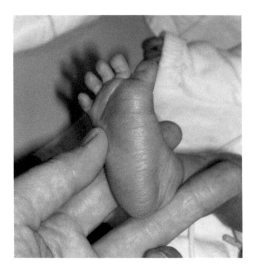

Babinski reflex

Reflex	Test and reaction	Physiological
Stepping reflex	Hold the child upright with both hands on the trunk, the upper body is slightly bent forward, pressure of the foot on the examining table causes the leg to be pulled up while the other leg is extended: apparent walking (automatic walking)	Up to 2 months
Glabella reflex	Pressure in the middle of the forehead causes the eyes to close	Up to 3 months
Rooting reflex	Stroke near the corner of the mouth with the finger and the child stretches the corner of their mouth toward the stimulus and follows with the head	Up to 3 months
Grasp reflex	When the inner surface of the hand is touched, the child grasps (palmar grasp reflex); when the sole of the foot is touched, the toes curl down (plantar reflex)	Up to 4 months
Galant reflex	Stroking the child with a finger paravertebrally along the back causes the child's body to curve in a direction concave to the touch	Up to 4 months
Bauer reaction	If the child is prone, pressure against the soles of the feet causes the child to make alternating crawling motions	Up to 4 months
Sucking reflex	Inserting a finger in the infant's mouth causes them to start sucking immediately	Up to 4 months
Moro reaction	In supine position triggered by suddenly releasing the head after it had been raised or by startle reaction (e.g., knock on the supporting surface); Phase I: Child opens mouth, arms are flung outward, hands opened Phase II: Mouth closed, arms are flexed and hugged in front of the chest	Up to 6 months
Babinski reflex (see Fig. Babinski reflex)	Stroking the lateral edge of the foot leads to dorsal extension of the great toe	Up to 12 months
Landau reflex	Hold the prone infant firmly by the trunk and raise them into the air; the infant extends their legs and raises their head	4–12 months

Comments

Problems in pediatric examination: Many doctors examining toddlers have the same experience as their colleague in the example case. Children often develop astonishing force and escape from almost any position. Parents protect their children and suffer with them. The physician becomes the "bad doctor," the adversary. Children do not understand the reason for procedures during the examination and do not tolerate unpleasant interventions. They react to the doctor, the unfamiliar surroundings, the glittering instruments with anxiety and resistance. Therefore, it is important to avoid anything that could add in any way to the child's fear. An attempt should be made to win the child's trust, or at least cooperation.

Creating trust: See answer to question 80.1. One should try to remain **friendly and patient** in all situations. Nowadays, many pediatricians no longer wear white coats because the child often connects unpleasant experiences such as painful immunizations or blood draws with that white coat. It is also useful, if the child's overall condition permits, not to start the admission examination immediately with the physical examination. The medical history conversation with the parents is the optimal starting point. The child can get accustomed to the doctor.

The doctor has this opportunity to observe the child and the parent–child interaction. Starting a contact with the child can then begin with the help of a stuffed animal or, as in the example case, involving the doll that the child brought along.

Caution: Do not make any false promises to the child (e.g., "There won't be any pinches," or "That doesn't hurt at all"). Children do not forgive lies.

Examination process: See answer to question 80.2. The examination should be as long as necessary and as short as possible, but never longer than 15 minutes.

Ask the parents to undress the child entirely, so that nothing can be overlooked (e.g., petechiae, skin rash). The child can be playfully drawn into the examination. The examination instruments can be examined; the child may want to "telephone" with the stethoscope. A doll or one of the parents can be examined first so that the child sees what will happen to them next. Often it is helpful for one parent to hold the child on their lap during the examination.

The examination cannot proceed according to a strict pattern. Unpleasant examinations like inspection of the throat or the auditory canal should come

→ Cases 80 Page 81

at the end of the examination, because auscultation and palpation are difficult with a screaming child. For inspection of the throat, a person holds the head in place by grasping the arms extended over the child's head (see Fig. Throat inspection).

However, the child's fear is sometimes so great that in spite of all the tricks, examination of the child is hardly possible. Then the examination should take place quickly, so that the child can soon calm down again. Evaluation of examination results for a screaming child is only possible to a limited extent.

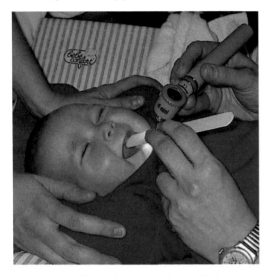

Throat inspection (fixating the arms over the head for throat examination)

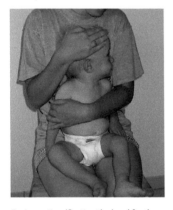

Ear inspection (fixating the head for the ear examination)

Drawing blood from a child: See answer to question 80.3. If drawing blood is absolutely necessary, everything should be well-organized in advance, i.e., all instruments must be laid out, and ready, experienced nursing personnel should hold the child and hand the instruments. To keep the stress as low

as possible for the child, the puncture site can be numbed with an anesthetizing patch. If an indwelling venous cannula must be placed, this is combined with the blood draw, to spare the child additional punctures. Good veins (see Fig. Venous puncture) can usually be found on the back of the hand (dorsal venous network of hand), in the crook of the elbow (basilic vein, cubital vein), on the head (superficial temporal vein, supratrochlear veins), on the inner side of the wrist (*Caution:* very painful), or on the dorsum of the foot (dorsal venous plexus of the foot), calf (great saphenous vein, small saphenous vein). *Note:* The better you search, the less you jab.

Normally, puncture is made with a size 1 cannula. For fine veins, it is possible to break off the cannula's cone (plastic end) ahead of time. This prevents formation of a clot in the cone. The suction of a syringe involves the danger of collapsing a vein. For this reason, the blood is allowed to drip into the test tube. Experience has shown that venous puncture, especially in infants and toddlers, is very difficult. Because of fat pillows, the veins can neither be seen nor palpated. If even the second attempt at puncturing the vein does not succeed, it is not necessary to give in to panic. Then it is important to ask a colleague for help. "New hands, new success!"

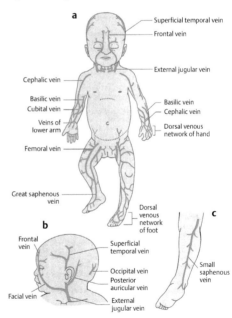

Veins suitable for venipuncture and infusion

ADDITIONAL TOPICS FOR STUDY GROUPS
- Health screening (birth to age 7 or 8)
- Examination of a newborn (see case 65)

→ Cases 80 Page 81

81.1 Your senior physician asks you which differential diagnoses you should consider with this finding.

The ultrasound findings show an enlarged liver with nodular, round foci. What differential diagnoses can be considered?

- Benign or malignant liver tumor: For example, hemangioma, hemangioendothelioma, hamartoma, hepatoblastoma, hepatocellular carcinoma
- Metastases of another solid tumor: For example, neuroblastoma, nephroblastoma, germ cell tumor

81.2 What is meant by a neuroblastoma? What other examinations must you order to confirm your suspected diagnosis?

- **Definition:** Neuroblastomas are malignant, solid tumors of the **autonomic nervous system** that develop from the cells of the neural crest, i.e., from the tissue of origin of the sympathetic trunk and the adrenal medulla. Thus they can arise everywhere that sympathetic nervous tissue is found: In the adrenal glands (approximately 50%), the sympathetic paraganglia, and in the cervical, thoracic, and abdominal sympathetic trunk. The tumor metastasizes early, especially in lymph nodes, bones, and bone marrow, liver, skin, and orbits.
- **Examinations:**
  - Careful medical history with questions about weight loss, restlessness, loss of appetite, weakness, fever, vomiting, constipation, diarrhea
  - Physical examination: Inspection of skin (paleness, skin metastases), auscultation of the lungs (stridor as indication of mediastinal tumor), palpation of the abdomen (palpable abdominal tumor, hepatosplenomegaly), palpation of all lymph node locations (lymph node metastases), neurological examination (paresis, Horner syndrome, cerebral pressure symptoms), blood pressure measurement (hypertension due to catecholamine production)
  - Blood examinations: Blood picture, liver function values (GOT, GPT, γGT, alkaline phosphatase, cholinesterase, Quick), creatinine, electrolytes, sedimentation rate, neuron-specific enolase (NSE) as tumor marker, LDH and ferritin as prognosis factors
  - Urinalysis: Homovanillylmandelic acid and vanillylmandelic acid in spontaneous urine
  - MRI of primary tumor: Location, extent of tumor, intraspinal involvement and relation to neighboring organs, operation planning, lymph node involvement
  - MIBG (metaiodobenzylguanidine) scintigraphy: MIBG is concentrated in catecholamine-producing tissue; evidence of primary tumor and distant metastases
  - Technetium bone scintigraphy in case of bone foci (to differentiate between skeletal and bone marrow involvement)

  - Bone marrow puncture at four sites (often focal infiltration) to prove bone marrow involvement; neuroblastoma cell nests in smear confirm the diagnosis. If the finding is positive, molecular genetic examination (examination for amplification of the N-myc oncogene, deletion at chromosome 1p) should be performed. If the bone marrow finding is negative, the diagnosis cannot be established with certainty preoperatively. In that case, for exact confirmation of diagnosis, it is necessary to wait for intraoperative tissue sampling and histological examination (exception: stage 4S; here it is possible to wait)
  - Sample biopsy of the primary tumor for confirmation of diagnosis and molecular genetic examination

81.3 What clinical symptoms can a neuroblastoma cause? Can the persistent diarrhea also be ascribed to the neuroblastoma?

- The clinical symptoms **depend on the location** of the tumor:
  - **Abdominal location of tumor:** Palpable or visible abdominal tumor, secondary vomiting, constipation, disorder of urine flow, hydronephrosis
  - **Intrathoracic tumor location:** Cough, stridor, dyspnea
  - **Sympathetic chain tumor:** Paraplegia symptoms caused by intraspinal growth (hourglass tumor), torticollis, Horner syndrome (miosis, ptosis, enophthalmus)
  - **Disseminated stage:** Hepatomegaly with liver metastasis, bone pain with bone metastases, livid skin nodes with skin infiltration, uni- or bilateral exophthalmos with spectacle hematoma with retrobulbar infiltration, cerebral pressure symptoms with cerebral involvement, changes in blood picture with anemia and thrombocytopenia with pronounced bone marrow infiltration, overall symptoms such as pain, fatigue, decreased productivity, weight loss, generalized lymph node swelling, fever
- The **therapy-resistant diarrhea** can be ascribed to the neuroblastoma: Neuroblastoma cells secrete vasointestinal **polypeptide** (VIP). VIP leads via cAMP or Ca^{2+}-mediated activation of Cl^- channels to increased fluid secretion into the intestines and thus to accelerated intestinal transit. The result is therapy-resistant secretory diarrhea.

81.4 What therapy does the tumor stage call for? What is the prognosis for the little patient? Are there factors that influence this prognosis?

- **Stage 4S** is a special stage of neuroblastoma that only occurs in infants. There can already be distant metastases in skin and liver, as in stage 4, but the bone marrow is only slightly involved (fewer than

10% malignant cells). The remarkable thing about this stage is **the high tendency for spontaneous remission**, even without chemotherapy. If there is no progress or no evidence of increase of N-myc oncogene, it is justifiable to begin with a waiting period. If tumor or metastases should lead to complications by their space-occupying growth or if increase of the N-myc oncogene is detected, chemotherapy or local radiation may be necessary to stimulate regression.

- The **prognosis** for patients with tumor stage 4S is good. The 5-year survival rate is 75%. Elevated LDH and ferritin serum levels and the detection of N-myc oncogene or a deletion on the short arm of chromosome 1 (1p deletion) are associated with rapid tumor progress and a worse prognosis.

Comments

Definition: Neuroblastoma is a malignant tumor that develops out of the embryonic tissue of the sympathetic crest and the adrenal medulla—the neural chain. It is one of the embryonic tumors characterized by their manifestation at an early age and by the typical cell morphology of embryonic precursor cells (neuroblasts). A neuroblastoma can arise anywhere that sympathetic nervous tissue is found: in the adrenal medulla, the sympathetic chain, and the sympathetic paraganglia.

Epidemiology: After the ALL, neuroblastoma is the second most frequently occurring malignant tumors in children. It constitutes 7% to 8% of all pediatric cancers. The incidence is approximately 1.1 cases in 100,000 children (< 15 years of age). In the United States, there are about 700 new cases each year; nearly 90% of cases are diagnosed by age 5. Most frequently affected are children aged 1 year (about 40% of cases). Ninety percent of cases are younger than 6 years. Boys are affected somewhat more frequently than girls.

Etiopathogenesis: The **etiology** of neuroblastoma is largely unclear; in very rare cases the occurrence of neuroblastoma is concentrated in families. One idiosyncrasy of neuroblastomas is that they can regress spontaneously. This is particularly true for tumor stage 4S or local tumor stages in early infancy. In patients with these tumors, diagnosis is often established on the basis of extensive liver metastases that cause enlargement of the liver. The size of the metastases can increase rapidly and become life threatening by compressing abdominal organs and the lungs. But then they regress either spontaneously or after chemotherapy at a mild dosage.

Especially in children beyond 1 year of age, neuroblastoma growth is often rapid and unobstructed. About half of neuroblastomas have already metastasized by the time the diagnosis is made. **Metastases** are observed in regional and distant lymph nodes, bone marrow, bones, liver, or as livid skin nodes. Rarely, metastases are found in the CNS; pulmonary metastases are rare.

Clinical aspects: See answer to question 81.3. In rare cases, **arterial hypertension** can be observed as the result of catecholamine metabolite action. A very rare but characteristic symptom is **opsomyoclonus syndrome** (dancing eye syndrome). This is a paraneoplastic syndrome with typical neurological symptoms: Myoclonus in the trunk and extremities, ataxia and short, rapid eye movements (opsoclonus).

Diagnostics:
- Ultrasound to search for the primary tumor (especially if it is located in the abdomen), as well as liver and lymph node metastases.
- Neuroblastoma cells, as well as chromaffin cells in the adrenal medulla, can produce catecholamine. For this reason, in patients with neuroblastoma, catecholamine metabolites (vanillin- and homovanillylmandelic acid) can be found in spontaneous urine. *Caution:* consumption of vanilla-containing foods within 3 days before the examination can lead to false-positive test results. The catecholamine metabolites can be used as tumor markers for the further course of the disease.
- **Neuron-specific enolase** (NSE) can also be used as a tumor marker. However, it is not as specific for neuroblastoma (elevated NSE values can also be detected for other tumors, e.g., Wilms tumor and leukemia). LDH and ferritin are decisive prognostic factors. In establishing the diagnosis, elevated values indicate a worse prognosis. They are an expression of the tumor burden and tumor activity.
- **Blood examinations, imaging diagnostics, MIBG- and skeletal scintigraphy, bone marrow puncture, and molecular genetics**: See answer to question 81.2.

Stage classification and therapy (see Tab.): Treatment is carried out in a controlled study at a pediatric oncology center. The rule is that every child (exception: infants in stage 4S without complication) is operated on, since it is only through surgery that the precise extent of the tumor (crossing the midline, affected lymph nodes) can be determined so that it can be assigned to a specific stage. In addition, this permits the sampling of tumor tissue for histological and molecular genetic study. Further procedure (pre-/postoperative chemo- and/or radiation therapy, immunotherapy, retinoic acid) depends on the stage of the disease, the child's age, location of the tumor, and molecular genetic markers (e.g., N-myc amplification, chromosome 1p deletion). The threat of paraplegia in hourglass tumors is an indication for **immediate surgery** (independent of the tumor stage).

→ Cases 81 Page 82

Stage	Description	Treatment
Stage 1	Localized tumor limited to original site, no lymph node involvement	Resection is the only therapy
Stage 2a	Localized tumor, can only be removed incompletely, no lymph node involvement	Resection
Stage 2b	Localized tumor, infiltrated environment without crossing the midline, possible homolateral lymph node invasion	Resection, with lymph node invasion additional chemotherapy[a] or local irradiation
Stage 3	Tumor crosses midline, regional lymph nodes can be affected bilaterally	Resection, intensified chemotherapy, possibly irradiation
Stage 4	Hematogenous distant metastases in bone, soft tissue, lymph nodes, etc.	Maximal therapy chemotherapy, resection, possibly irradiation, high-dose chemotherapy with stem cell transplantation, immunotherapy, administration of retinoic acid
Stage 4S	Like stage 1 or 2, but with distant metastases in liver and skin; bone marrow may only be minimally invaded; occurs only in infants, can regress spontaneously	Possibly spontaneous regression → wait and observe, if appropriate (mild) chemotherapy or local irradiation and resection if there is excessive tumor growth with signs that organs are being compressed

[a] Cyclophosphamide, ifosfamide, vincristin, cisplatin, etoposide, adriamycin, daunorubicin, or dacarbazine.

Staging neuroblastoma: (according to International Neuroblastoma Staging System [INSS])

Complete tumor removal in stage 4S should only be performed if it causes no extensive sequelae (e.g., development of short bowel syndrome with extensive intestinal resection, primary nephrectomy). If complete removal of the tumor is not possible, other treatment measures are taken (chemotherapy or radiation). In the **advanced stages** (from stage 3), before surgery on large primary tumors, chemotherapy is generally administered before the operation to reduce the size of the primary tumor (= **neoadjuvant therapy**). If MIBG-concentrating tumor remnants are detected after the operation, an additional therapy with ¹³¹Iodine-marked metaiodobenzylguanidine is initiated (this is intravenously injected to destroy tumor tissue). Patients in stage 4 have an

unfavorable prognosis in spite of intensive therapy (5-year survival range only 30%–40%). New methods are applied here: In **immunotherapy** the patient is given antibodies directed against the ganglioside GD2 (antigen-to-cell surface of neuroblastoma cells → a certain marker for neuroblastoma). The objective is for the body's intrinsic immune system to fight independently against the neuroblastoma cells by means of antibody-mediated cellular toxicity. **Retinoic acid** induces the ripening of the neuroblastoma cells into benign ganglion cells.

Prognosis: The 5-year survival rate for all stages is 65%. For patients with localized, non-metastasized tumors in stages 1 and 2 it is up to 95%. In stage 3, about 75% survive; in stage 4, only 30% to 40%. Infants in disseminated stage 4S have a good prognosis. In 75% of cases, there is spontaneous tumor regression.

82 Meningococcal sepsis/Waterhouse–Friderichsen syndrome

82.1 What clinical picture is meant? Please give a short definition and name the cause and prognosis of the clinical picture.
- **Waterhouse–Friderichsen syndrome:** The most severe form of peracute meningococcal sepsis with septic shock, fulminant purpura (bleeding into the skin, mucosa, and internal organs), disseminated, intravascular clotting with consumption of clotting factors and bilateral adrenal bleeding.
- **Cause:** Invasive infection with *Neisseria meningitidis* (*Meningococci*).
- **Prognosis:** Lethality is between 50% and 70%.

82.2 What differential diagnoses can be considered? What do you do next?
- **Differential diagnoses:** Particularly other diseases associated with petechiae, such as hemolytic–uremic syndrome (see case 59), idiopathic thrombocytopenic purpura (see case 83), leukemia (see case 45), Schoenlein–Henoch purpura (see case 8), endocarditis, acute allergic vasculitis.
- **Further procedure: Every minute counts!** For this reason diagnostic measures cannot be allowed to delay the start of treatment; every delay worsens the chance of survival. Order immediate transfer to intensive care unit.

82.3 How do you interpret the blood values? What supplementary studies must still be performed?

- **Laboratory values:**
  - Leukopenia: Evidence of a (bacterial) infection
  - Elevated CRP: Evidence of infection
  - Clotting parameters: Thrombocytopenia, quick lowered, PTT elevated, fibrinogen lowered, anti-thrombin III lowered→ consumption of platelets and clotting factors by elevated intravascular coagulation (consumption coagulopathy)
- **Supplementary examinations:** Possibly lumbar puncture to rule out meningitis. If no blood culture was taken, order antigen determination in blood, cerebrospinal fluid (or skin biopsy)

82.4 Are there measures to prevent further spread of the disease?

Meningococci are transmitted by droplet infection. Therefore, it is important to learn how close the contact to the sick person was. **Close contact persons** (this includes members of the household, contact persons in community facilities, persons with close contact to the patient and who had nasopharyngeal secretions, including treating personnel in the clinic) have a 500 to 1,000-fold elevated risk of infection. They should, therefore, receive chemoprophylaxis as soon as possible (only useful within 10 days after contact with the patient).

All other persons who have had contact with the patient must be informed of the symptoms of a meningococcal disease and receive close clinical monitoring. At the first signs of infection (e.g., rising fever), antibiotic treatment must begin immediately after taking a blood culture.

- **Chemoprophylaxis:**
  - First-line medications: Rifampicin (20 mg/kg/d in two individual doses for 2 days) p.o.
  - Alternatives: Ceftriaxone (125 mg for children under 12, from the age of 12 years 250 mg) i.v. or i.m.
  - For adults, a one-time dose of ciprofloxacin (500 mg) p.o. can be given

To prevent a wider spread, the specific illness must be reported to the competent health authority within 24 hours, which will initiate further prophylactic measures. In addition, the patient must be isolated for 24 hours. After this, if antibiotic treatment has been properly carried out, there is no longer a risk of infection.

Treatment algorithm for Waterhouse-Friderichsen Syndrome

Monitoring (blood pressure, ECG, pulse-oximetry)
Administration of oxygen
Airway management, if necessary early intubation, establishment of a large-bore i.v. line, two if possible.

↓

Blood draw with blood culture

↓

Fluid replacement: NaCl 0.9% or Ringer solution 20 mL/kg body weight as short-term infusion (20 min or faster), repeat if necessary

↓

Antibiotics: Cefotaxim initially 100 mg/kg body weight, Then 200 mg/kg body weight in 3 separate doses

↓

Acidosis compensation with pH < 7.15 with NaHCO3 (8.4% solution),
Calculate requirement according to formula:
Requirement NaHCO3 in mmol = BE x kg body weight x f
(f = age-dependent constant:
newborn 0.5; infant 0.3;
toddler 0.25; school-age child 0.2)
calculated amount1:1 diluted with distilled water, infused as short infusion

↓

Steroids: hydrocortisone 3-4 mg/kg body weight/d in 3 to 4 individual doses or as an extended infusion

↓

In volume-refractory shock:
Catecholamine through central port
- Adrenaline: 0.1-1-(5) µg/kg body weight/min
- noradrenaline 0.1-1-(5) µg/kg body weight/min
Keep in mind: all the corticoids and catecholamines in the world will not help a patient who is still hypovolemic.

↓

Treatment of disseminated intravascular coagulation:
- Protein C concentrate (50-100 IU/kg body weight 2-3 x/d)
- AT III (50 IU/kg body weight)
- Low-dose heparinization: 100 IU/kg body weight/d

↓

If necessary, treatment with blood products:
- Platelet transfusion (in thrombocytopenia < 50,000/µl): 15 mL/kg body weight
- Erythrocytes transfusion: 10-15 mL/kg body weight
- FFP (fresh frozen plasma): 10-15 mL/kg body weight

↓

Stress ulcer prophylaxis:
omeprazole 0.25-0.5 mg/kg body weight /d i.v. in one single dose

↓

If necessary, **renal dialysis**

Treatment algorithm for Waterhouse–Friderichsen syndrome

→ Cases 82 Page 83

Definition: See answer to question 82.1.

Etiology and pathogenesis: The cause of Water-house–Friderichsen syndrome is usually a systemic infection with *Neisseria meningitidis*; in rare cases *Pneumococci* or *Hemophilus influenzae* can trigger this clinical picture. *Meningococci* are Gram-negative, encapsulated *Diplococci* with a characteristic bun-shaped appearance. It is an exclusively human patho-gen, transmitted in droplets. The incubation time is 1 to 10 days. It is important to differentiate between a usually symptomatic colonization of the nasophar-ynx with *Meningococci* and an invasive meningococ-cal illness. About half of all invasive meningococcal infections present as purulent meningitis (see case 1); 25% proceed as meningococcal sepsis and 25% as a mixed form of the two types. Ten percent to 15% of the forms with a septic course have a peracute course as Waterhouse–Friderichsen syndrome.

Meningococci are endotoxin producers. The release of endotoxins leads to circulatory shock with arterial hypotension, respiratory insufficiency, oliguria, and activation of the coagulation system with consump-tion of coagulation factors and platelets (consump-tion coagulopathy). This causes microthrombosis of the vessels with undersupply to peripheral areas of the systemic circulation, bleeding into skin (intra-vital lividity), mucosa, and internal organs (fulmi-nating purpura, see Fig.) which ends in multiorgan failure. A characteristic finding for Waterhouse–Friderichsen syndrome is bilateral bleeding into the adrenal glands, which results in necrosis.

Epidemiology: In the United States, over 50% of *N. meningitidis* infections in infants younger than 1 year of age are caused by serogroup B, and sero-groups C, Y, and W135 cause 75% of meningococ-cal disease in those 11 years of age and older. The incidence of invasive meningococcal infections is 0.3–0.5/100,000 population.

The first infection peak is in infancy; a second peak is observed between the ages of 15 and 19 years. Males and females are affected in equal numbers. **Reporting is obligatory** in case of suspicion of ill-ness, manifest illness, and death. Any evidence of pathogen in otherwise sterile examination material must be reported to the competent health authority.

Clinical aspects:
- **Meningococcal sepsis:** Sudden onset, high fever, chills, nausea, vomiting, and increasing apathy. Shock symptoms as well as petechial skin and mucosal bleeding develop within a few hours. In full-blown Waterhouse–Friderichsen syndrome, there is copious bleeding into skin, mucosa, and

internal organs with consumption coagulopathy and adrenocortical insufficiency.
- **Meningitis:** See case 1 Petechial bleeding is typical for meningococcal meningitis.

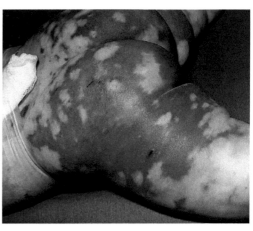

Fulminating purpura in Waterhouse–Friderichsen syndrome

Diagnostics:
- Blood picture: Leukocytosis or leukocytopenia (→ Infection), thrombocytopenia (→ consumption coagulopathy)
- Inflammation parameters: CRP, BSG, possibly Inter-leukin 6 (↑), Procalcitonin (↑)
- Kidney function parameters: Sodium, potassium, creatinine, urea (↑) with shock kidneys
- Liver values: GOT, GPT, γGT, Bilirubin (↑) with shock liver
- Coagulation tests: Quick ↓, PTT ↑, TZ ↑, Fibrinogen and AT III ↓, D-Dimers (Fibrin degradation products) ↑ suggest disseminated intravascular coagulation)
- Blood sugar ↓
- Blood gas analysis: Metabolic acidosis through peripheral hypoxia with elevated lactate
- Blood culture: For identification of pathogen
- LP for examination of cerebrospinal fluid: Cell count, spinal fluid sugar, lactate, and microscopy (*Diplo-cocci*?) to rule out meningitis, spinal fluid culture (for identification of pathogens)
- If necessary *Meningococcus* antigen evidence is pos-sible from blood, spinal fluid, skin biopsy

Treatment: The key to successful treatment of the dramatic clinical picture is the earliest diagnosis possible, and rapid and consistent intensive care treatment that concentrates not only on fighting the infection but also especially on controlling the shock event and coagulopathy (see therapy algorithm).

Prognosis: The prognosis for invasive meningococ-cus infections depends strongly on age, the patient's overall condition on admission, and the germ count when the diagnosis is established. The lethality of all invasive meningococcal disease is on average 0% and of Waterhouse–Friderichsen syndrome, 50% to 70%! **Long-term damage** after meningitis includes particularly hearing disorders, cerebral nerve paralysis, hemiplegia, seizures, psychomotor developmental disorders, and hydrocephalus. Waterhouse–Friderichsen syndrome often leaves behind scar formation on the skin and amputation of extremities.

Prophylaxis: See Comments to question 82.4. Patients who become ill with invasive meningococcus infections must remain isolated for 24 hours. According to the United States Centers for Disease Control and Prevention, all 11- to 12-year-olds should be vaccinated with a quadrivalent (serogroups A, C, W, and Y) conjugate vaccine (see case 35). Vaccines for serogroup B were licensed by the Food and Drug Administration in 2014 and 2015.

👤👤👤 ADDITIONAL TOPICS FOR STUDY GROUPS
- Hemophilus influenzae and Pneumococci infections
- Endocarditis

---

83   Idiopathic thrombocytopenic purpura (ITP)

83.1   What important differential diagnoses should you consider in this case?
- Coagulation disorders: Coagulopathy, vasculopathy or thrombocytopenia; the petechial hemorrhagic type points to a disorder or decrease in thrombocytes
- Child abuse: See case 75

83.2   What causes of thrombocytopenia do you know? What further tests are necessary?
- Autoimmune thrombocytopenia: Idiopathic thrombocytopenic purpura (ITP)
- Drug-induced thrombocytopenia: For example, through phenytoin, trimethoprim sulfamethoxazole, carbamazepine, cytostatics, heparin, etc.
- Associated thrombocytopenia in sepsis, hemolytic–uremic syndrome (see case 59), congenital infections (e.g., connatal CMV), hepatitis
- Transient bone marrow depression in a viral infection: In this case, the other cell lines are also affected so that leukocytopenia and anemia are also seen (pancytopenia)
- Bone marrow invasion in hematological-oncological diseases: Leukemia, neuroblastoma, aplastic anemia
- Hereditary thrombocytopenia such as Fanconi anemia, TAR syndrome (thrombocytopenia with radius aplasia), Wiskott–Aldrich syndrome
- Thrombocytopenia in hypersplenism: In this case, there is usually pancytopenia also
- Necessary examinations:
  - Blood picture with manual differential and where necessary cell counting of platelets, determination of LDH and uric acid (elevated values point to a malignancy), liver values (hepatitis?), and kidney values (elevated, for instance, in HUS); inflammation parameters
  - Possibly bone marrow puncture to rule out a malignancy and to determine the megakaryocyte count

83.3   Can the symptoms—persistent nosebleed and hematomas—be attributed to the decreased thrombocyte count? Which symptoms can generally occur in thrombocytopenia?
Since there is an elevated risk of hemorrhaging at platelet counts < 30,000/µL, the hemorrhagic symptoms described in the example case (hematomas and nosebleed) can be ascribed to the thrombocytopenia. When the platelet count is > 30,000/µL, an elevated tendency to bleeding need not be expected if the patient is not taking anticoagulants (e.g., ASA) or suffering from a disorder of the coagulation system (e.g., thrombocytopathy, coagulopathy). The characteristic type of bleeding for thrombocytopenia is petechiae (punctiform skin bleeding that does not disappear with pressure). Hematomas and mucosal bleeding (nosebleed, bleeding gums) are also observed. Depending on the degree of severity, there can also be gastrointestinal bleeding, more copious menstrual bleeding, bleeding in internal organs and muscles, as well as, very rarely, intracerebral hemorrhaging. If the thrombocytopenia lasts longer than 6 months, the condition is a chronic ITP.

83.4   Idiopathic thrombocytopenic purpura (ITP) is the most frequent cause of thrombocytopenia in children. Please speak briefly about the etiology, therapy, and prognosis of ITP.
- The **etiology** of ITP is largely unexplained. Days to weeks after a virus infection, autoantibodies against platelets are formed. Bonding of immunoglobulins to the surface of the thrombocytes leads to premature degradation of the thrombocytes in the hepatolienal system.
- **Treatment:** In most cases, the thrombocyte count normalizes in a matter of days to months
  - A pressure bandage or tamponade for local, external bleeding

→ Cases 83 Page 84

- Thrombocyte count > 30,000/μL and absence of bleeding tendency: outpatient follow-up, restriction of sport activities
- Thrombocyte counts between 10,000 and 30,000/μL without bleeding tendency: Inpatient observation
- Thrombocytes < 5,000/μL or marked signs of bleeding: corticosteroids (prednisone 2–5 mg/kg body weight/d or dexamethasone 0.6 mg/kg body weight/d) until the thrombocyte count rises; alternatively, immunoglobulins (400 mg/kg body weight for 5 days or 1 g/kg body weight/d for 1–2 days).

- In life-threatening emergency situations (severe gastrointestinal or intracerebral hemorrhaging) combination therapy with high-dose corticosteroids (prednisone 10–20 mg/kg body weight) and immunoglobulin (1 g/kg body weight/d) and thrombocyte concentrate (15 mL/kg body weight)
- **Prognosis:** Usually self-limiting course with normalization of all symptoms and thrombocyte count within a few weeks. In chronic ITP, spontaneous remissions without treatment are rare, one-third of chronic cases are refractory to treatment. Acutely life-threatening hemorrhages are very rare; the risk of mortality is less than 1%.

Comments

Definitions: Thrombocytopenia is a decrease of the thrombocyte count to below 150,000/μL. ITP (idiopathic thrombocytopenic purpura) is defined as an acutely presenting autoimmune thrombocytopenia in an otherwise healthy child. The bone marrow exhibits a normal or increased number of megakaryocytes; on palpation, the spleen is not enlarged.

Etiology: In ITP, for unexplained reasons, usually 1 to 4 weeks after a viral infection, thrombocyte antibodies are formed that bond to antigen structures at the surface of thrombocytes. The antibody-loaded platelets are prematurely degraded in the hepatolienal system, which significantly shortens the thrombocyte survival time.

Epidemiology: Acute ITP occurs with a frequency of 1–4/100,000; all age groups are affected. The peak age is between the ages of 2 and 4 years. Boys and girls are affected with the same frequency. Children over the age of 10 and girls are particularly affected with chronic ITP (about 20% of cases).

Symptoms: The occurrence of spontaneous bleeding is significantly dependent on the thrombocyte count. When the thrombocyte count is > 30,000/μL there is usually no increased tendency to bleed. In thrombocytopenia < 10,000/μL, spontaneous bleeding is frequently a symptom. The patient's general condition is usually not impaired. Depending on the degree of severity, there are petechiae and hematomas over the whole body. There can be mucosal bleeding such as nosebleed, bleeding gums, gastrointestinal bleeding, and intensified menstrual bleeding. Very rare complications are severe internal and intracerebral bleeding. Severe hemorrhages in the nose and gastrointestinal tract can lead to anemia (sometimes with a need for transfusions). In 20% of cases, the symptoms last longer than 6 months. This is considered chronic ITP; 5% of cases have a chronic-relapsing course.

Differential diagnoses of thrombocytopenia: See answer to question 83.1.

Diagnostics:
- Medical history: Of special interest here are virus infections in prior history, tendency to bleed, medications taken, and prior diseases.
- Detailed physical examination: Special attention should be given to hepatosplenomegaly (→ possible indication of malignancy), evidence of bleeding, and anemia symptoms (paleness, low energy, dyspnea).
- Blood examinations: Complete blood count with manual differential and if applicable, manual platelet count, LDH, uric acid, GOT, GPT, γGT, CRP, sedimentation rate.
- Urine study to rule out micro- or macrohematuria.
- **If necessary, bone marrow puncture:** With typical clinical picture and medical history, bone marrow puncture can be omitted; however, with abnormal findings like splenomegaly, lymphadenopathy, atypical blood picture or differential, as well as LDH or uric acid elevation, it is urgently necessary to rule out malignancy. If it is done, it should in every case be done before the start of steroid therapy (steroid therapy complicates establishment of a malignancy diagnosis).

Treatment: The primary goal of the treatment is to **prevent bleeding** or treat it appropriately. Normalization of the thrombocyte count is only of secondary urgency because ITP often exhibits a self-limiting course. If there is no severe or life-threatening bleeding, the first indicated measure is to wait. Low platelet counts with no symptoms also do not absolutely require treatment.
- Corticosteroids and/or immunoglobulins are used for acute bleeding; platelet concentrates are only administered in emergencies. For therapy schedule and dosages, see answer to question 83.3.
- In chronic, treatment-refractory courses with an illness course of over 1 year, with frequent, severe bleeding, a splenectomy can be considered. To protect against invasive pneumococcus infections (OPSI), the patient should be immunized against *Pneumococci* preoperatively. Postoperatively, long-term antibiotic prophylaxis with penicillin is required.

Prognosis: See answer to question 83.4.

→ Cases 83 Page 84

84.1 What can you do to quiet the situation down?

Try to establish eye contact with the boy, use body contact (e.g., touch on the shoulder) and give simple instructions in a quiet but firm tone: e.g., "Stop kicking and hitting the furniture. Please be quiet now so that I can talk to your mother."

If it is not possible to establish quiet in this way, it can be helpful to send the mother out of the room for a short time and first gather the medical history from the boy. Here too, it is important to speak with the boy calmly and firmly. The mother will probably not like going out and leaving you alone with the boy. A short explanation of why this is necessary will reassure the mother.

84.2 What disorder seems to be present here? Please describe the clinical picture.

This is probably **attention deficit hyperactivity disorder** (ADHD); rationale: decreased ability to concentrate, motor unrest, tantrums, aggressivity as evidence of disturbed impulse control

Definition: ADHD is characterized by the cardinal symptoms of attention deficit (significant impairment of the ability to concentrate and attention span, increased distractibility), **increased impulsiveness, and large (motor) restlessness.** If hyperactivity is missing, the condition is called ADD (attention-deficit disorder).

84.3 How is the diagnosis generally established?

- **Detailed medical history** regarding course of pregnancy, developmental milestones, sleep habits, snoring, medication history, prior diseases, family history (psychological disorders, drug/medication abuse, family stress/crises, upbringing, quality of parent–child relationship), social environment
- **Questionnaire** for parents, teachers/childcare workers with questions about ADHD/ADD-typical abnormalities in the child's behavior in various situations
- **Physical examination** to rule out organic causes with particular attention to developmental and grooming conditions, check of cerebral nerves and reflex status, fine motor skills and coordination, blood pressure, if appropriate, vision and hearing tests

- **EEG** to rule out a seizure disorder or organic cerebral diseases
- **Psychological examination:** Intelligence test (to rule out excessive and insufficient challenges), test of ability to concentrate, attention, attention span, memory retention, and developmental status (to determine severe developmental deficits)
- **Before the start of drug therapy:** ECG, laboratory tests (blood picture with differential, liver values, thyroid values, creatinine), measure height and weight, rule out drug abuse

84.4 What therapeutic possibilities are available?

Multimodal treatment plan with combination of various forms of therapy individually adapted to the patient: psychoeducation, i.e., counseling of parents (always!), the child (only useful once the child has reached school age), caregivers/teachers (only with parents' permission); behavioral therapy interventions in kindergarten/school; parent training; cognitive behavioral therapy for child; if appropriate, drug therapy (see Comments). Close cooperation of all disciplines involved (pediatricians and adolescent health specialists, psychologists, parents, teachers/caregivers) is useful.

84.5 The boy's grandmother considers hyperactivity "newfangled nonsense." The boy's behavior is just a matter of bad upbringing, she says. What do you think of that statement?

Case descriptions of "hyperactive" children are already known from the 19th century (among others, Zappelphilipp [Fidgety Philipp] in the book "Der Struwwelpeter" [Shockheaded Peter] by the neurologist Heinrich Hoffmann, 1845). Extensive research about the disease has been going on since the 1950s.

ADD is a disease with demonstrable functional impairment of the brain. "Poor upbringing" (e.g., lack of attention, inconsistency, lack of rules, difference of parenting styles between the two parents) can intensify ADHD but is never the cause of the problem. But upbringing can also regulate and have a positive influence on ADHD symptoms.

Comments

Definition: See answer to question 84.2.

Etiology: There are many factors inducing the disease. Family clustering suggests that there is a **genetic predisposition. Pre- and perinatal problems** such as mother's smoking, alcohol and drug consumption during pregnancy, as well as pregnancy and birth complications and low birth weight elevate the risk of ADHD. An underlying problem of

ADHD is **functional impairment of certain areas of the brain** (especially frontal lobes, basal ganglia). Imbalance in neurotransmitter metabolism (dopaminergic system) influences the self-regulation of affected persons. Because of genetic changes in dopamine receptors and presynaptic dopamine transporter, dopamine is more rapidly transported out of the synaptic gap back into the presynaptic nerve endings so that less dopamine is available for information exchange. The result is a constant flooding of stimuli expressed in the typical ADHD symptoms of impaired attention, motor hyperactivity, and impulsive behavior.

Epidemiology: ADHD is one of the most frequent psychiatric diseases in childhood and adolescence. It occurs at all social levels, with almost the same frequency all over the world. Three percent to 6% of all children between 4 and 16 years of age are affected, boys more frequently than girls. The disorder can persist into adulthood; approximately 1% to 6% of all adults are affected.

Symptoms: Children with ADHD/ADD have a diminished attention span not adequate to their age: they are agitated and distracted, do not finish a game, leave things lying around, fail to find things although they are lying directly in front of them, and forget the simplest orders. In school the children seem far away, work extremely slowly or disrupt the class, fidget, make noises, interrupt, or play the class clown. Their handwriting is illegible, their notebooks are messy, and their schoolwork is bad. The problems are often aggravated by associated impairment of individual skills (weakness in reading, spelling, and arithmetic). Homework is a daily battle between parents and child.

As a result of increased impulsivity, affected children have a tendency to tantrums and mood swings. Aggressive behavioral tendencies, leading them to injure schoolmates, are possible. And yet the aggression is not intentional; their emotions are on a rollercoaster and in the momentary rage, the child is unable to step on the brakes. For this reason, patients with this disorder are not well-liked, have no friends, and increasingly lead a life of social isolation. The basic mood of affected persons is unhappy and self-confidence dwindles. Frequent failures and conflicts often lead to secondary comorbidities: aggressive behavioral disorders, impaired social behavior, delinquency, depression, anxiety, tics (involuntary muscle twitches, usually in the face, e.g., blepharospasm).

Untreated, patients often turn to alcohol and drugs; the risk of addiction is elevated.

Differential diagnoses:
- Age-appropriate behavior of active children (especially in young children, the boundary between a still-normal urge for movement and hyperactivity is hard to define)
- Medication-induced disorders, e.g., by antiasthmatic agents, anticonvulsive agents, antihistamines, etc.
- Physical causes: Visual and hearing disorders, epilepsy, lack of sleep caused by sleep apnea syndrome, result of concussion, result of traumatic brain injury,

meningitis/encephalitis, metabolic disorder, hyperthyroidism, intoxication, allergies, asthma
- Profound developmental disorders, partial performance disorders, cognitive impairment
- Other psychological disorders: Dysfunctional social behavior, depressive diseases, oppositionally defiant behavior

Treatment: There are no hard and fast rules for the treatment of ADHD. The treatment must be adapted to the individual problems of each patient. A multimodal therapy concept is used for this purpose, based on several pillars:
- **Psychoeducation:** Extensive information and counseling for parents, patient, teachers/caregivers about the clinical picture (causes, course, treatment possibilities). The objective is to structure the patient's environment in such a way as to exert a positive effect on the ADHD.
- In **parent training**, parents receive practical tips on bringing up the child and learn behavioral treatment techniques to deal with their child. This includes the introduction of rules and their consistent application, and the use of incentive systems (e.g., token system) that reinforce the desired behavior with rewards and decrease undesirable behavior by withdrawing rewards that have already been granted. In the "downtime," children are sent out of the room for a short time if they exhibit undesirable behavior or are made to sit on a designated "quiet chair" in order to de-escalate the situation. These behavioral interventions should also be used at school and in the kindergarten, to the extent that cooperation is available.
- **Cognitive behavioral therapy** for the child: at kindergarten age, play training is used to improve play intensity and perseverance. School-age children learn self-instruction training and self-management methods. With the help of self-instruction training, they will learn how attention can be focused on real tasks and impulses can be better controlled. Action plans are developed for finding improved solutions to assigned tasks. The goal of self-management is to observe one's own behavior and to exhibit appropriate behavior in critical situations through abiding by fixed rules.
- If necessary, **drug therapy**: If the ADHD symptoms do not improve sufficiently with the above-mentioned measures, drug therapy is indicated. **Psychostimulants** (methylphenidate, amphetamine, fenethylline, etc.) are the most frequently used medications. Dopamine is sufficient for information transfer, acting by blockade of the presynaptic dopamine transporter. **Methylphenidate** is the first-line medication; it is subject to the controlled substance guidelines and may only be ordered with a controlled substance prescription. Although it does not have an intrinsic addiction potential, in combination with hard drugs, it has a stimulant effect. Contraindications include manifest psychoses, disturbed

cardiac rhythm, epilepsy, arterial hypertension. The dosage and number of daily doses are determined by the treatment objective (decrease of hyperkinetic symptoms only in school or also in the family environment?). The individual dosage is determined by titration, beginning with the lowest possible dose (daily dose usually < 1 mg/kg body weight). The most significant side effects include difficulty in falling asleep, loss of appetite, and tics. There is no risk of addiction. On the contrary: the risk of addiction in untreated patients is decreased through

stimulant therapy. **Atomoxetine**, a noradrenaline reuptake inhibitor can be used as an alternative to methylphenidate. The action and side-effect profiles correspond to those of methylphenidate. Since atomoxetine is not a stimulant, it is not subject to the controlled substance law. Other medications that can be used as first-line medications in case of contraindication or depending on symptoms are **antidepressants** (e.g., imipramine, desimipramine, bupropion), **carbamazepine**, and clonidine.

---

85   Acute hematogenous osteomyelitis

85.1 **The boy says there was no trauma. What else could be the cause of the complaint? What do you do next?**
- **Possible causes:**
  - Phlegmonous skin infection; rationale: redness, swelling, pain, slight fever
  - Osteomyelitis; rationale: pain, fever, no trauma
  - Arthritis; rationale: limited motion, pain, swelling, fever, no trauma
  - Benign or malignant bone tumor; rationale: swelling, pain, no trauma
  - Leukemia; rationale: fever, pain, no trauma
- **Further procedure:**
  - Admission of patient for further investigation
  - Blood examinations: Blood picture with differential, CRP, sedimentation rate, LDH, alkaline phosphatase
  - X-ray of the foot in two planes

85.2 **Is the mother's fear justified? Please give a brief overview of the two most frequent malignant bone tumors.**
In the differential diagnosis, a bone tumor must be ruled out (see Tab.). However, malignant bone tumors are very rare. More frequent causes such as arthritis or

osteomyelitis (frequency 3–20/100,000 persons/year) are therefore more likely.

85.3 **Please describe and interpret the abnormalities in the findings. What is your diagnosis now? Are any further studies necessary?**
- **MRI findings:** A strong signal enhancement is seen over the entire calcaneal tuberosity, caused by bone marrow edema. This finding suggests incipient osteomyelitis. In addition to medical history (pain, acute onset, missing pathogens) and clinical examination findings (slight fever, intense pain on touch, swelling, limited motion), the elevated inflammation parameters (leukocytosis, elevated sedimentation rate, and CRP) suggest an infectious source of the symptoms. A space-occupying lesion and a fracture were reliably ruled out in the X-ray. But it was not possible to rule out osteomyelitis in the normal X-ray since the typical changes (simultaneous occurrence of osteolysis and sclerosing, periostal bone neogenesis, defects in spongiosa and cortex) in this disease can only be seen radiologically from the fifth day of illness.
- **Further tests:** Two, or possibly three blood cultures before the start of treatment; if pus is found, aspiration.

	Osteosarcoma	Ewing sarcoma
Definition	Highly malignant, spindle cell tumor of the bone forming matrix	Small cell, malignant bone tumor
Epidemiology	5/1,000,000 children/year; peak age 13.5–14.5 years; m > w	2/1,000,000 children/year; peak age 10–14 years; m > w
Location	In 85% of cases, metaphysis of the long, hollow bones, usually in the knee region (distal femur, proximal tibia), proximal humerus, ilium, rarely involvement of the trunk	Usually proceeding from the diaphysis and skeleton of the trunk; the most frequent primary locations are pelvis, femur, and thoracic wall
Symptoms	Intermittent pain and swelling, possibly redness and overly warm, limited function	Swelling, pain, signs of local inflammation, possibly leukocytosis, anemia, fever, elevated LDH

	Osteosarcoma	Ewing sarcoma
Metastases	Early hematogenous in lungs, skeleton	Early hematogenous in lungs, skeleton, bone marrow
Primary diagnostics	**X-ray:** Osteosarcoma: Destruction, irregular bone neogenesis, spicules (infiltration of surrounding soft tissue), Codman triangle (periosteum raising) Ewing sarcoma: Bone necroses resembling moth holes, onion-skin calcifications **MRI:** Extent of tumor **Laboratory:** Elevated LDH and AP (→ indication of poor prognosis) **Bone biopsy:** Confirmation of diagnosis	
Staging	Thoracic X-ray Spiral-CT (Thorax) Skeletal scintigraphy Ewing sarcoma in addition: Bone marrow puncture at two sites outside the primary tumor with histology, cytology, and molecular biology	
Treatment	Combination of neoadjuvant chemotherapy, local surgical treatment and adjuvant polychemotherapy; unsuccessful radiation, since osteosarcoma is not sensitive to radiation	Combination of chemotherapy, radiation, and/or surgical treatment
Prognosis	5-year survival rate 60%, poor in the presence of metastasis	5-year survival rate 60%–70%, worse with disseminated disease

85.4 How is the disease treated?

- **Intravenous antibiotic therapy:** Begins with calculated antibiotic treatment with a good combination of antibiotics commonly used for bone (e.g., clindamycin), later change after antibiogram over a course of 2 to 4 weeks
- If needed, **surgical interventions:** Drainage, debridement of foci, necrosectomy
- Supportive decrease **in load bearing and elevation** of the extremity
- **Pain therapy**

Comments

Definition: Osteomyelitis is an infection of the bone marrow and the surrounding bone tissue caused by bacteria or, more rarely, fungi. A distinction is made between acute (duration of disease < 14 days) and the chronic form (duration of disease > 14 days).

Etiology: The **pathogen invasion** into the bone marrow is usually blood-borne, starting, e.g., from inflammation in the nasopharyngeal area, pneumonia, or skin infection, and in newborns, navel infection. Osteomyelitis can also occur post-traumatically, e.g., after (open) fractures, operations, or introduced foreign bodies. The chief manifestation site is the metaphysis of the long trabecular bones (especially femur and tibia): the phalanges (3% of cases) are more rarely affected. Osteomyelitis can also occur in the vertebral bodies. Up to 2 years of age, osteomyelitis is very frequently associated with purulent arthritis because of certain anatomical relationships. At this age, the epiphysis does not yet have a barrier function because it is supplied by the same blood vessels as the metaphysis. As a result, there is a direct spread of the infection from the metaphysis to the joint.

The **pathogen spectrum** is age-dependent. After infancy, osteomyelitis is primarily caused by *Staphylococci*, followed by *Streptococci*, *Pneumococci*, and *Kingella kingae*. Fungi or specific pathogens such as *Mycobacterium tuberculosis* (especially in vertebral body osteomyelitis) can occasionally be identified as pathogens. *Hemophilus influenzae* is only of importance in infants since the introduction of Hib immunization. In newborns, there are also the typical pathogens of newborn sepsis (*B streptococci, E. coli*), in premature babies, coagulase-negative *Staphylococci*, fungi, and Gram-negative pathogens can also be detected.

Symptoms: Signs of **local inflammation** such as redness, swelling, excess heat with limited function and pain must suggest osteomyelitis. These signs can be associated with reduced overall condition and fever, running as far as sepsis-like symptoms. In advanced or **chronic courses** with periostal abscesses, formation of fistulas to the skin can be observed.

→ Cases 85 Page 86

In newborns and infants, the symptoms are often less characteristic: Possibly lack of motion in the affected extremity can be observed, especially with associated septic arthritis. Passive movement causes pain. In 50% of cases, osteomyelitis in infants presents multifocally.

Diagnostics:
- **Laboratory:** CRP and sedimentation rate are usually markedly elevated, leukocytosis is found in only about half the cases, but a left-shift in the blood picture is almost always present.
- **Evidence of germs:** Before the start of antibiotic therapy. In half of cases, this succeeds with (two to three) blood cultures but there are better results with pathogen detection in puncture material. A puncture should be done where there is evidence of pus and in any case where there is no response to therapy or a chronic disease course.
- **X-ray** (obligatory): To demarcation of malignant processes and fracture and to monitor the course of the disease. In the early phase of the infection, the radiograph can often still be unremarkable; changes are seen approximately after 5 days at the earliest (with adequate and early therapy, it may be that the changes are completely invisible in the X-ray).
- **Sonography:** Especially suitable for early diagnosis. Soft tissue edema, subperiostal abscess formation, and possibly associated septic arthritis can be well visualized with this technique.
- **MRI:** Because of high sensitivity and specificity, technique of first choice for early diagnosis. The bone marrow edema of the early phase and the displacement of the marrow-containing bone marrow by inflammatory exudate can be reliably visualized.
- ^{99m}Tc scintigraphy (optional): This is particularly suitable for detection of multilocal foci.

Differential diagnoses: In addition to trauma (aseptic and septic) arthritis, and phlegmonous skin infections, benign and malignant bone tumors in particular must be ruled out. The most frequently occurring bone tumors in children and adolescents are osteosarcoma and Ewing sarcoma (see Tab.).

Treatment of acute hematogenous osteomyelitis: The diagnosis must be established as early as possible so that an **adequate antibiotic therapy** can be rapidly started. Delays can mean transition to chronic osteomyelitis and make surgical interventions necessary. Antibiotic therapy is more difficult and protracted than for many other infections since only a few antibiotics can penetrate into the bone and accumulate to sufficiently effective levels of activity. The first-line preparation is **clindamycin** (40 mg/kg body weight in three individual doses for 2–4 weeks). Because of the increasing resistance of *Staphylococcus aureus*, clindamycin can be combined with **rifampicin** (10–15 mg/kg body weight in one dose) or **fosfomycin** (3 × 50–80 mg/kg body weight/d).

Alternatively, **Staphylococcus-active cephalosporins** at high doses (e.g., cefuroxime 150–200 mg/kg body weight/d in three individual doses) can be used as monotherapy.

In infants, clindamycin is not sufficient because of the insufficient efficacy against *Haemophilus influenzae* and other Gram-negative germs. Here combinations with cefotaxim or aminoglycosides are useful. In newborns, the treatment should be like that for an amniotic infection syndrome (see case 69). Thought must be given to the medication's ability to penetrate bone, and selection of an appropriate antibiotic combination. If it is possible to detect a pathogen, the antibiotic treatment must be adapted to the resistance determination. Depending on the course, a **surgical intervention** may be necessary in order to clear osteomyelitic foci or remove necrotic material. Particularly in a chronic course, the instillation-suction technique may have to be applied. Often, several revisions are necessary. Septic joint involvement requires primary surgical intervention in order to unburden the joint and prevent permanent joint damage. Adjuvant therapy consisted of local cooling measures, unburdening or immobilization and elevation of the affected extremity and analgesia.

Prognosis: The prognosis of acute hematogenous osteomyelitis is usually good; 80% of cases heal with consistent antibiotic treatment with no sequelae. If the epiphysis is involved, there can be growth impairment in the affected extremity. If the antibiotic treatment is insufficient, transition into chronic osteomyelitis with sequester formation and fistula development is a possibility.

ADDITIONAL TOPICS FOR STUDY GROUPS
- Osteomyelitis caused by specific pathogens
- Benign bone tumors
- Chronic relapsing multifocal osteomyelitis (CRMO)

Appendix

Source of Images

Table of Contents, Section opener Cases
Deichmann, A., Herbolzheim, Germany

Case 1
Kurz, R., Roos, R., Checkliste Pädiatrie, 2. Auflage, Georg Thieme Verlag, Stuttgart, New York, 2000

Case 4
Niessen, K.-H., Pädiatrie, 6. Auflage, Georg Thieme Verlag, Stuttgart, New York, 2001

Case 6
Baumann, T., Atlas der Entwicklungsdiagnostik, Georg Thieme Verlag, Stuttgart, New York, 2002

Case 7
Kayser, F. H. et al., Medizinische Mikrobiologie, 9. Auflage, Georg Thieme Verlag, Stuttgart, New York, 1998
Toppe, E., GK3 Dermatologie, 15. Auflage, Georg Thieme Verlag, Stuttgart, New York, 2003

Case 8
Siegenthaler, W., Differentialdiagnose innerer Krankheiten, 18. Auflage, Georg Thieme Verlag, Stuttgart, New York, 2000

Case 9
Hertl, M., Der Gesichtsausdruck des Kranken, Georg Thieme Verlag, Stuttgart, New York, 1993
Kurz, R., Roos, R., Checkliste Pädiatrie, 2. Auflage, Georg Thieme Verlag, Stuttgart, New York, 2000

Case 11
Neurath, M., Lohse, A., Checkliste Anamnese und klinische Untersuchung, Georg Thieme Verlag, Stuttgart, New York, 2002
Probst, R. et al., Hals-Nasen-Ohren-Heilkunde, Georg Thieme Verlag, Stuttgart, New York, 2000

Case 12
Jung, E. G., Moll, I., Duale Reihe Dermatologie, 5. Auflage, Georg Thieme Verlag, Stuttgart, New York, 2003

Case 13
Kayser, F. H. et al., Medizinische Mikrobiologie, 9. Auflage, Georg Thieme Verlag, Stuttgart, New York, 1998

Sitzmann, F. C., Duale Reihe Pädiatrie, 2. Auflage, Georg Thieme Verlag, Stuttgart, New York, 2002

Case 15
Sitzmann, F. C., Duale Reihe Pädiatrie, 2. Auflage, Georg Thieme Verlag, Stuttgart, New York, 2002

Case 16
Benz-Bohm, G., Kinderradiologie, Georg Thieme Verlag, Stuttgart, New York, 1997

Case 17
Hoehl, M., Kullick, P. (Hrsg.), Kinderkrankenpflege und Gesundheitsförderung, 2. Auflage, Georg Thieme Verlag Stuttgart, New York, 2002

Case 19
Betke K. et al. (Hrsg.), Lehrbuch der Kinderheilkunde, 6. Auflage, Georg Thieme Verlag, Stuttgart, New York, 1991

Case 20
Hertl, M., Der Gesichtsausdruck des Kranken, Georg Thieme Verlag, Stuttgart, New York, 1993
Pfleiderer, A. et al., Gynäkologie und Geburtshilfe, 3. Auflage, Georg Thieme Verlag, Stuttgart, New York, 2000

Case 22
Niessen, K.-H., Pädiatrie, 6. Auflage, Georg Thieme Verlag, Stuttgart, New York, 2001

Case 24
Dörner, K., Klinische Chemie und Hämatologie, 4. Auflage, Georg Thieme Verlag, Stuttgart, New York, 2001

Case 25
Emmrich, P. et al., Notfälle im Kindesalter, 12. Auflage, George Thieme Verlag, Stuttgart, New York, 1998
Sitzmann, F. C., Duale Reihe Pädiatrie, 2. Auflage, Georg Thieme Verlag, Stuttgart, New York, 2002

Case 26
Rossi, E. et al., Pädiatrie, 3. Auflage, Georg Thieme Verlag, Stuttgart, New York, 1997

274

→ Table of Contents, Section opener Cases Continued ▶

Case 27

Remschmidt, H., Kinder- und Jugendpsychiatrie, 3. Auflage, Georg Thieme Verlag, Stuttgart, New York, 1999

Case 29

Rettenmaier, G., Seitz, K. (Hrsg.), Sonographische Differentialdiagnostik Band 1, Georg Thieme Verlag, Stuttgart, New York, 2000

Case 30

Mach, K., Dermatologie, Ferdinand Enke Verlag, Stuttgart, 1995

Case 31

Frey, G., GK3 Pädiatrie, 14. Auflage, Georg Thieme Verlag, Stuttgart, New York, 2001

Case 32

Murken, J., Cleve, H., Humangenetik, 6. Auflage, Ferdinand Enke Verlag, Stuttgart, 1995
Rossi, E. et al., Pädiatrie, 3. Auflage, Georg Thieme Verlag, Stuttgart, New York, 1997

Case 33

Baumann, T., Atlas der Entwicklungsdiagnostik, Georg Thieme Verlag, Stuttgart, New York, 2002
(2×) Ebel, K.-D. et al. (Hrsg.), Differenzialdiagnostik in der Pädiatrischen Radiologie, Bd. 1, Georg Thieme Verlag, Stuttgart, New York, 1995
Sitzmann, F. C., Duale Reihe Pädiatrie, 2. Auflage, Georg Thieme Verlag, Stuttgart, New York, 2002

Case 34

Hof, H., Dörries, R., Duale Reihe Mikrobiologie, 2. Auflage, Georg Thieme Verlag, Stuttgart, New York, 2002

Case 39

Hof, H., Dörries, R., Duale Reihe Mikrobiologie, 2. Auflage, Georg Thieme Verlag, Stuttgart, New York, 2002
Mach, K., Dermatologie, Ferdinand Enke Verlag, Stuttgart, 1995

Case 40

Murken, J., Cleve, H., Humangenetik, 6. Auflage, Ferdinand Enke Verlag, Stuttgart, 1995

Case 41

Jung, E. G., Moll, I., Duale Reihe Dermatologie, 5. Auflage, Georg Thieme Verlag, Stuttgart, New York, 2003

(2X) Sterry, W., Paus, R., Checkliste Dermatologie, 3. Auflage, Georg Thieme Verlag, Stuttgart, New York, 1999

Case 44

Benz-Bohm, G., Kinderradiologie, Georg Thieme Verlag, Stuttgart, New York, 1997
Merkle, W. (Hrsg.), Duale Reihe Urologie, Georg Thieme Verlag, Stuttgart, New York, 1997

Case 45

Dörner, K., Klinische Chemie und Hämatologie, 4. Auflage, Georg Thieme Verlag, Stuttgart, New York, 2001
Rossi, E. et al., Pädiatrie, 3. Auflage, Georg Thieme Verlag, Stuttgart, New York, 1997

Case 47

Niessen, K.-H., Pädiatrie, 6. Auflage, Georg Thieme Verlag, Stuttgart, New York, 2001
Siegenthaler, W. (Hrsg.), Klinische Pathophysiologie, 7. Auflage, Georg Thieme Verlag, Stuttgart, New York, 1994

Case 48

Baenkler, H.-W. et al., Duale Reihe Innere Medizin, Georg Thieme Verlag, Stuttgart, New York, 1999

Case 49

Masuhr, K. F., Neumann, M., Duale Reihe Neurologie, 3. Auflage, Hippokrates Verlag GmbH, 1996

Case 51

Laer, L. von, Frakturen und Luxationen im Wachstumsalter, 3. Auflage, Georg Thieme Verlag, Stuttgart, New York, 1996
Schumpelick, V. et al. (Hrsg.), Kurzlehrbuch Chirurgie, 6. Auflage, Georg Thieme Verlag, Stuttgart, New York, 2003

Case 55

Roos, R. et al., Checkliste Neonatologie, Georg Thieme Verlag, Stuttgart, New York, 2003

Case 57

Niessen, K.-H., Pädiatrie, 6. Auflage, Georg Thieme Verlag, Stuttgart, New York, 2001

Case 59

Dörner, K., Klinische Chemie und Hämatologie, 4. Auflage, Georg Thieme Verlag, Stuttgart, New York, 2001

→ Table of Contents, Section opener Cases Continued ▶

Case 60

(2×) Hofmann, V. et al., Ultraschalldiagnostik in Pädiatrie und Kinderchirurgie, 2. Auflage, Georg Thieme Verlag, Stuttgart, New York, 1996
(4×) Sitzmann, F. C., Duale Reihe Pädiatrie, 2. Auflage, Georg Thieme Verlag, Stuttgart, New York, 2002

Case 62

Schmidt, G. (Hrsg.), Checkliste Sonographie, 2. Auflage, Georg Thieme Verlag, Stuttgart, New York, 1999

Case 65

Schulte am Esch, J. et al., Duale Reihe Anästhesie und Intensivmedizin, Georg Thieme Verlag, Stuttgart, New York, 2000

Case 68

Füßl, H. S., Middeke, M., Duale Reihe Anamnese und körperliche Untersuchung, 2. Auflage, Georg Thieme Verlag, Stuttgart, New York, 2002
Kruse, K., Pädiatrische Endokrinologie, 2. Auflage, Georg Thieme Verlag, Stuttgart, New York, 1999

Case 74

Niessen, K.-H., Pädiatrie, 6. Auflage, Georg Thieme Verlag, Stuttgart, New York, 2001

Case 75

Baumann, T., Atlas der Entwicklungsdiagnostik, Georg Thieme Verlag, Stuttgart, New York, 2002

Case 76

Hirner, A., Weise, K., Chirurgie Schnitt für Schnitt, Georg Thieme Verlag, Stuttgart, New York, 2003
Schumpelick, V. et al. (Hrsg.), Kurzlehrbuch Chirurgie, 6. Auflage, Georg Thieme Verlag, Stuttgart, New York, 2003

Case 79

Abeck, D., Fölster-Holst, R., Was hilft meinem Kind bei Neurodermitis? Georg Thieme Verlag, Stuttgart, New York, 2003
Sterry, W., Paus, R., Checkliste Dermatologie, 3. Auflage, Georg Thieme Verlag, Stuttgart, New York, 1999

Case 80

Kurz, R., Roos, R., Checkliste Pädiatrie, 2. Auflage, Georg Thieme Verlag, Stuttgart, New York, 2000
Neurath, M., Lohse, A., Checkliste Anamnese und klinische Untersuchung, Georg Thieme Verlag, Stuttgart, New York, 2002

Case 81

Hofmann, V. et al., Ultraschalldiagnostik in Pädiatrie und Kinderchirurgie, 2. Auflage, Georg Thieme Verlag, Stuttgart, New York, 1996

Case 82

Sitzmann, F. C., Duale Reihe Pädiatrie, 3. Auflage, Georg Thieme Verlag, Stuttgart, New York, 2007

→ Table of Contents, Section Opener Cases

Forms of juvenile idiopathic arthritis (JIA)

	Clinical signs	Laboratory	Peak age	Characteristics
Still syndrome	• High fever • Exanthema • Lymphadenopathy • Organ involvement (esp. hepato-/splenomegaly, polyserositis, perimyocarditis) • No joint involvement until disease progresses	• Inflammatory parameters (leukocytes, CRP, sedimentation rate) ↑ ↑ ↑ • Platelets ↑ • RF negative • ANA negative	1–4 years	• f > m • 10–20% of all JIA
RF-negative polyarthritis	• More than five or five joints affected over a period of 6 months • Symmetrical involvement of large and small joints	• Inflammatory parameters (leukocytes, CRP, sedimentation rate) ↑ ↑ ↑ • RF negative • ANA positive in 25% of cases	2–5 years	• f >> m • 20–25% of all JIA can be cured
RF-positive polyarthritis	• More than five or five joints affected over a period of 6 months • Symmetrical involvement of large and small joints • Early destructive arthritic nodes • Organ involvement (hepatomegaly, polyserositis)	• Inflammatory parameters (leukocytes, CRP, sedimentation rate) ↑ ↑ ↑ • RF positive • ANA positive in 75% of cases	More than 12 years	• f >> m • 5–10% of all JIA are not cured
Oligoarthritis	• Less than four or four joints involved over a period of 6 months • Asymmetrical involvement of large joints	• Inflammatory parameters ↑ • ANA positive	2–4 years	• f >> m • Accounts for 50–60% of all JIA • After 6 months, classification as persistent (< five joints) and extended oligoarthritis (> five joints; caution: often iridocyclitis)

Psoriatic arthritis	• 1. Arthritis + psoriasis or
	• 2. Arthritis + at least 2 of the following criteria:
	  – Dactylitis
	  – Abnormal fingernails
	  – Confirmed psoriasis in a first degree relative
		• Inflammatory parameters ↑
		• RF negative
		• ANA positive
		• HLA B27 frequently positive
			6–14 years	• f > m
				• Accounts fir 5–10% of all JIA

JIA with enthesitis	• 1. Arthritis in one or more joints and enthesitis or
	• 2. Arthritis + at least two of the following criteria:
	  – Inflammatory lumbago/sacroileitis
	  – Onset of the arthritis in boys < 8 years
	  – HLA B27 positive
	  – Anterior uveitis
	  – HLA B27-associated disease in a first degree relative
		• Inflammatory parameters ↑
		• RF negative
		• ANA negative
		• HLA B27 frequently positive
			6–14 years	• w > m
				• Accounts for 5–10% of all JIA

Abbreviations: ANA, antinuclear antibodies; CRP, C reactive protein; HLA, human leukocyte antigen; RF, rheumatoid factor.

→ Forms of juvenile idiopathic arthritis (JIA)

Viral infections

Disease	Pathogen	Incubation time	Symptoms	Treatment	Complications
Varicella	Varicella zoster virus	14–16 (21) days	Numerous efflorescences (papules, blisters, pustules, scabs) in various stages ("star map") on skin and mucosa, associated fever and catarrh symptoms possible	• Symptomatic: zinc- or tannin-containing anti-itch suspensions, antihistamines • In case of immunodeficiency or complications acyclovir (30–45 mg/kg body weight/d i.v.) • In case of bacterial superinfection, antibiotic therapy	Secondary bacterial infections (impetigo, abscesses, phlegmones, necrotizing fasciitis), cerebellitis, encephalitis, meningitis, cerebral vasculitis hepatitis, arthritis, myocarditis, a severe course in patients with poor resistance and newborns
Measles	Measles virus	8–12 days	Two-phase course: prodromal stage with fever, catarrhal symptoms, conjunctivitis, Koplik spots on cheek mucosa, enanthem, repeated rise in fever after 3 to 4 days with outbreak of typical exanthema	• Symptomatic • Antibiotic therapy in case of bacterial superinfection	Transitory decrease in immunity, secondary bacterial infection (pneumonia, otitis media), croup, measles encephalitis, subacute sclerosing panencephalitis
Mumps	Mumps virus	12–25 days	Fever, uni- or bilateral parotitis, inflammation of other salivary glands, possibly pancreatitis	• Symptomatic • Antibiotic therapy in case of bacterial superinfection	Aseptic meningitis, encephalitis, orchitis, epididymitis, myocarditis
Rubella	Rubella virus	14–21 days	Prodromal stage with flu-like symptoms, discrete maculopapulous exanthema, starting in the face and spreading over the body and extremities, associated lymph node swelling retroauricular and occipital, sometimes slight fever, arthralgia	• Symptomatic	Thrombocytopenic purpura, encephalitis, danger of rubella embryopathy (Gregg's syndrome) in case of first infection during pregnancy
Erythema infectiosum	Parvovirus B19	4–14 days	Influenza-like prodromal stage, very variable, maculopapulous exanthema, starting at the cheeks ("slapped cheek disease"), spreading over the body and extremities, typical wreath or screen pattern (duration 1–7 weeks), occasionally associated arthralgia	• Symptomatic	Rarely hepatitis, myocarditis, aseptic meningitis and encephalitis, polyarthritis, aplastic crises in patients with hemolytic anemia In case of first infection during pregnancy, there is danger of miscarriage, stillbirth, hydrops fetalis, fetal myocarditis
Three-day fever (exanthema subitum)	Human herpes virus 6	5–15 days	Usually in infants and young toddlers, high fever for 3 (to 5) days; when fever subsides, maculopapulous exanthema, frequently associated with gastroenteritis, eyelid edema, cough, cervical lympadenopathy, bulging fontanelle; in older children mononucleosis–like clinical picture	• Adequate antipyretic therapy	Fever seizures, rarely, meningoencephalitis, Guillain–Barre syndrome

→ Childhood Diseases Continued ▶

Bacterial infections

Scarlet fever	β-hemolyz-ing group A streptococci	2–4 days	High fever, reduced general condition, possible vomiting, pharyngeal enanthem, tonsillopharyngitis, raspberry tongue, small-spotted, sand paper-like exanthema, especially in the groin, absent periorally, coarsely lamellar scaling on hands and feet	Penicillin V (50,000–100,000 IU/kg body weight/d) for 10 days, alternatively cephalospo-rine, macrolides	Peritonsillar and retropharyngeal abscess, otitis media, sinusitis, purulent lymphad-enitis colli, acute rheumatic fever, acute glomerulonephritis, chorea minor
Whoop-ing cough (pertussis)	Bordetella per-tussis, Bordetella parapertussis	7–10 days	Stages: • Catarrhal stage: lasts 1–2 weeks, mild respiratory symptoms such as rhinitis and cough • Convulsive stage: lasts 4–6 weeks; typical, staccato cough attacks, usu-ally at night, followed by inspiratory wheezing, regurgitation of thick mucus, and vomiting • Fading stage: gradual decrease of symptoms, atypical course in youths and adults	• For infants younger than 6 months, in-pa-tient monitoring (assessment of apnea) • Antibiotic treatment with erythromycin (40–60 mg/kg body weight/d in three doses) affects the course only if administered early (catarrhal stage and start of convulsive stage), patient's infectiousness is terminated with antibiotic administration in all stages	Secondary infection such as pneumonia and otitis media, danger of life-threatening apnea in newborns and younger infants with risk of encephalopathy

→ Childhood Diseases

Body mass index (BMI [kg/m²]) girls

Age (years)	N	Mean value	Standard deviation	Min	3%	10%	25%	50%	75%	90%	97%	Max
Birth	112	13.19	1.270	9.81	10.55	11.66	12.50	13.21	14.03	14.80	15.25	16.45
1 mo	108	13.36	0.945	11.08	11.44	12.10	12.82	13.33	13.95	14.53	14.99	15.88
3 mo	108	15.30	1.011	13.01	13.56	14.03	14.56	15.36	15.87	16.67	17.52	17.76
6 mo	111	16.45	1.234	13.62	14.25	15.01	15.57	16.43	17.30	17.88	19.02	19.42
9 mo	109	16.84	1.324	13.77	14.56	15.03	15.99	16.88	17.73	18.36	19.50	20.51
1	108	17.14	1.335	13.63	14.71	15.35	16.19	17.20	18.00	18.80	19.75	20.49
1.5	107	16.83	1.351	14.08	14.75	15.16	15.94	16.62	17.65	18.53	19.36	21.44
2	107	16.16	1.242	13.10	14.11	14.74	15.46	16.11	16.87	17.58	18.65	20.66
2.5		15.85	1.224	13.06	13.80	14.33	15.08	15.77	16.51	17.42	18.20	19.98
3	110	15.54	1.206	13.02	13.49	13.92	14.70	15.43	16.15	17.26	17.75	19.30
3.5		15.38	1.200	12.63	13.45	13.84	14.55	15.28	16.01	17.00	17.59	19.38
4	110	15.22	1.194	12.25	13.41	13.76	14.40	15.12	15.88	16.75	17.42	19.47
4.5		15.19	1.197	12.29	13.36	13.74	14.37	15.09	15.86	16.67	17.46	19.46
5	110	15.16	1.200	12.33	13.30	13.71	14.35	15.06	15.85	16.60	17.49	19.45
5.5		15.16	1.226	12.18	13.25	13.69	14.33	15.06	15.86	16.59	17.65	18.99
6	111	15.16	1.252	12.03	13.19	13.67	14.32	15.06	15.87	16.58	17.81	18.54
6.5		15.23	1.309	12.02	13.18	13.70	14.34	15.12	15.94	16.68	18.11	19.43
7	112	15.29	1.365	12.01	13.16	13.72	14.36	15.18	16.01	16.78	18.41	20.33
7.5		15.41	1.447	11.87	13.18	13.80	14.42	15.28	16.15	17.02	18.77	20.52
8	112	15.53	1.528	11.74	13.20	13.88	14.47	15.38	16.29	17.26	19.13	20.70
8.5		15.71	1.629	11.99	13.27	13.98	14.59	15.53	16.49	17.61	19.59	21.27
9	111	15.90	1.730	12.25	13.35	14.08	14.70	15.68	16.69	17.96	20.04	21.84
9.5	111	16.12	1.841	12.39	13.46	14.20	14.84	15.88	16.96	18.35	20.56	22.91
10	111	16.37	1.950	12.25	13.59	14.33	15.00	16.10	17.27	18.77	21.06	23.14
10.5	111	16.65	2.052	12.12	13.71	14.49	15.18	16.36	17.61	19.21	21.51	23.03
11	109	16.96	2.149	12.71	13.84	14.69	15.38	16.67	18.02	19.70	21.91	22.87
11.5	112	17.31	2.240	13.00	14.00	14.94	15.62	17.04	18.49	20.22	22.27	24.68
12	111	17.69	2.315	13.19	14.22	15.23	15.89	17.47	19.01	20.71	22.60	24.63
12.5	109	18.10	2.372	13.53	14.51	15.56	16.20	17.91	19.52	21.17	22.93	25.57
13	112	18.50	2.412	13.64	14.87	15.92	16.57	18.35	20.01	21.61	23.32	25.78
13.5	110	18.90	2.441	13.93	15.25	16.28	16.97	18.74	20.46	21.99	23.76	28.10
14	112	19.27	2.464	14.24	15.60	16.63	17.37	19.09	20.84	22.33	24.27	27.47
14.5	110	19.59	2.483	14.44	15.88	16.94	17.75	19.37	21.12	22.60	24.81	27.55
15	111	19.85	2.501	14.60	16.10	17.19	18.07	19.57	21.30	22.81	25.34	28.90
15.5	104	20.05	2.517	15.07	16.25	17.39	18.33	19.72	21.40	23.00	25.75	28.63
16	108	20.20	2.530	15.28	16.37	17.55	18.53	19.84	21.44	23.22	26.00	29.56
16.5		20.30	2.537	15.54	16.46	17.66	18.64	19.93	21.44	23.40	26.02	29.01
17	109	20.40	2.543	15.80	16.55	17.78	18.75	20.03	21.45	23.59	26.04	28.46
17.5		20.44	2.561	15.88	16.61	17.83	18.77	20.10	21.45	23.63	25.94	28.85
18	110	20.48	2.579	15.95	16.67	17.88	18.79	20.17	21.45	23.67	25.83	29.23
18.5		20.49	2.607	15.94	16.73	17.88	18.77	20.20	21.48	23.63	25.68	31.74
19	109	20.50	2.636	15.93	16.79	17.88	18.75	20.22	21.51	23.60	25.53	34.25
19.5		20.49	2.644	15.94	16.86	17.85	18.72	20.21	21.56	23.53	25.41	34.25
20	108	20.49	2.652	15.95	16.94	17.83	18.69	20.20	21.61	23.46	25.28	34.25
Adult	111	20.47	2.631	15.95	17.07	17.79	18.69	20.14	21.73	23.32	25.12	34.25

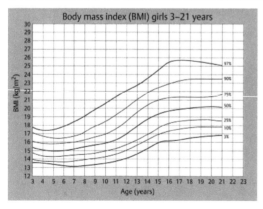

Body mass index (BMI) girls 3–21 years

→ Body Mass Index Continued ▶

Body mass index (BMI [kg/m²]) boys

Age (years)	N	Mean value	Standard deviation	Min	3%	10%	25%	50%	75%	90%	97%	Max
Birth	119	12.95	1.27	9.88	10.33	11.47	12.16	12.99	13.70	14.38	15.25	16.37
1 mo	114	13.45	0.93	10.99	11.79	12.36	12.80	13.45	14.03	14.51	14.97	16.70
3 mo	114	15.51	1.39	12.02	12.70	13.81	14.78	15.50	16.41	17.27	18.03	18.92
6 mo	118	16.54	1.33	13.43	14.10	14.51	15.65	16.67	17.52	18.15	18.73	19.19
9 mo	115	17.11	1.38	14.25	14.73	15.33	16.18	17.15	18.12	18.76	19.39	21.50
1	118	17.41	1.50	13.98	14.87	15.59	16.43	17.36	18.26	19.41	20.26	22.83
1.5	118	17.27	1.38	14.23	14.97	15.40	16.23	17.31	18.14	18.98	19.83	21.98
2	115	16.51	1.23	13.97	14.43	15.02	15.60	16.40	17.37	18.14	18.82	20.43
2.5		16.16	1.18	13.43	14.17	14.65	15.27	16.15	16.98	17.72	18.28	19.72
3	117	15.80	1.12	12.89	13.91	14.29	14.94	15.90	16.59	17.31	17.74	19.01
3.5		15.60	1.13	12.75	13.68	14.12	14.74	15.66	16.41	17.15	17.59	18.52
4	117	15.39	1.13	12.62	13.45	13.95	14.54	15.42	16.22	16.98	17.43	18.03
4.5		15.35	1.13	12.53	13.42	13.93	14.53	15.34	16.19	16.91	17.36	17.87
5	117	15.30	1.12	12.44	13.38	13.90	14.52	15.25	16.15	16.85	17.28	17.72
5.5		15.29	1.14	12.37	13.35	13.89	14.51	15.20	16.14	16.82	17.33	17.76
6	117	15.28	1.15	12.29	13.32	13.88	14.50	15.14	16.12	16.80	17.38	17.80
6.5		15.31	1.19	12.38	13.32	13.91	14.51	15.15	16.14	16.84	17.56	18.52
7	118	15.34	1.23	12.47	13.31	13.93	14.52	15.15	16.16	16.88	17.74	19.23
7.5		15.42	1.28	12.51	13.34	13.98	14.57	15.22	16.23	17.02	18.02	19.62
8	120	15.50	1.33	12.56	13.38	14.02	14.61	15.28	16.29	17.17	18.29	20.00
8.5		15.63	1.40	12.59	13.45	14.11	14.70	15.40	16.44	17.41	18.66	20.70
9	119	15.76	1.46	12.62	13.53	14.19	14.79	15.51	16.58	17.64	19.02	21.39
9.5		15.94	1.55	12.78	13.63	14.31	14.91	15.66	16.79	17.95	19.44	21.47
10	118	16.12	1.63	12.94	13.72	14.42	15.03	15.81	17.01	18.26	19.86	21.56
10.5	118	16.33	1.72	12.70	13.81	14.55	15.1·8	15.99	17.25	18.61	20.31	23.18
11	120	16.55	1.80	13.10	13.90	14.69	15.35	16.17	17.52	18.97	20.75	23.18
11.5	117	16.79	1.89	13.16	14.01	14.85	15.53	16.38	17.81	19.35	21.15	23.22
12	120	17.04	1.96	13.44	14.14	15.02	15.74	16.60	18.12	19.72	21.50	23.54
12.5	119	17.32	2.01	13.47	14.31	15.21	15.97	16.86	18.46	20.07	21.78	23.33
13	119	17.62	2.05	13.52	14.50	15.44	16.23	17.17	18.83	20.41	22.03	26.00
13.5	120	17.95	2.06	13.50	14.75	15.73	16.53	17.53	19.24	20.73	22.29	24.13
14	120	18.30	2.06	13.81	15.06	16.06	16.86	17.91	19.66	21.03	22.60	23.28
14.5	120	18.67	2.06	13.73	15.41	16.42	17.21	18.30	20.09	21.32	22.97	25.16
15	120	19.03	2.06	13.87	15.80	16.78	17.55	18.67	20.50	21.62	23.34	25.08
15.5	120	19.37	2.07	13.67	16.18	17.13	17.88	19.00	20.87	21.92	23.67	25.89
16	119	19.69	2.09	14.16	16.51	17.45	18.17	19.29	21.20	22.25	23.98	27.02
16.5		19.95	2.13	14.41	16.75	17.70	18.40	19.51	21.47	22.61	24.31	26.57
17	120	20.22	2.17	14.65	16.99	17.95	18.63	19.74	21.74	22.96	24.64	26.12
17.5		20.43	2.24	15.09	17.15	18.13	18.80	19.90	21.95	23.30	25.05	27.47
18	119	20.63	2.32	15.53	17.30	18.30	18.97	20.06	22.15	23.65	25.45	28.83
18.5		20.79	2.39	15.67	17.39	18.40	19.11	20.19	22.31	23.90	25.78	29.87
19	119	20.95	2.46	15.82	17.48	18.51	19.24	20.33	22.46	24.15	26.11	30.91
19.5		21.07	2.49	15.70	17.50	18.56	19.36	20.46	22.60	24.33	26.20	30.66
20	112	21.19	2.53	15.58	17.52	18.62	19.47	20.59	22.73	24.51	26.29	30.41
Adult	117	21.40	2.54	15.58	17.60	18.70	19.71	20.86	22.97	24.77	26.22	29.98

281

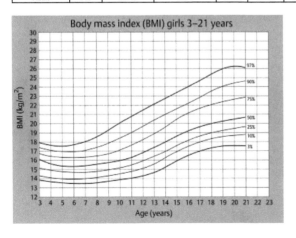

Body mass index (BMI) girls 3–21 years

→ Body Mass Index

Important reference values				
Laboratory values				
Blood parameters	**Newborns**	**Infants**	**Young children**	**School-aged children**
Electrolytes				
• **Sodium** (mmol/L)	130–148	←	135–146	→
• **Potassium** (mmol/L)	4–6.5	3.8–5.3	3.4–5.3	3.4–5.0
• **Chloride** (mmol/L)	90–115	←	95–110	→
• **Calcium** (mmol/L)	2.2–2.8	2.2–2.5	2.2–2.8	2.4–2.8
• **Magnesium** (mmol/L)	0.5–0.8	0.7–1.1	←	0.7–0.9 →
• **Inorganic phosphate**				
(mg/dL)	4.8-9	4.9–7	←	3.4–4.8 →
(mmol/L)	1.55–2.9	1.58–2.26	←	1.1–1.9 →
Urinary excreted substances				
• **Urea**				
(mg/dL)	14–28	20–30	24–38	20–40
(mmol/L)	2.5–10	3.3–5.0	4.0–6.3	3.3–6.7
• **Creatine**				
(mg/dL)	0.2–0.4	0.2–0.6	0.3–0.7	0.5–0.9
(µmol/L)	18–35	18–53	27–62	44–80
• **Uric acid**				
(mg/dL)	2.6–5	1.0–1.8	3–6	3–6
(mmol/L)	135–295	59–106	177–354	177–354
Other				
• **Blood glucose**				
(mg/dL)	45–60	50–90	50–100	70–110
(mmol/L)	1.67–3.33	2.78–4.9	2.78–5.56	3.9–6.1
	Premature			
	20–50			
	(1.1–2.78)			
• **Total protein** (g/dL)	4.8–7.3	5–7.2	5.2–7.5	5.8–7.6
	Premature			
	3.0–5.6			
• **C-reactive protein (CRP)**	< 2.0 mg/dL (<20 mg/L) (first to third day of life)			
	<1.0 mg/dL (<10 mg/L) (> fourth day of life)			
Serum enzymes (mU/mL)				
• **GOT (ASAT)**	8–38[a]	7–25	5–20	5–20
• **GPT (ALAT)**	5–33	6–25	5–20	5–20
• **γ-GT**	40–120	10–30	5–20	5–20
• **CK**	17–150	28–80	16–70	15–80
• **CK-MB**	2–12	0.5–5	0.5–5	0.4–4
• **LDH (total)**	300–600	200–350	160–260	120–260
• **Cholinesterase**	2880–6900	3660–9600	5220–10500	← →
• **Lipase**[b]	5–27	←	2–80 →	–190
• **Amylase**	5–65	←	50–300 →	

[a] Higher levels in breast-fed babies
[b] Different reference values, depending on the method

→ Reference Values **Continued** ▶

Blood gas analysis	Newborns	Infants	Young children	School-aged children
pH	7.25–7.45	←	7.35–7.45	→
Base excess (mmol/L)	–7bis+0.5	←	– 3.00 – + 3.00	→
Standard bicarbonate (mmol/L)	17.8–25.3	←	20–25	→
P_{CO2} (mm Hg or torr)	28.5–45	28–42	32–44	→
(kPa)	3.8–6.0	3.75–5.60	4.3–6.0	→
PO_2 (mm Hg or torr)	80–40/90–55 (first hour postpartum/24 hours)	95–65	95–65	100–70
(kPa)	10.7–5.35/ 12–7.35	12.0–8.7	12.7–8.0	13.3–9.35
S_aO_2				
(%)	80–100	86–100	90–100	91–98
(mol/mol)	0.89–1.0	0.86–1.0	0.9–1.0	0.91–0.98

Coagulation				
Partial thromboplastin time (PTT) intrinsic system	33 – 60	← – – –	35 – 70	– – – →
Prothrombin time (PT) extrinsic system (%)	20 – 80	← – – –	75 – 110	– – – →
Fibrinogen (mg/dL)	100 – 250	← – – –	50 – 500	– – – →
Antithrombin III (%)	45 – 80	← – – –	60 – 120	– – – →

CSF parameters	Newborns	Infants	Beyond infancy
Number of cells (number/μL = 10^6/L)	0–30 10–30% lymphocytes 50–80% monocytes	0–10	0–5
Protein (mg/dL)	20–110	16–35	15–40
Glucose			
(mg/dL)	30–60	4.5–8.0	4.5–8.0
(mmol/L)	1.66–3.33	2.5–4.4	2.5–4.4
Lactate			
(mg/dL)	11–19	12–17	11–18
(mmol/L)	1.2–2.1	1.3–1.9	1.2–2.0

→ Reference Values Continued ▶

Erythrogram	Red blood cells (million/µL = 10¹²/L)	Reticulo-cytes (%)	Hb (g/dL)	MCV (µm³)	MCH (pg)	MCHC (p/dL)	Hct. (%)	White blood cells (number/µL = 10⁹L)	Platelets (number/µL = 10⁹L)
Birth								9,000–30,000	1,00,000–3,50,000
1 Day	4.6–6.5	1.0–8	14.5–23	95–121	31–37	29–37	45–72	9,000–30,000	1,00,000–350 000
2 Days	4.0–6.6	1.0–8	14–22	94–120		29–38	43–65	9,000–30,000	1,00,000–350 000
7. Days	3.9–6.2	0.5–1	15–22	88–126	28–40	28–38	42–60	5,000–21,000	1,00,000–3,50,000
1 month	3.0–5.4	<2–8	12–18	85–123	26–34	29–37	31–55	5,000–19,500	1,00,000–3,50,000
1 year	4.0–5.5	<1.6	12–16	70–86	25–35	30–36	37–54	6,000–17,000	1,50,000–3,50,000
2–6 years	3.8–5.2	<1.5	13–15	75–87	24–30	31–37	34–40	5,000–13,000	1,50,000–3,50,000
7–12 years	4.5–5.5	<1.5	11.9–14.7	69–93	22–34	32–36	32–43	5,000–13,000	2,00,000–3,50,000
13–17 years	4.8–5.7	<1.5	11.9–14.7	69–93	22–34	32–36	39–43	5,000–13,000	2,00,000–3,50,000

Weight	Age	Neutrophils (N) (number/µl)	Bands (B) (number/µL)	B/N
below 2.500 g	0–96 h	<12,000	<1400	<0.17
	>96 h	2,000–4,700	<500	<0.14
above 2.500 g	0–96 h	<14,000	<1400	<0.17
	>96 h	2,400–4,500	<400	<0.14

→ Reference Values Continued ▶

Nomogram

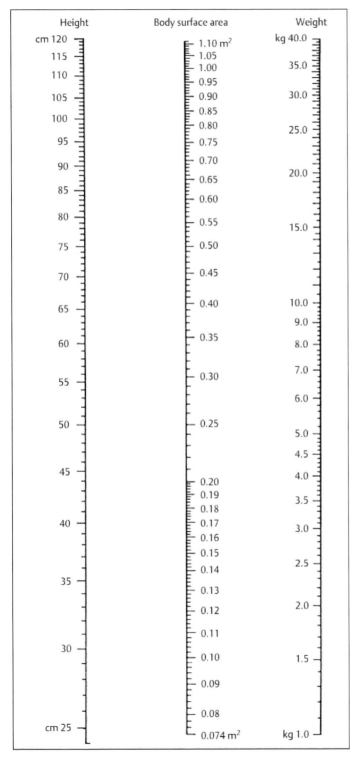

Height	Body surface area	Weight
cm 120	1.10 m²	kg 40.0

Nomogram to calculate body surface area. The intersection of the straight lines (between the subject's height and weight) with the average scale yields the body surface area (m²) (according to Dubois et al.). Body surface area [m²] = 0.007184 × height [cm]$^{0.725}$ × weight [kg]$^{0.425}$

→ Reference Values Continued ▶

Blood pressure, heart rate and respiratory rate

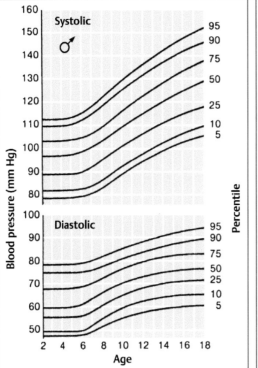

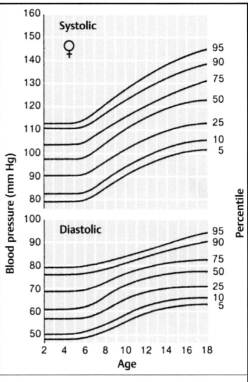

	Newborns	Infants	Young children	School-aged children
Breathing rate	45–35	40–25	30–20	25–15
Heart rate	140–120 (postpartum up to 200)	120–100	110–90	110–70
Blood pressure (mm Hg ± 10)	70/45	80/50	100/60	115/70
(kPa)	9.33/6.00	10.6/6.65	13.3/8.0	15.29/9.31
Cuff width (cm)	5–6	8–9	12–14	12–14
Cuff length (cm)	13	20	25	25

→ Reference Values

Drugs		
Drug	**Indication**	**Dosage**	**Major side effects**
Acetylcysteine	Paracetamol intoxication	150 mg/kg BW in glucose 5% IV for15 min, then 50 mg/kg BW in glucose 5% IV for 3 h, then100 mg/kg BW in glucose 5% IV for 16 h	Allergic reactions, rash, nausea
	Secretolysis	<2 y: 3 × 50 mg/d; 2–6 y: 3 × 100 mg/d 6–14 y: 2 × 200 mg/d;> 14 y: 3 × 200 mg/d PO	
Acetylsalicylic acid	Analgesic, antipyretic, anti-inflammatory	10–15 mg/kg BW PO every 4–6 h (maximum: 60–80 mg/kg BW/d)	Elevated bleeding tendency, hepatotoxic in high doses, gastrointestinal ulcers
Aciclovir	Antiviral	5–10 (to 15) mg/kg BW/single dose 3–5 times daily 250–500 mg/m² body surface every 8 h	Temporary kidney function impairment
Ambroxol	Secretolytic	<2y: 2 × 7.5 mg; 2–5 y: 3 × 7.5 mg > 5 y: 2–3× 15 mg	Allergic reactions, rash, nausea, blockage of secretory ducts in the event of concomitant administration of antitussives
Amoxicillin	Antibiotic	50–100 mg/kg BW PO in 3 single doses	Gastrointestinal complaints, rash, allergic reactions
Ampicillin	Antibiotic	Newborns: 100–200 mg/kg BW IV in 3 single doses Infants: 100–300 mg/kg BW IV in 3 single doses > 1 y: 50–100 mg/kg BW PO or 100–300 mg/kg BW IV in three single doses	Gastrointestinal complaints, rash, allergic reactions
Budesonide	Inhaled form of corticosteroid for management of asthma	Aerosol: 2 × 1 (to 2) sprays/d Suspension: < 12 y: 2 × 0.5–1 mg/d > 12 y: 2 × 1–2 mg/d	Hoarseness, oral thrush
Butylscopolamine	Parasympatholytic for spasmolysis	0.3–0.5 (to 1) mg/kg BW PO 3 times daily 0.3–0.6 mg/kg BW IV up to 3 times daily	Tachycardia, voiding disorders, gastrointestinal disorders, dizziness
Carbamazepine	Anticonvulsant	20–25 mg/kg BW/d PO in 3–4 single doses	Allergic rash, fatigue, nausea, leukopenia, thrombopenia, elevated transaminase levels
Activated charcoal	Primary poisoning antidote; not effective for poisoning with lithium, thallium, heavy metals, alcohols and glycols; contraindicated for ingestion of acids and lyes	0.5–1 g/kg BW PO	Reduces the effect of medication
Cefaclor	Second-generation oral cephalosporin	30–50 mg/kg BW/d PO in 3 single doses	Gastrointestinal complaints, allergic reactions, urticaria, flush
Cefadroxil	First-generation oral cephalosporin	50–100 mg/kg BW/d PO in 3 single doses	Gastrointestinal complaints, allergic reactions, urticaria, flush
Cefotaxime	Parenteral third-generation broad-spectrum cephalosporin	100–200 mg/kg BW/d in 3 single doses IV	Gastrointestinal complaints, allergic reactions, urticaria, flush
Cefpodoxime proxetil	Third-generation oral cephalosporin	5–12 mg/kg BW/d in 2 single doses IV	Gastrointestinal complaints, allergic reactions, urticaria, flush, blood count changes

→ Drugs Continued ▶

Drugs

Drug	Indication	Dosage	Major side effects
Ceftriaxone	Parenteral third-generation broad-spectrum cephalosporin	50–80 (to 100) mg/kg BW/d in 1 single dose IV	Gastrointestinal complaints, allergic reactions, urticaria, flush, reversible sludge in bile ducts and urinary tract, blood count changes
Cefuroxime axetil	Second-generation oral cephalosporin	20–30 mg/kg BW/d in 2 single doses PO	Gastrointestinal complaints, allergic reactions, urticaria, flush, blood count changes
Cefuroxime	Parenteral third-generation broad-spectrum cephalosporin	75–150 mg/kg BW/d in 3 single doses IV	Gastrointestinal complaints, allergic reactions, urticaria, flush, blood count changes
Chloral hydrate	Sedative	10–15 mg/kg BW every 6–8 h rectally, PO	Paradoxical reaction
Clarithromycin	Macrolide antibiotic	10–15 mg/kg BW in 2 single doses PO	Nausea, vomiting, rash, itching, urticaria, elevated transaminase levels
Diazepam	Anticonvulsant, sedative	0.2–0.8 mg/kg BW/d PO in 3–4 single doses 0.05–0.3 mg/kg BW IV every 2–4 h 0.3–0.5 mg/kg BW rectally	Hypertension, respiratory depression, fatigue, sleepiness
Diclofenac	Anti-inflammatory	1–2 mg/kg BW in 2 to 3 single doses PO	Rash, gastrointestinal ulcers, bronchospasm
Dimenhydrinate	Antiemetic for vomiting	5 mg/kg BW PO/rectally in 3–4 single doses 1–2 mg/kg BW IV/IM in 1 single dose	Rash, sedation, agitation, voiding disorder
Dimetindene	Antihistamine	0.05–0.1 mg/kg BW PO 3 times daily 0.025–0.05 mg/kg BW IV up to 3 times daily	Fatigue, dry mouth, visual disorders
Erythromycin	Macrolide antibiotic	40–60 mg/kg BW in 3 single doses PO/IV	Gastrointestinal complaints, rash, allergic reactions, elevated transaminase levels, venous irritation when administered by IV infusion
Ethambutol	Tuberculostat	850 mg/m² body surface area PO	Optic neuropathy, in rare cases, hyperuricemia
Fenoterol	Sympathomimetic beta 2 for treating bronchospasm	1–2 sprays 3 to 4 times per day inhaled	Tremor, restlessness, tachycardia, nausea, in high doses, hypocalcemia
Furosemide	Diuretic	1–2 (to 6) mg/kg BW/single dose PO every 6–8 h 0.5–1 (maximum: 5) mg/kg BW/single dose IV/IM every 2–3 h	Rash, dizziness, electrolyte loss (sodium, potassium, calcium, magnesium), hyperglycemia
Gentamicin	Aminoglycoside antibiotic	3–5 mg/kg BW IM/IV in 1–2 single doses	Nephrotoxicity and ototoxicity
Ibuprofen	Analgesic, antipyretic, anti-inflammatory	20–30 mg/kg BW in 3–4 single doses PO	Rash, peptic ulcers, headache, fatigue, dizziness
Syrup of ipecac	Emetic for primary treatment of poisoning	1–2 y: 10 mL; 2–3 y: 20 mL; > 3 y: 20–30 mL	Prolonged vomiting, nausea, pallidness, cardiotoxicity in high doses
Ipratropium bromide	Parasympatholytic for treating bronchospasm	1–2 sprays 3–4 times per day inhaled	Tachycardia, nervousness, fatigue, hypotension

→ Drugs Continued ▶

Drug	Category/Indication	Dosage	Side effects
Isoniazid	Tuberculostat	200 mg/m² body surface area in 1 (to 2) single doses PO	Elevated transaminase levels, gastrointestinal complaints, polyneuritis, rash, headache, fever
Lactulose	Constipation, laxative	< 1 y: 5 (to 15) mL; 1–6 y: 20–30 mL < 6 y: 30–90 mL PO in 1 (to 3) single doses	Tympanites, flatulence, stomachache, nausea, vomiting, diarrhea
Mebendazole	Anthelmintic for nematode infestations	>2 y: 100–200 mg/kg BW PO in 1 (to 2) single doses	In the case of high dosage or long-term treatment of gastrointestinal disorders, neutropenia
Meropenem	Carbapenem antibiotic, drug of last resort for treating severe infections	30–60 (to 80) mg/kg BW IV in 3 single doses	Gastrointestinal disorders, local thrombophlebitis, allergic reactions, elevated transaminase levels
Metamizole	Analgesic, antipyretic, (drug of last resort for children)	10–15 mg/kg BW PO/IV/rectally/IM every 6–8 h	Allergic reactions, agranulocytosis, if administered intravenously drop in BP, interstitial nephritis
Metoclopramide	Antiemetic, reflux esophagitis	>2 y: 0.1 mg/kg BW PO/IV in 3–4 single doses (maximum: 0.5 mg/kg BW/d)	CNS disturbances, dyskinetic syndrome, tardive dyskinesia, elevated prolactin levels, diarrhea
Metronidazole	Antibiotic	20–30 mg/kg BW/d IV/PO in 2 (to 3) single doses	Rash, urticaria, CNS-related symptoms, gastrointestinal disorders, leukopenia, allergic reactions, candidiasis
Netilmicin	Aminoglycoside antibiotic	4–9 mg/kg BW/d IV in 2 to 3 single doses	Muscle ache, ototoxicity and nephrotoxicity, allergic reactions, elevated transaminase levels
Nifedipine	Calcium antagonist for treating arterial hypertension	0.3–1.0 mg/kg BW PO 0.5–1 (to 4) mg/kg BW IV	Flush, headache, tachycardia, hypotension, edema, dizziness
Nystatin	Antifungal medication	< 1 y: 3 × 100,000–150,000 IU/d PO > 1 y: 1.6–2.4 million IU/d PO in 4 single doses	Gastrointestinal disorders, allergic reactions
Omeprazole	Proton pump inhibitor for treating gastritis, gastrointestinal ulcer, reflux esophagitis, helicobacter pylori eradication therapy (triple therapy with amoxicillin and clarithromycin)	> 1 y: 0.5–1 (to 3) mg/kg BW/d in 3 single doses 0.25 mg/kg BW/single dose IV 1 times daily	Nausea, diarrhea, constipation, elevated transaminase levels, allergic reactions, blood count changes, pancreatitis
Paracetamol	Analgesic, antipyretic	10–15 mg/kg BW PO every 4–6 h (maximum: 50–75 mg/kg BW/d)	In the case of intoxication, hepatotoxic and nephrotoxic; in the case of long-term use, analgesic nephropathy, allergic reactions
Paraffinum liquidum	Laxative for regulating bowel movements in patients with constipation	Initially 20–30 mL/m² body surface area in 3–4 single doses, then taper	In the case of long-term use, impaired absorption of fat-soluble vitamins, when aspirated, chemical pneumonitis
Penicillin C/ benzylpenicillin	Antibiotic	(50,000 to) 100,000–500,000 IU/kg BW in 4–6 single doses IV/IM	Rash, urticaria, neurotoxicity, gastrointestinal disorders, taste disturbance, dry mouth, vasculitis, leukopenia, thrombocytopenia, allergic reactions
Penicillin V	Antibiotic	50,000–100,000 IU/kg BW/d PO in 3–4 single doses	Rash, urticaria, neurotoxicity, gastrointestinal disturbances, taste disturbance, dry mouth, vasculitis, leukopenia, thrombocytopenia, allergic reactions
Phenobarbital	Sedative, anticonvulsant/ antiepileptic	Loading dose 20 mg/kg BW as single dose, then 10 mg/kg BW in 3 single doses IV or PO	Fatigue, dizziness, ataxia, confusion, paradoxical reaction, rash, nausea, vomiting, respiratory depression, allergic reactions

→ Drugs Continued ▶

→ Drugs

Drugs

Drug	Indication	Dosage	Major side effects
Prednisone/ Prednisolone	Glucocorticoid	Systemic: bolus 5 (to 10) mg/kg BW, then 1–2 (to 5) mg/kg BW in 1–3 single doses PO/IV or 100 mg rectally, repeat after 4 h, as needed	Cushing syndrome, peptic ulcer, leukocytosis, polyglobulia, impaired growth, immunosuppression, increased risk of blood clots, hyperglycemia
Promethazine	Antihistamine, sedative, antiemetic, neuroleptic	0.1–0.5 (to 1) mg/kg BW IV/PO up to 4 times daily	Dizziness, tachycardia, pallidness, extrapyramidal symptoms, cholestasis, agranulocytosis
Pyrazinamide	Tuberculostat	20–30 (to 35) mg/kg BW/d in 1 single dose PO	Photosensitivity, gastrointestinal complaints, hepatotoxicity, arthralgia, hyperuricemia
Rifampicin	Tuberculostat, meningococcal prophylaxis	10–20 mg/kg BW in 1–2 single doses PO/IV	Flush, itching, urticaria, elevated transaminase levels, gastrointestinal disorders, allergic reactions, yellowish-red discoloration of body secretions
Roxithromycin	Macrolide antibiotic	5–7.5 mg/kg BW/d in 1–2 single doses PO	Gastrointestinal complaints, rash, allergic reactions, elevated transaminase levels
Salbutamol	Sympathomimetic ß2 for treating asthma and bronchospasm	Inhaled, 1 drop/y old/single dose or 1 drop/3 kg BW/single dose depending on symptoms, up to 10 times daily	Agitation, tachycardia, tremor, restlessness, nausea, headache
Theophylline	Bronchodilator	Initially 2–6 mg/kg BW in 20 min IV, then continuous infusion with 10–15 mg/kg BW/d	Agitation, tachycardia, tremor, restlessness, nausea, headache, seizures, rapid or uneven heartbeats, hypotension
Valproic acid	Antiepileptic	20–30 mg/kg BW/d, can be increased as needed up to 120 mg/kg BW/d PO	Severe to lethal impaired liver function, temporary alopecia, leukopenia and thrombocytopenia, hyperammonemia, fatigue, paresthesia, disturbed appetite

Emergency medications for resuscitation

Drug	Indication	Dosage	Major side effects
Adrenaline (0.1 % solution = 1:10,000 diluted)	Cardiopulmonary resuscitation	Initially: 10 mg/kg BW = 0.1 mL of the solutions diluted to 1:10,000 IV/IO, follow-up dose 100 mg/kg BW = 1 mL/kg BW IV/IO, endotracheal 100 mg/kg BW = 1 mL/kg BW	Vasoconstriction, cardiac arrhythmia, ventricular fibrillation
Atropine	Anticholinergic, treatment of bradycardia, antidote for poisoning with cholinergic substances	0.02 mg/kg IV/IO/ET	Underdosing leads to paradoxical bradycardia, tachycardia
Calcium carbonate (10% solution)	Last resort for electromechanical decoupling	1–2 mL/kg BW slowly IV/IO	Bradycardia if injected too quickly, deterioration of blood flow leads to ischemic areas of the brain and heart
Lidocaine (2% solution)	Class Ib antiarrhythmic drug	1–2 mg/kg BW as bolus, then 0.5 mg/kg BW IV/IO	
Sodium bicarbonate (8.4% solution)	Only in the case of cardiac arrest and after prolonged resuscitation	1 mmol/kg BW/dose IV/IO	Exacerbation of respiratory and cerebral acidosis, hypernatremia, hyperosmolarity, alkalosis

Abbreviations: BW, body weight; CNS, central nervous system; ET, endotracheal; IO, intraosseous; IV, intravenous; PO, peroral.

Index

A

Abdominal pain, 51, 235–239
– acute, 236–237
– and anal itching, 27
– basic tests for, 236
– causes, 236
– chronic, 237–238
– diagnosis, 238–239
– functional, 238
– intense, 57
– patient assessment, 235
– physical examination, 235–236
– recurrent, 74
– and weight loss, 55
Abdominal sonography, 6f
Abdominal tuberculosis, 232–233
Abnormal appearance, girl with, 69
Abrasion, 36
Activated charcoal, 38, 155
Active immunization, 149
Acute appendicitis
– causes, 177–178
– clinical aspects, 178–179
– complications, 178
– definition, 178
– diagnosis, 178, 179
– differential diagnoses, 178
– treatment, 179
Acute epiglottitis, 91, 92
Acute hematogenous osteomyelitis, 267–270
– definition, 268
– diagnosis, 267, 268
– differential diagnosis, 267, 268
– etiology, 268–269
– prognosis, 270
– symptoms, 269
– treatment, 268, 269

Acute lymphatic leukemia
– classification, 169
– clinical aspects, 169–170
– definition, 169
– diagnosis, 170
– diagnostic measures, 168
– epidemiology, 169
– etiopathogenesis, 169
– risk factors, 169
– symptoms, 170t
– treatment, 168–169, 170–171, 171f
Acute otitis media
– causes, 110
– clinical aspects, 110
– complications, 110
– definition, 110
– diagnosis, 110–111
– epidemiology and etiopathogenesis, 110
– prognosis, 111
– treatment, 110, 111, 111f
Acute Salmonella enteritis, 210
Acute sinusitis, 125
Acyanotic heart defects, 198–199
Adenoid hyperplasia, 224–225, 225f
Adult behavior, 251
Aggressive behavior, 85
Alcohol intoxication and alcohol abuse, 152–154
– diagnosis, 151
– diagnostics, 152
– kinetics and metabolism, 152
– reasons, 151
– smptoms of, 152
– sources, 151–152
– treatment, 152–153
Allergen avoidance, 107
Anorexia nervosa
– causes, 133
– clinical aspects, 134

– definition and epidemiology, 134
– diagnosis, 133, 134
– prognosis, 135
– treatment, 133–135
Antibiosis, 14
Anti-HAV-IgM antibodies, 146
Anuria, 60
Apathetic infant with persistent skin folds, 5
Asymmetrical screaming face, 124, 124f
Ataxia telangiectasia. See Louis-Bar syndrome
Atopic dermatitis, 32
Attention deficit hyperactivity disorder (ADHD), 265–267

B

"Babbling" speech, 53
Bacterial infections of neonate, 221–224
Barking cough
– and dyspnea, 3
– hoarseness, and inspiratory stridor, 91
Birth trauma injuries, 123–124
Blood alcohol concentration BAC), 152
Blood gas analysis, 66, 70
Blood smear, 49f
Body mass index (BMI), 240
Bone tuberculosis, 233
Booster shots, 149–150
Bourneville–Pringle disease, 139
Brachial plexus, damage to, 124
Breastfeeding
– advantages, 226, 228
– problems, 228–229

Bronchial asthma
- classification, 108
- clinical aspects, 108
- definition, 108
- diagnosis, 106–107, 108
- etiopathogenesis, 108
- pathogenesis, 107
- prognosis, 110
- treatment, 107, 108–109
Bronchiolitis
- causes, 115
- definition and epidemiology, 116
- diagnosis, 115
- etiopathogenesis, clinical aspects, and diagnosis, 116
- pathogens, 115
- treatment, 115
- treatment and prophylaxis, 116
Burns, 26, 26f
- classification, 131
- definition, 131
- diagnosis, 131–132
- etiopathogenesis and clinical aspects, 131
- extent, determining, 130
- first aid measures, 130
- prophylaxis, 132
- severity, degrees of, 131
- treatment, 131, 132

C

Caput succedaneum, 123, 123f
Carbohydrate malabsorption, 237
Cardiopulmonary resuscitation of newborn, 214–215
Celiac disease
- clinical aspects, 122
- definition and pathogenesis, 122
- diagnosis, 121
- differential diagnoses, 121
- epidemiology and etiology, 122
- prognosis, 123
- treatment, 122–123, 122f

Cephalhematoma, 123, 123f
Cerebral concussion, 128
Cerebral hemorrhage, 190–191, 191t
Cerebrospinal fluid diagnosis, 88
Cesarean section, newborn delivered by, 66
Changing table, infant fallen from, 76, 242–245
Chassaignac's "paralysis," 180–181
Chemoprophylaxis, 260
Chicken pox, 13. See Varicella (chicken pox)
Child abuse, 243–245
Childhood diseases, 126–127
Chorionic villus sampling, 160
Chromosome analysis, 159–160
Clavicle fracture, 124
Colic-like stomach pains and vomiting, 6
Congenital deformities, 77
Congenital heart defects
- classification, 198–199
- diagnosis, 198
- endocarditis, 198
- epidemiology, 199
- etiology, 199
- persistent ductus arteriosus botalli, 201–202, 201f
- risk groups, 198
- tetralogy of Fallot, 200–201, 200f
- transposition of great arteries (TGA), 199, 199f
- treatment, 198
- ventricular septum defect (VSD), 199–200, 200f
Congenital hip joint luxation and dysplasia, 145
Congenital hypothyroidism, 100
Connatal infections, 78, 247
Conspicuous genitals, newborn boy with, 68
Constipation, 191–193
Contagious impetigo, 140–141
Cortisone-containing medications, 80
Cough, 15, 73
Coxitis fugax, 142, 142f
Craniocerebral trauma

- classification, 242–243
- definition, 242
- examination, 242
- Glasgow Coma Scale and, 242–243, 243t
Cryptorchism, 184
Cyanosis, newborn with persistent, 61
Cyanotic heart defects, 199
Cystic fibrosis (CF), 204–206
Cytomegaly virus (CMV) infection, 249–250

D

Dehydration, 94
Development status assessment, 98–99
Diabetes mellitus Type I
- clinical aspects, 186
- complications, 186
- definition, 186
- diagnosis, 185, 186
- epidemiology, 186
- etiology, 185
- pathogenesis, 186
- prognosis, 187
- treatment, 185, 186–187
Diabetic (embryo-) fetopathy, 135–136
Diarrhea, 6, 60
Disposition prophylaxis, 149
Down syndrome, 159–160
Drug and nicotine abuse during pregnancy, 248–249
Duplex ultrasonography, 118–119

E

Early stage food, 72, 226
Eat, refusing to, 40
Ectopic testis, 183
Encephalotrigeminal angiomatosis. See Sturge–Weber syndrome
Epileptic seizure, 64, 206–209
- causes, 206
- clinical aspects, 207

– definition, 207
– diagnosis, 208
– etiology, 207
– prognosis, 208–209
– treatment, 207, 208
– types, 206–207
Ewing sarcoma, 268t
Exasperated parents, 72
Exposure prophylaxis, 149

F

Facial nerve palsy, 124
Facial swelling, 48
Falling from jungle gym, 24
Fatigue, 16, 71
Febrile respiratory infection, 9,
    54
Febrile seizure
– diagnosis, 92–93
– diagnostic measures, 93
– etiopathogenesis, 93
– immediate measures for, 93
– treatment and prophylaxis,
    93–94
Febrile tonsillitis, 62
Femoral epiphysis, 143, 144
Fever, 88. See also High fever
– and exanthema, 47
Fever curve, 65f, 209
First care and first examination
    of neonate, 211–215
– APGAR score, 212–213, 213t
– blood gas analysis, 211
– cardiopulmonary resuscitation
    of newborn, 214–215
– first measures, 212
– mother–child–father relations,
    213
– by pediatrician, 212
– physical examination, 213–
    214
– preparation for, 212
– suction, 212
– transfer from delivery room,
    214
– umbilical artery pH, 213
– vitamin K prophylaxis, 214
Fluoride prophylaxis, 230
Foreign body aspiration, 17,
    117–118

Fructose malabsorption, 237
Functional abdominal pain, 238

G

Gastroenteritis, 6, 65
Gingivostomatitis herpetica
    (ulcerative), 157–158
Glomerular hematuria,
    119–120
Glucocorticoids, 107
– bronchiolitis, 115
– for Krupp syndrome, 92
– nephrotic syndrome, 173
Gluten-sensitive enteropathy. See
    Celiac disease
Grade I traumatic brain injury,
    128
Grand mal seizure, 206–207
Growth retardation, 248

H

Hand surface rule, 130
Headache, 53
– and abnormal behavior, 50
– high fever and, 22
Head and neck pain, 88
Head lice. See Pediculosis capitis
Health log, 99
Health screenings
– premature birth, 7
– procedure, 99–100
– – 1 day of age, 100
– – 3 to 10 days of age, 100
– – 6 to 7 months of age, 101
– – 10 to 12 months of age, 101
– – 21 to 24 months of age, 101
– – 33 to 36 months of age,
    101–102
– – 43 to 48 months of age, 102
– – 60 to 64 months of age, 102
– – 3 to 4 weeks of age, 100–101
– – 4 to 6 weeks of age, 100
– – 10 to 14 years of age, 102
– purpose of, 98
– usual course of, 98
Helicobacter pylori infections,
    238
Hematomas, 60

Hematopoietic system and
    infectious mononucleosis,
    116
Hematuria, 30
Hemolytic–uremic syndrome
    (HUS), 195t, 196–197
Hepatitis A, 145–146
Hereditary spherical cell anemia,
    175–176
Herpes simplex viruses (HSV),
    158
Herpes simplex virus infection,
    158
High fever, 65
– and abdominal pain, 44
– and headache, 22
– and joint pain, 67
– and rash, 23
– rash, and swollen joints, 58
– and seizure, 4
– sucking weakness, and
    vomiting, 25
High fever, vomiting, and
    headache, 2
Hip diseases in childhood
– congenital hip joint luxation
    and dysplasia, 145
– coxitis fugax, 142, 142f
– femoral epiphysis, 143, 144
– Perthes disease, 142–143,
    143f, 144
– transient synovitis, 144
Hippel–Lindau syndrome, 139
Hyperbilirubinemia. See
    Neonatal icterus
Hypertonic dehydration, 94
Hypertrophic pyloric stenosis, 10
– clinical aspects, 106
– definition, 106
– diagnosis, 105
– epidemiology, 106
– pathogenesis, 105
– symptoms, 105
– treatment, 105, 106
– ultrasound, 105f
Hypochromic anemia, 121
Hyponatremia, 70
Hypospadia, 217–218
Hypothermia, 37
Hypotonic dehydration, 94
Hypotrophic newborn with
    abnormal phenotype, 33

I

Ibuprofen, 93
Icterus
– pathogenesis of, 146
– and sucking weakness,
  newborn with, 39
Idiopathic thrombocytopenic
  purpura (ITP), 84, 263–265
Immune system and infectious
  mononucleosis, 116
Immunizations, 100
– active and passive, 149
– adverse effects, 147
– basic, 149
– contraindications, 150
– contraindications for, 147
– generally recommended, 150
– hepatitis A, 146
– 15-month-old child, 149
– parents' permission for, 147
– procedure, 150
– schedule for infants, children,
  adolescents, and adults, 148t
– steps for, 147
– unwillingness for, 150
Induction therapy, 168
Infant foods, 72
Infection prophylaxis, 149
Infectious mononucleosis,
  116–117
Influenza (flu), 215–217
Influenza viruses, 216
Infusion therapy, 131
– for gingivostomatitis herpetica
  (ulcerative), 157
– for hyperbilirubinemia, 156
Ingestion of unknown fluid, 38
Inguinal hernia, 195–196, 195f
Inguinal swelling, 59
Inguinal testis, 183
Inhalation therapy, 115
Intoxications
– amount of active agent
  consumed, 153
– classification of severity of,
  154t
– clinical aspects, 154
– diagnosis, 154–155
– information about, 153
– prevention, 155–156
– symptoms, 153
– treatment measures, 153–154
– – at accident site, 155
– – in hospital, 155
Intrahepatic cholestasis, 146
Intrauterine growth, retardation
  of, 249t
Invagination
– clinical aspects, 97
– complications, 97
– diagnosis, 97, 97f, 98
– epidemiology, 97
– etiopathogenesis, 97
– prognosis, 98
– treatment, 98
Isotonic dehydration, 94
Itching and eczematous skin
  changes on neck and head,
  42

J

Jaw angle, swollen, 14
Joint tuberculosis, 233
Jones diagnostic criteria, 62, 202,
  202t

K

Kawasaki syndrome, 171–173
Kernicterus, 156–157
Knee pain and protective
  limping, 34
Krupp syndrome, 91t
– clinical aspects, 91–92
– definition, 91
– diagnosis, 90, 92
– differential diagnosis, 90, 92
– etiology, 91
– etiopathogenesis, 91
– prognosis, 92
– treatment, 92

L

Laparoschisis, 245–247
Laryngeal diphtheria, 92
Lindane-containing products,
  161

Lobar pneumonia
– clinical aspects, 165
– definition, 165
– diagnosis, 164, 165
– etiology, 165
– forms, 165
– pathogens, 164–165
– prognosis, 166
– treatment, 165–166
Louis–Bar syndrome, 139
Lower plexus paralysis, 124
Lumbar puncture, 88
Lyme borreliosis
– diagnosis, 103
– epidemiology:, 103
– etiopathogenesis, 103
– prognosis, 104
– prophylaxis, 103–104
– skin finding, 102
– symptoms, 102–103
– treatment, 103
Lymphadenitis colli, 140, 202
– causes, 113–114
– clinical aspects, 114
– definition, 114
– diagnosis and treatment,
  114–115
– etiopathogenesis, 114
– treatment, 114
Lymph node tuberculosis, 233

M

Macrohematuria, 19, 119
Macrosomal newborn, 21
Macrosomia, 135
Maintenance therapy, 169
Malignant
  laryngotracheobronchitis, 91
Measles, 126, 127
Medicamentous treatment, 132
Medulloblastoma, 176–177
Meningitis
– clinical aspects, 89
– clinical examination, 88
– definition and forms, 89
– diagnosis, 88, 89–90, 89f
– etiopathogenesis, 89
– forms of, 88–89
– prognosis, 90
– reporting, 90

– treatment, 90
Meningitis serosa, 88–89
Meningococcal sepsis. *See*
    Waterhouse–Friderichsen
    syndrome
Migraine
– diagnosis, 181
– epidemiology, 182
– etiopathogenesis, 182
– prognosis, 183
– prophylaxis with drugs, 183
– treatment, 181–183
miliary tuberculosis, 232
morphological abnormalities,
    newborn with, 41
Mosaic trisomy 21, 159
Mother's milk, 228
Mother's milk substitute, 229
Mumps, 126, 127

N

Necrotizing enterocolitis, 190
Neonatal diseases caused by pre-
    birth injuries, 247–250
Neonatal herpes infection, 158
Neonatal icterus, 156–157
Neonatal reflexes, 254–257, 255*t*
Nephritic syndrome, 120
Nephroblastoma, 137–138, 138*t*
Nephrotic syndrome, 173–174
Neuroblastoma, 82, 257–260
– clinical aspects, 259
– clinical symptoms, 258
– definition, 257, 258
– diagnosis, 257–259
– differential diagnoses, 257
– epidemiology, 258
– etiopathogenesis, 259
– prognosis, 260
– stage classification and
    therapy, 259–260, 259*t*
– staging, 260
Neurodermatitis, 80
Neurodermitis, 252–254, 253*f*
– clinical aspects, 252–253
– definition, 252
– diagnosis, 253
– epidemiology, 252
– etiology and pathogenesis, 252

– prognosis, 254
– prophylaxis, 253–254
– treatment, 253
Neurofibromatosis, 138–139
Non-glomerular hematuria, 120
Noonan syndrome. *See* Ullrich–
    Turner syndrome
Nosebleed and hematomas, 84
Nutrient requirement of infant,
    228
Nutrition plan for first year of
    child's life, 227

O

Obesity, 239–241
Ocular fundus, 88
Omphalocele, 245–247
Orchitis, 119
Orofacial herpes, 158
Osteosarcoma, 268*t*
Overweight, 239–241
Oxyuriasis, 132–133
Oxyuris vermicularis, 132*f*, 133

P

Pale skin and splenomegaly, 49
Palpitations, 79
Paracetamol, 93
– poisoning, 38, 153
Passive immunization, 149
Paul–Bunnell test, 117
Pediatric admission examination,
    81
Pediatric examination, anomalies
    in, 254–257
Pediculosis capitis
– clinical aspects, 161
– diagnosis, 160, 161
– etiopathogenesis, 161
– prognosis, 162
– recommendations for, 161
– treatment, 160, 161–162
Peptic gastrointestinal diseases,
    238
Percentile curves, 20, 121
Peritonitis tuberculosa, 233
Peritonsillar abscess, 203

– with acute tonsillitis, 202
Persistent ductus arteriosus
    botalli, 201–202, 201*f*
Perthes disease, 142–143, 143*f*,
    144
Pertussis. *See* Whooping cough
Petechiae, 83
Petechial dermatorrhagie, 9
Pfeiffer glandular fever. *See*
    Infectious mononucleosis
Phenylketonuria (PKU), 100
Phototherapy, 156, 157
Physical therapy, 99, 100
Pigment spots, 31, 31*f*
Plexus paralysis treatment, 124
Pneumonia and bone pain, 46
Postenteritis syndrome, 237
Post-infectious
    glomerulonephritis, 140
Postnatal period physiology, 214
Postpartum care of child, 245
Postprimary tuberculosis, 232
Post-streptococcal
    glomerulonephritis, 119–121
Premature baby with acute
    deterioration of general
    condition, 70
Premature birth, 56, 189
Premature development of
    puberty, 220
Premature thelarche, 219
Prenatal diseases, 248*t*
– of TORCH complex, 249–250
Primary nephrotic syndrome,
    174
Primary vaccination and booster
    shots, 149–150
Projectile vomiting, 10
Prophylactic measures, 29
Psychosomatic complaints, 251
Pubertal gynecomastia, 220
Pubertas praecox, 220
Pubertas praecox vera, 220
Pubertas tarda, 220
Puberty, 251
– normal and pathological
    development of, 219–221
– signs of progressing, 75
Purulent meningitis, 90
Purulent (bacterial) meningitis,
    88

R

Rash and high fever, 23
Rattling breath and
   hypersalivation, 62
Rectal pain, 57
Recurrent pulmonary infections,
   63
Recurrent urinary tract
   infections, 45
Red urine, 120
Reinduction therapy, 168
Respiratory distress syndrome,
   56, 188–191
Retinopathy of immaturity, 190
Retractile testis, 183
Retrograde amnesia, 24
Rheumatic fever, 202, 203
Ribavirin, 115
Right arm, protective posture
   of, 52
Right lower abdomen, pain in, 51
Rubella virus infection, 249
Rule of Nines, 130, 130f
"Runny ear," 12

S

Salmonella enteritis, 209–210
Scarlet fever, 126–127
Schoenlein–Henoch purpura
– clinical aspects, 104–105
– definition, 104
– diagnosis, 104, 105
– differential diagnoses, 104
– etiopathogenesis, 104
– prognosis, 105
– treatment, 104, 105
Scleral icterus, 35
Screaming child, consultation for,
   72, 226–228
Scrotum, 54
Scrotum, swelling of, 18, 18f
Secondary meningitis, 89
Secondary nephrotic syndrome,
   174
Septic shock, 210
Serous (aseptic) meningitis,
   88–89
Severe exsiccosis/toxicosis in
   acute gastroenteritis

– classification, 95
– clinical aspects, 95–96
– diagnosis, 94, 96
– etiology, 95
– pathogenesis, 95
– prognosis, 97
– treatment, 94–95, 96–97
Shock therapy, 97
Shortness of breath, 79
– cough and, 15
– recurrent, 11
Shoulder dystocia, 21
Sinusitis, 125
Skin changes, 31, 31f
Sliding testis, 183
Small for Gestational Age (SGA),
   248
Small intestine biopsy, 121
Soft high-parietal swelling, 21
Soft swelling on head, 123–124
Solid food, 229–230
Somatization syndrome, 250–
   251
Somatogram, 20, 121
Spasmodic or recurrent croup,
   91
Speech disorder, 53
Spherocytosis. See Hereditary
   spherical cell anemia
Stage 1, and stage 2 food, 72,
   226–227
Staphylogenic Lyell syndrome,
   140
Stem cell transplantation, 169
Streptococcal angina, 62, 202
Sturge–Weber syndrome, 139
Sudden infant death, 163f
– definition, 162
– diagnosis, 162
– differential diagnoses, 164
– epidemiology, 163
– etiology, 163
– prophylaxis, 164
– risk assessment, 162
– risk factors, 163–164
– risk reduction measures, 162
Sudden infant death syndrome
   (SIDS), 43
Swallowing, difficulty, 16
Swelling of right foot, 86
Swelling of right knee, 8
Symptomatic treatment, 115

Systemic juvenile chronic
   arthritis (Still syndrome),
   193–194

T

Testicular torsion, 118–119
Testis, undescended, 54
Tetanus vaccination, 36
Tetralogy of Fallot, 200–201,
   200f
Theophylline, 107
Therapy-resistant diarrhea, 82
Thoracic X-ray, 11f, 15f, 17f, 44f,
   73f
Throat pain, 16
Thrombocyte count, 84
Thrombocytopenia, 84
Tingling paresthesia, 53
Toddler burned by boiling water,
   26, 26f
Tonsillitis, 202–203
Tonsillogenic sepsis, 202
Tonsils and infectious
   mononucleosis, 116
Torticollis, 124
Toxoplasmosis, 249–250
Transient synovitis, 144
Translocation trisomy, 159
Transposition of great arteries
   (TGA), 199, 199f
Trisomy 21. See Down syndrome
True precocious puberty, 220
Tuberculin skin test, 233
Tuberculosis, 230–235
– course of, 230, 232
– definition, 231
– diagnosis, 230, 233–234, 234t
– epidemiology, 231
– etiopathogenesis, 231–232
– mandatory reporting, 235
– prognosis, 235
– prophylaxis recommendations,
   231, 235
– stages of, 232t
– treatment, 231, 234, 234t
Tuberculous meningitis
   tuberculosis, 232
Tuberculous pleuritis, 233
Tuberous cerebral sclerosis. See
   Bourneville–Pringle disease

Type 1 diabetes during
   pregnancy, 29
Type 1 diabetic mother, newborn
   of, 29

U

Ullrich–Turner syndrome, 141–
   142, 142f
Unconscious patient, 37
Undescended testis, 183–185
Upper plexus paralysis, 123
Urinary tract infection, 128–129
– classification, 166, 167t
– clinical aspects, 167
– course of examination, 166
– definition, 167
– diagnosis, 167–168
– etiopathogenesis, 167
– prognosis, 168
– treatment, 166–168
Urine, microscopic examination
   of, 25f
Urogenital tuberculosis, 233
Urosepsis, 128–129

V

Vaccination. See Immunizations
Varicella (chicken pox)
– clinical aspects, 113
– complications, 112
– definition and epidemiology,
   113
– diagnosis, 113
– etiopathogenesis, 113
– immunization for, 112
– prognosis, 113
– prophylaxis, 113
– symptoms, 112
– treatment, 113
Venous puncture, 255f
Ventricular septum defect (VSD),
   199–200, 200f
Vesicoureterorenal reflux,
   166–168
Viral croup, 91
Vojta physiotherapy, 7
Vomiting, 88
von Recklinghausen disease. See
   Neurofibromatosis

W

Waterhouse–Friderichsen
   syndrome, 260–263
– clinical aspects, 262
– diagnosis, 260, 262
– differential diagnoses, 260
– epidemiology, 262
– etiology and pathogenesis, 262
– measures to prevent spread
   of, 260
– prognosis, 263
– prophylaxis, 263
– treatment, 262
– treatment algorithm, 261f
Weight loss and social
   withdrawal, 28
Whooping cough, 126, 127
Wiedemann–Beckwith
   syndrome, 246
Wilms tumor. See
   Nephroblastoma
Wound care, 131
Wry neck. See Torticollis

Z

Ziehl–Neelsen stain, 14f